Depression in
Neurologic Disorders:
Diagnosis and Management

I wish to dedicate this book to all the academicians of the Universities in Israel, who through their creativity and accomplishments have been a constant inspiration to me throughout my professional career.

I also wish to dedicate this book to my wife Hilary and my daughters Lesley Anne and Lauren Amanda who through their unconditional love and support have filled my life with joy.

Depression in Neurologic Disorders: Diagnosis and Management

EDITED BY

Andres M. Kanner, MD

Professor of Neurological Sciences and Psychiatry
Rush Medical College at Rush University
Director, Laboratory of Electroencephalography and Video-EEG-Telemetry
Associate Director, Section of Epilepsy and Rush Epilepsy Center
Rush University Medical Center
Chicago, IL, USA

⟨W⟩WILEY-BLACKWELL

A John Wiley & Sons, Ltd., Publication

This edition first published 2012 © 2012 by Blackwell Publishing Ltd.

Blackwell Publishing was acquired by John Wiley & Sons in February 2007. Blackwell's publishing program has been merged with Wiley's global Scientific, Technical and Medical business to form Wiley-Blackwell.

Registered office: John Wiley & Sons, Ltd, The Atrium, Southern Gate, Chichester, West Sussex, PO19 8SQ, UK

Editorial offices: 9600 Garsington Road, Oxford, OX4 2DQ, UK
The Atrium, Southern Gate, Chichester, West Sussex, PO19 8SQ, UK
111 River Street, Hoboken, NJ 07030-5774, USA

For details of our global editorial offices, for customer services and for information about how to apply for permission to reuse the copyright material in this book please see our website at www.wiley.com/wiley-blackwell

Library of Congress Cataloging-in-Publication Data

Depression in neurologic disorders : diagnosis and management / edited by
Andres M. Kanner. – 1st ed.
       p. ; cm.
   Includes bibliographical references and index.
   ISBN 978-1-4443-3058-8 (hardback : alk. paper)
   I. Kanner, Andres M.
   [DNLM: 1. Depressive Disorder–complications.   2. Nervous System
Diseases–complications.   3. Brain Injuries–complications.   4. Depressive
Disorder–diagnosis.   5. Depressive Disorder–therapy.   WM 171.5]
   616.85'27–dc23

                           2012014817

A catalogue record for this book is available from the British Library.

Wiley also publishes its books in a variety of electronic formats. Some content that appears in print may not be available in electronic books.

Cover image: © iStockphoto/artfromthefringe
Cover design: Meaden Creative

Set in 8.75/11.75 pt Utopia by Toppan Best-set Premedia Limited
Printed and bound in Singapore by Markono Print Media Pte Ltd

01   2012

Contents

Color plate section is found facing page 20

Contributors

John J. Barry, MD, Department of Psychiatry, Stanford School of Medicine, Stanford, CA, USA

Julián Bustin, MD, MRCPsych, Head of Geriatric Psychiatry and Co-Head of The Memory Clinic, Institute of Cognitive Neurology (INECO); Institute of Neuroscience, Favaloro University, Buenos Aires, Argentina

Rochelle Caplan, MD, Department of Psychiatry, David Geffen School of Medicine, UCLA Semel Institute for Neuroscience and Human Behavior, Los Angeles, CA, USA

Alan B. Ettinger, MD, Neurological Surgery P.C., Lake Success, NY, USA

Christopher L. Grote, PhD, Department of Behavioral Sciences, Rush University Medical Center, Chicago, IL, USA

Hrvoje Hecimovic, MD, PhD, Zagreb Epilepsy Center, Department of Neurology, University Hospital, Zagreb, Croatia

Erica J. Kalkut, PhD, Department of Neurology, Medical College of Wisconsin, Milwaukee, WI, USA

Andres M. Kanner, MD, Departments of Neurological Sciences and Psychiatry, Rush Medical College at Rush University; Laboratory of EEG and Video-EEG-Telemetry; Section of Epilepsy and Rush Epilepsy Center, Rush University Medical Center, Chicago, IL, USA

Michael P. Kerr, MD, Welsh Centre for Learning Disabilities, Cardiff University, Cardiff, UK

Joan Roig Llesuy, MD, Neuropsychiatry and Addiction Institute, Hospital del Mar, Barcelona, Spain

Facundo Manes, MD, Director, Institute of Neuroscience, Professor of Neurology and Cognitive Neuroscience, Favaloro University; Director, Institute of Cognitive Neurology (INECO), Buenos Aires, Argentina; Co-President, World Federation of Neurology, Research Group on Aphasia and Cognitive Disorders

Seth A. Mensah, MB, ChB, DPM, MSc, MRCPsych, Consultant Neuropsychiatrist, Welsh Neuropsychiatry Service, Whitchurch Hospital, Cardiff, UK

Marco Mula, MD, PhD, Department of Clinical and Experimental Medicine, Amedeo Avogadro University; Division of Neurology, University Hospital Maggiore della Carità, Novara, Italy

Pablo Richly, MD, Co-Head of The Memory Clinic, Institute of Cognitive Neurology (INECO), Buenos Aires, Argentina

Dana J. Serafin, BS, Department of Neurology, Stony Brook University Medical Center, Stony Brook, NY, USA

Angela Strobel Parsons, Chicago College of Osteopathic Medicine, Midwestern University, Downers Grove, IL, USA

Yukari Tadokoro, Department of Neuropsychiatry, School of Medicine, Aichi Medical University, Aichi-ken, Japan

Ludger Tebartz van Elst, MD, Section of Experimental Neuropsychiatry and Psychotherapy, Department of Psychiatry and Psychotherapy, University of Freiburg Medical Center, Freiburg, Germany

Oliver Tüscher, MD, Section of Experimental Neuropsychiatry and Psychotherapy, Department of Psychiatry and Psychotherapy; Department of Neurology, University of Freiburg Medical Center, Freiburg, Germany; Department of Psychiatry and Psychotherapy, University of Mainz Medical Center, Mainz, Germany

Deborah M. Weisbrot, MD, Department of Psychiatry and Behavioral Sciences, Stony Brook University Medical Center, Stony Brook, NY, USA

Foreword

There is a new buzzword in neurologic circles, which is *comorbidity*. Sometimes mistaken for denoting any separate medical problem found to be increased in frequency with an index disorder, and defined as the co-occurrence of two disorders at above chance levels, the term usefully should relate to where there is a direct or a heuristic proposition of a biological or sociological link between the conditions. In other words, where the substrate of condition x presupposes condition y or vice versa. There needs to be some dependent endogenous link between two disorders, such that the causal link between them can be explored.

There is little to be pursued in trying to understand why people with tetraplegia develop sacral ulcers or have urinary infections, or why someone with epilepsy has head injuries. However, where a common organ is involved in two diagnostically separate disorders, then an increased comorbidity between the two will have both biological relevance and may lead to improved patient management. Since psychiatric and neurologic disorders both share the brain as the font of symptomatology, it is hardly surprising that overlapping syndromes are frequently noted in clinical practice.

The description of psychiatric symptoms in neurologic disorders has a long history, dating back to the times of Hippocrates, but such interest accelerated in the European literature of the 19th century, when the distinction between neurology and psychiatry as separate medical disciplines was not countenanced. With the growing rift between an organically based neurology and a psychologically based psychiatry in the first six decades of the 20th century, interest in such comorbidities waned, in spite of such obvious clinical presentations of, for example,

postictal psychoses, or the dementias seen in conditions such as Parkinson's disease or multiple sclerosis.

However, we are now in a different era, not only of shifting paradigms, with disciplines such as behavioral neurology and neuropsychiatry ready to embrace a more holistic view of brain–behavior associations, but with an understanding of neurobiology based on sophisticated technology, both for exploring the intricacies of brain structure and function, but also for bringing the live brain to life with differing imaging modalities. This timely book has been edited by Andres M. Kanner, who has not only made the psychiatric comorbidities of epilepsy a central area of research, but who has also the requisite clinical experience to envisage a wider perspective, embracing a spectrum of neurologic disorders and a frequently encountered but often ignored clinical problem, namely depression.

The observation that patients with various neurologic disorders develop depression is nothing new, except that few investigators have expressed much interest in the association until recently. The renewed importance of the comorbidity arises from several factors. Some decade or two ago, measuring quality of life (QOL) in various disorders became fashionable, and not surprisingly most neurologic conditions investigated compromised this important variable. However, closer inspection of QOL assessments revealed that much of the variance could be explained by the presence of depression. The growing understanding of the neuroanatomical and neurochemical substrates of depression, revealing interlinks between neural circuits and neurotransmitters common to both neurologic and psychiatric disorders, led the curious minded to reexplore the clinical situation, and the therapeutically minded to pursue treatments for the psychiatric comorbidity, thus going beyond that required for the index condition. Even more recently, the acknowledged link between certain neurologic disorders and their treatment and suicidal behaviors, including completed suicide, has placed all neurologists in the challenging position to explore the affective state of their patients, and if depression is suggested, to either manage it themselves or to refer to a competent associate.

Andres M. Kanner sets the scene by asking, "Why should neurologists care?" The rest of the book develops this theme, and helps with an even more important question: "How should neurologists care?"

Michael Trimble
Professor of Behavioral Neurology
Institute of Neurology, Queen Square
London, UK
January 2012

Preface

The lack of communication between psychiatrists and neurologists is one of the most incomprehensible phenomena in modern medicine, as most (if not all) neurologic disorders affecting the central nervous system are associated with a psychiatric comorbidity, of which depression is the most common. And yet, in a majority of patients, depression remains unrecognized and untreated, as most neurologists focus only on the identification of neurologic signs and symptoms and their treatment.

Nevertheless, the impact of a comorbid depressive disorder in the life of these patients can be as devastating as and often more disabling than the actual neurologic disorder. When investigated, a lifetime history of depression can be identified in one out of every three to four patients suffering from any of the major neurologic conditions including epilepsy, stroke, migraine, multiple sclerosis, dementia, movement disorders and traumatic brain injury.

Contrary to old assumptions, depression is not simply a "reactive process" to the limitations and obstacles caused by the underlying neurologic disorder. In fact, there is a complex relation between depression and several neurologic disorders, as evidenced by the existence of a bidirectional relation between depression and conditions like epilepsy, stroke, migraine, Parkinson's disease and possibly also dementia. In other words, not only are patients with these neurologic conditions at higher risk of developing depression, but patients with depression are at a higher risk of developing one of these neurologic disorders. This bidirectional relation does not establish causality but suggests the existence of common pathogenic mechanisms operant in the psychiatric and neurologic conditions.

The complex relation between depression and neurologic disorders has significant clinical implications that should be of great concern to neurologists, as the existence of a comorbid depressive disorder is associated with a worse course and poorer response to treatment of the neurologic disorder. Furthermore, comorbid depression has been found to be an independent risk factor for a poor quality of life and increased suicidal risk. It accounts for higher medical costs (not related to the psychiatric treatment) and lesser compliance with the neurologic treatment. Accordingly, one would expect to find a plethora of data on the impact of the treatment of depression on the course of the neurologic disorder. Alas, nothing is further from the truth! In fact, a review of the literature reveals a paucity of studies on the treatment of depression in most neurologic disorders. This problem is compounded by the limited access of patients to psychiatric treatment because of financial reasons, reluctance on the part of patients and their family to seek psychiatric evaluations, and a discomfort on the part of psychiatrists to treat patients with neurologic disorders.

The aim of this book is to start overcoming these serious shortcomings in the management of patients with neurologic disorders and facilitate the dialogue among neurologists, psychiatrists, neuropsychologists and other mental health providers. I was extremely fortunate to count with a group of international experts in the field to make this book a reality. The task given to each author was to review the available data in the literature and to provide practical strategies for the identification and treatment of comorbid depressive disorders in the major neurologic conditions.

The book is introduced by a chapter that makes the case of why neurologists should care about depression in neurologic patients by reviewing its impact on the course and treatment response of the neurologic disorder. In the other chapters of the book's first section, we review the neurobiologic aspects of primary depression (Chapter 2), its clinical characteristics and treatment strategies (Chapter 3), and the use of screening instruments of depression in various neurologic disorders (Chapter 4). Suicide is more frequent in neurologic patients than in the general population. This important topic is reviewed with a focus on the prevalence and variables associated with its occurrence in the major neurologic conditions (Chapter 5). Cognitive disturbances are key clinical manifestations of depression, but they may result as well from the underlying neurologic condition. Distinguishing one from the other poses a significant diagnostic dilemma, which can be resolved with neuropsychological testing. The indications, diagnostic yield and limitations of this diagnostic modality are discussed in patients with primary depression as well as in neurologic patients with comorbid depression (Chapter 6). The diagnosis and management of depression in pediatric patients poses particular challenges which frequently limit its recognition and its management. Accordingly, a chapter is dedicated to review the principal aspects of this topic (Chapter 7). The last chapter of the first section (Chapter 8) provides a review of the basic principles in the management of depression in neurologic disorders.

The second section of the book focuses on the specific aspects of depression in the major neurologic disorders, including migraine (Chapter 9), stroke (Chapter 10), epilepsy (Chapter 11), movement disorders (Chapter 12), multiple sclerosis (Chapter 13), Alzheimer's disease (Chapter 14) and traumatic brain injury (Chapter 15). Each one of these seven chapters reviews the epidemiologic aspects of depression in the respective neurologic condition, the potential pathogenic mechanisms that may explain the high comorbid prevalence and bidirectional relation, the clinical manifestations, with special emphasis on the clinical differences of depression in each particular neurologic disorder (relative to primary depression) and, finally, the treatment strategies that can be considered.

My hope is that this book will provide clinicians the necessary data to understand the need to identify and treat comorbid depression in neurologic disorders, and make available the necessary tools to achieve those goals. While I do not expect or believe that neurologists should treat the depressive disorders in all their patients, they should ensure that their existence is investigated in every evaluation and, when possible and appropriate, treated by them or referred to a mental health professional.

Andres M. Kanner, MD

Acknowledgments

I wish to acknowledge the invaluable assistance
of Mr. Jacob Wolff in the editing of this book.

Part One

General Considerations

Depression in Neurologic Disorders: Why Should Neurologists Care?

Andres M. Kanner
Departments of Neurological Sciences and Psychiatry, Rush Medical College at Rush University; Laboratory of EEG and Video-EEG-Telemetry; Section of Epilepsy and Rush Epilepsy Center, Rush University Medical Center, Chicago, IL, USA

Introduction

Depressive disorders are the fourth medical disorder with a significant burden on the individual, the family, and society worldwide. In the general population, their lifetime prevalence has been estimated to be 26% for women and 12% for men [1, 2]. In patients with neurologic disorders, the lifetime prevalence of depressive disorders ranges between 30% and 50%. For example, in patients with epilepsy, a lifetime prevalence of 34.2% (25.0–43.3%) was identified in a Canadian population-based study [3]. In a population-based study of 115,071 subjects aged 18 and older a 12-month prevalence rate of major depression of 25.7% was found among people with multiple sclerosis (compared with only 8.9% of those without) [4]. In a review of the literature, Robinson and Spalletta found an overall prevalence of major depression of 21.7% and minor depression of 19.5% based on pooled data [5]. Reijnders et al. conducted a systematic review of the literature of the prevalence of depressive disorders in Parkinson's disease (PD) and found major depressive disorder in 17%, minor depression in 22%, dysthymia in 13%, and significant symptoms of depression not meeting any *Diagnostic and Statistical Manual of Mental Disorders*, Fourth Edition (DSM-IV) diagnostic criteria in 35% of patients [6].

Yet, despite their high prevalence rates, depressive disorders remain underrecognized and undertreated in patients with neurologic disorders. For example, in a study of 100 consecutive patients with epilepsy, 69 patients were found to experience symptoms of depression severe enough to warrant referral for treatment; 63% of patients with spontaneous depression and 54% of patients with an iatrogenic depression had been symptomatic for more than 1 year before treatment was initiated [7].

Failure to recognize depression in patients with neurologic disorders is the result of various problems: (1) poor, if not lack of communication between neurologists and psychiatrists; (2) limited training of psychiatric disorders in neurology residency programs and vice versa; and (3) limited access of patients to psychiatric care due to insurance-related obstacles and other economic factors. Thus, can neurologists continue ignoring the comorbid depressive disorders affecting their patients and can they just focus on the management of the neurologic disorder at hand? The aim of this chapter is to set up the

Depression in Neurologic Disorders: Diagnosis and Management, First Edition.
Edited by Andres M. Kanner.
© 2012 Blackwell Publishing Ltd. Published 2012 by Blackwell Publishing Ltd.

case for why neurologists must care about the existence of comorbid depressive disorders and ensure of their timely treatment as part of a comprehensive management of their patients.

Neurologists must care about the presence of comorbid depressive disorders for various reasons. These include:

1. Depressive disorders are a risk factor for the development of neurologic disorders.
2. The presence of depressive disorders is associated with a worse course and outcome of the neurologic disorder.

These points are reviewed in some detail in most of the chapters of this book.

Are depressive disorders a risk for the development of neurologic disorders?

Stroke

Since the last decade of the 20th century, various studies were published in the literature suggesting that a history of depression or the mere presence of depressive symptoms were associated with a two- to threefold higher risk of developing a stroke [8–10]. These data were confirmed in a recent meta-analysis of 28 prospective cohort studies that included a total of 317,540 subjects and 8478 stroke cases during a follow-up period ranging from 2 to 29 years [11]. An increased risk was found for total stroke (hazards ratio [HR] = 1.45; 95% confidence interval [CI] = 1.29–1.63), fatal stroke (HR = 1.55; 95% CI = 1.25–1.93), and ischemic stroke (HR = 1.25; 95% CI = 1.11–1.40). The pathogenic mechanisms associated with the increased risk of stroke in people with depression are reviewed in detail in Chapter 10.

Migraine

Patients with depression have been found to be at increased risk of developing migraine and vice versa. For example, in a prospective study of 496 subjects aged 25–55 years with migraine, 151 subjects with other types of headaches of comparable severity and 539 healthy controls were followed for a 2-year period. The presence of major depression at baseline predicted the first onset migraine during the 2-year follow-up period (odds ratio [OR] = 3.4; 95% CI = 1.4, 8.7) but not other severe headaches (OR = 0.6; 95% CI = 0.1,

4.6). Likewise, migraine at baseline predicted the first onset major depression during follow-up (OR = 5.8; 95% CI = 2.7, 12.3) [12]. Of note, this risk was limited to migraines and did not include other types of headache (see also Chapter 9).

Epilepsy

Hippocrates was the first clinician to identify the increased risk of epilepsy associated with depressive disorders when he wrote 26 centuries ago that "epileptics become melancholics and melancholics epileptics." In the last two decades, three population-based studies have shown that patients with a depressive disorder have a three- to sevenfold higher risk of developing epilepsy [13–15]. The pathogenic mechanisms that may explain the increased risk of epilepsy in subjects with depression are reviewed in detail in Chapters 2 and 11.

Dementia

A history of depression has been associated with an increased risk of developing Alzheimer's dementia (AD). For example, a meta-analysis of 20 studies that encompassed 102,172 subjects in eight countries revealed a positive relation between a history of depression and a risk for developing AD in 19 of the 20 studies [16]. Symptoms of depression may often be the initial clinical manifestation of AD. Thus, studies that investigate the relation between depressive disorders and the risk of developing AD may be biased by this temporal relation of psychiatric and cognitive symptoms. Yet, in this meta-analysis, the interval between the diagnosis of depression and that of AD was positively and significantly related to the odds of developing AD. In other words, the longer the timing between depressive episodes and the onset of AD was significantly associated with the risk of developing this type of dementia. Furthermore, in a study of 1003 elderly subjects (all with a Mini-Mental State score of more than 26), the presence of significant depressive symptoms at baseline predicted a higher risk of cognitive decline 4 years later [17]. The severity of a mood disorder was also associated with the risk of developing dementia. Also, data from a case register study of almost 23,000 patients with an affective disorder suggested that increasing severity, expressed as the number of major depressive episodes leading to an inpatient admission, increased the risk of developing dementia [18]. Thus, patients with three admissions had close to a threefold increased risk of dementia (95% CI: 0.64–13.2), compared with patients with only one admission.

Whether a history of depression in individuals with mild cognitive impairment is predictive of an increased risk of developing AD or is only an expression of the temporal association between depressive symptomatology and the onset of the dementing process remains to be established. This dilemma is illustrated in a study of 114 patients with amnesic mild cognitive impairment who were followed for a 3-year period; 41 patients (36%) displayed a depressive disorder at baseline. After 3 years, 35 (85%) of these patients had developed AD, in comparison with 32% of the nondepressed subjects, yielding a relative risk of developing AD of 2.6 (95% CI: 1.8–3.6) [19].

Parkinson's disease

As in the case of dementia, depressive episodes may be the initial clinical manifestations of PD. However, there are data suggestive that depressive disorders may increase the risk of developing PD. These data are illustrated in two population-based studies. In the first one, conducted in The Netherlands, all subjects diagnosed with depression between 1975 and 1990 were included and matched with subjects with the same birth year who were never diagnosed with depression. Follow-up ended at April 30, 2000. Among the 1358 depressed subjects, 19 developed PD, and among the 67,570 nondepressed subjects, 259 developed PD, yielding an HR of 3.13 (95% CI: 1.95–5.01) for depressed versus nondepressed in multivariable analysis [20]. In the second study that included 105,416 subjects, investigators compared the lifetime incidence of depressive disorders in patients later diagnosed with PD with that of a matched control population. At the time of their diagnosis of PD, 9.2% of the patients had a history of depression, compared with 4.0% of the control population; the OR for a history of depression for these patients was 2.4 (95% CI: 2.1–2.7) [21].

The data outlined in the previous two sections illustrate a bidirectional relation between depressive disorders and these neurologic conditions.

These data do not establish causality, however, but rather suggest the existence of common pathogenic mechanisms operant in depressive and neurologic disorders. These mechanisms are reviewed in great detail in the respective chapters of this book.

A comorbid depression is associated with a worse course of the neurologic disorder

If there is one reason for neurologists to care about recognizing and ensuring the treatment of comorbid depression in patients with neurologic disorders, this is it. Here are some concrete examples:

Stroke

Poststroke depression (PSD) has been found to have a negative impact on the recovery of cognitive deficits, on the ability to perform activities of daily living (ADL), and in the mortality risks in patients with stroke. For example, one study demonstrated that patients with major PSD had significantly more cognitive deficits than patients without depression who experienced a similar location and size of left-hemisphere (but not right-hemisphere) stroke [22]. In another study of 140 patients, the presence of major PSD was associated with greater cognitive impairment 2 years after a stroke [23]. Likewise, one study found that in-hospital PSD was the most important variable predicting poor recovery in ADL over a 2-year period. In fact, the score of in-hospital ADL was not associated with the 2-year recovery [24].

There is also an increased mortality risk in patients with stroke associated with the presence of comorbid depressive disorders [25–27]. For example, in a population-based study, 10,025 subjects were followed over 8 years; 1925 deaths were recorded. Mortality rate per 1000 person-years of follow-up was highest in the group with both a history of stroke and depression (HR: 1.88; 95% CI: 1.27, 2.79) versus only depression present (HR: 1.23; 95% CI: 1.08, 1.40) versus only stroke (HR: 1.74; 95% CI: 1.06, 2.85) [25]. However, the combined effect of depression and stroke is less than additive. Furthermore, in another study, patients with PSD had a 3.4-fold higher risk of dying during a 10-year follow-up period than patients without depression independently of other stroke risk factors [26]. Finally, a higher mortality risk was found over a 3-year follow-up period in patients with PSD even though these patients were younger and suffered from fewer chronic conditions [27].

Epilepsy

A history of depression preceding the onset of epilepsy or identified at the time of diagnosis of the seizure disorder has been associated with a worse response to pharmacotherapy. For example, in a study of 780 patients with newly diagnosed epilepsy who were followed over a median period of 79 months, seizures were controlled in 462 patients, while in 318 patients epilepsy remained refractory to antiepileptic drug (AED) therapy [28]. Univariate and multivariate logistic regression analyses demonstrated that a psychiatric history, and in particular a history of depression preceding the diagnosis of epilepsy, was associated with a twofold higher risk of pharmacoresistance. In a more recent study of 138 patients with new onset epilepsy, those with symptoms of depression at the time of diagnosis were significantly less likely to be seizure free after a 12-month follow-up period [29]. Likewise, in a study of 100 consecutive patients with treatment-resistant temporal lobe epilepsy who underwent an anterotemporal lobectomy, a lifetime history of depression was found to be associated with a worse postsurgical seizure outcome [30]. Indeed, a history of depression was recorded in only 12% of patients who became free of auras and disabling seizures in contrast to 79% of patients with persistent disabling seizures.

Parkinson's disease

The presence of depression in patients with PD has been associated with a more rapid deterioration of motor and cognitive functions, especially executive function [31]. In a study that compared cognitive functions between 45 patients with PD with current depression and 45 patients without depression matched for age, education, gender, age at disease onset, disease duration, and disease severity, patients with depression were significantly more impaired cognitively. While cognitive functions were impaired in both groups, impaired memory was found only in patients with PD with depression [32]. Another study compared neuropsychological functions among patients with PD and major depression, patients with PD without depression, patients with major depression but without PD, and age-comparable healthy controls. More severe cognitive deficits were identified in patients with major depression, with or without PD, than both healthy controls and patients with PD without depression on tests of verbal fluency and auditory attention [33]. In addition, more severe deficits on tasks of abstract reasoning and set alternation were found in patients with PD and major depression than the other three groups.

Alzheimer's dementia

As in the case of epilepsy, there are data suggesting that a history of depression may be associated with a worse course of AD. For example, in a study of 43 patients with AD who had a mild to moderate cognitive impairment, 22 were found to have a history of a major depressive disorder before the onset of any cognitive impairment. None of these patients were suffering from a depressive episode at time of cognitive assessment. After controlling for age, education, duration of illness, gender, and medication status, subjects with a history of major depressive disorder had significantly lower scores on neuropsychological tests, which included the Mini-Mental State Exam, Wechsler Adult Intelligence Scale (WAIS) Full-Scale and Verbal Scale IQ, and the Initiation/Perseveration subscale of the Mattis Dementia Rating Scale [34]. These subjects also developed symptoms of dementia at a significantly earlier age than the subjects without a prior history of a depressive disorder.

The presence of comorbid depressive disorders in patients with AD is associated with a faster cognitive deterioration, worse deterioration in ADL [35], an earlier placement in a nursing facility [36], and it is also associated with a faster decline in cognitive functions [37].

Is depression a neurologic disorder with psychiatric symptoms?

The pathogenic mechanisms that explain the bidirectional relation between depression and various neurologic disorders and the mechanisms mediating the negative impact of comorbid depression on their course are multiple and complex and are reviewed in great detail in the corresponding chapter of this book. Accordingly, they do not need to be discussed here. Yet neuroimaging and neuropathologic abnormalities in primary depressive disorders suggest that depression is in fact a neurologic disorder. Here is a very brief summary of the evidence: Neuroimaging studies with volumetric measurements of various neuroanatomical brain structures conducted in patients with primary major depressive disorders have revealed the presence of atrophy of hippocampal formations and frontal lobes, including cingulate gyrus and orbitofrontal and dorsolateral cortex [38–41]. The presence of neuropathologic abnormalities further supports our contention that depressive disorders are a neurologic disorder. These are manifested by: (1) decreased glial densities and neuronal size in the cingulate gyrus; (2) decreased neuronal sizes and neuronal densities in layers II, III, and IV in the rostral orbitofrontal cortex, resulting in a decrease of cortical thickness; (3) a significant decrease of glial densities in cortical layers V and VI, associated with decreases in neuronal sizes in the caudal orbitofrontal cortex; and (4) a decrease of neuronal and glial density and size in all cortical layers of the dorsolateral prefrontal cortex [42–46].

Concluding remarks

The data reviewed in this chapter clearly illustrate the negative impact of comorbid depressive disorders on the course and response to treatment of neurologic disorders. If for no other reasons, these are the ones which should make neurologists care about the early recognition and treatment of depressive disorders. This topic is discussed in great detail in the chapters of this book. Yet, if we are to believe in these data, we must start thinking on how to overcome the obstacles that have been responsible for the indifference of neurologists toward psychiatric comorbidities, beginning by expanding the training of medical students and neurology and psychiatry residents on the psychiatric comorbidities of neurologic disorders and the neurologic comorbidities of psychiatric disorders. Finally, if a bidirectional relation between psychiatric and neurologic disorders appears to be well established, isn't it time for neurologists and psychiatrist to establish a bidirectional relation?

> ### 💡 PEARLS TO TAKE HOME
>
> - A history of depression is associated with a two- to threefold higher risk of developing a stroke.
> - Poststroke depression has been found to have a negative impact on the recovery of cognitive deficits, ability to perform activities of daily living, and in the mortality risks of patients with stroke.
> - Patients with depression have been found to be at increased risk of developing migraines and vice versa.
> - Patients with a depressive disorder have a three- to sevenfold higher risk of developing epilepsy.
> - A history of depression preceding the onset of epilepsy or identified at the time of diagnosis of the seizure disorder has been associated with a worse response to pharmacotherapy, while a lifetime history of depression is associated with a worst postsurgical seizure outcome in temporal lobe epilepsy.
> - A history of depression has been associated with an increased risk of developing AD.
> - A history of depression is associated with a worse course of AD.
> - Depressive disorders may increase the risk of developing PD.
> - The presence of depression in patients with PD has been associated with a more rapid deterioration of motor and cognitive functions.

References

1. Akiskal H. Mood disorders. In: *Comprehensive Textbook of Psychiatry*, eds. B Sadock and V Sadock. New York: Lippincott Williams & Williams, pp. 1559–1575, 2005.
2. Barry JJ. The recognition and management of mood disorders as a comorbidity of epilepsy. *Epilepsia*, 44, Suppl. 4: 30–40, 2003.
3. Tellez-Zenteno JF, et al. Psychiatric comorbidity in epilepsy: a population-based analysis. *Epilepsia*, 48: 2336–2344, 2007.
4. Patten SB, et al. Major depression in multiple sclerosis: a population-based perspective. *Neurology*, 61(11): 1524–1527, 2003.

5. Robinson RG, Spalletta G. Poststroke depression: a review. *Can J Psychiatry*, 55(6): 341–349, 2010.

6. Reijnders JS, et al. A systematic review of prevalence studies of depression in Parkinson's disease. *Mov Disord*, 23(2): 183–189, 2008.

7. Kanner AM, et al. The use of sertraline in patients with epilepsy: is it safe? *Epilepsy Behav*, 1(2): 100–105, 2000.

8. May M, et al. Does psychological distress predict the risk of ischemic stroke and transient ischemic attack? The Caerphilly Study. *Stroke*, 33: 7–12, 2002.

9. Larson SL, et al. Depressive disorder, dysthymia, and risk of stroke. Thirteen-year follow-up from the Baltimore Epidemiological Catchment Area Study. *Stroke*, 32: 1979–1983, 2001.

10. Colantonio A, et al. Depressive symptoms and other psychosocial factors as predictors of stroke in the elderly. *Am J Epidemiol*, 136: 884–894, 1992.

11. Pan A, et al. Depression and risk of stroke morbidity and mortality: a meta-analysis and systematic review. *JAMA*, 306(11): 1241–1249, 2011.

12. Breslau N, et al. Comorbidity of migraine and depression: investigating potential etiology and prognosis. *Neurology*, 60(8): 1308–1312, 2003.

13. Forsgren L, Nystrom L. An incident case-referent study of epileptic seizures in adults. *Epilepsy Res*, 6: 66–81, 1990.

14. Hesdorffer DC, et al. Major depression is a risk factor for seizures in older adults. *Ann Neurol*, 47: 246–249, 2000.

15. Hesdorffer DC, et al. Depression and attempted suicide as risk factors for incident unprovoked seizures and epilepsy. *Ann Neurol*, 59: 35–41, 2006.

16. Ownby RL, et al. Depression and risk for Alzheimer disease: systematic review, meta-analysis, and metaregression analysis. *Arch Gen Psychiatry*, 63(5): 530–538, 2006.

17. Paterniti S, et al. Depressive symptoms and cognitive decline in elderly people. Longitudinal study. *Br J Psychiatry*, 181: 406–410, 2002.

18. Kessing LV, Andersen PK. Does the risk of developing dementia increase with the number of episodes in patients with depressive disorder and in patients with bipolar disorder? *J Neurol Neurosurg Psychiatry*, 75: 1662–1666, 2004.

19. Modrego PJ, Fernandez J. Depression in patients with mild cognitive impairment increases the risk of developing dementia of Alzheimer's type: a prospective cohort study. *Arch Neurol*, 61: 1290–1293, 2004.

20. Leentgens AFG, et al. Higher incidence of depression preceding the onset of Parkinson's disease: a register study. *Mov Disord*, 18: 414–418, 2003.

21. Nilsson FM, et al. Increased risk of developing Parkinson's disease for patients with major affective disorder: a register study. *Acta Psychiatr Scand*, 104: 380–386, 2001.

22. Starkstein SE, et al. Comparison of patients with and without post-stroke major depression matched for age and location of lesion. *Arch Gen Psychiatry*, 45: 247–252, 1988.

23. Robinson RG, et al. A two year longitudinal study of post-stroke mood disorders: findings during the initial evaluation. *Stroke*, 14: 736–744, 1983.

24. Parikh RM, et al. The impact of post-stroke depression on recovery in activities of daily living over two year follow-up. *Arch Neurol*, 47: 785–789, 1990.

25. Ellis C, et al. Depression and increased risk of death in adults with stroke. *J Psychosom Res*, 68(6): 545–551, 2010.

26. Morris PL, et al. Association of depression with 10-year poststroke mortality. *Am J Psychiatry*, 150: 124–129, 1993.

27. Williams LS, et al. Depression and other mental health diagnoses increase mortality risk after ischemic stroke. *Am J Psychiatry*, 161: 1090–1095, 2004.

28. Hitiris N, et al. Predictors of pharmacoresistant epilepsy. *Epilepsy Res*, 75: 192–196, 2007.

29. Petrovski S, et al. Neuropsychiatric symptomatology predicts seizure recurrence in newly treated patients. *Neurology*, 75: 1015–1021, 2010.

30. Kanner AM, et al. A lifetime psychiatric history predicts a worse seizure outcome following temporal lobectomy. *Neurology*, 72: 793–799, 2009.

31. Starkstein SE, et al. Cognitive impairment in various stages of Parkinson's disease. *J Neuropsychiatry*, 1: 243–248, 1989.

32. Tröster AI, et al. The influence of depression on cognition in Parkinson's disease: a pattern of impairment distinguishable from Alzheimer's disease. *Neurology*, 45(4): 672–676, 1995.

33. Kuzis G, et al. Cognitive function in major depression and Parkinson's disease. *Arch Neurol*, 54: 982–986, 1997.

34. Cannon-Spoor HE, et al. Effects of previous major depressive illness on cognition in Alzheimer disease patients. *Am J Geriatr Psychiatry*, 13(4): 312–318, 2005.

35. Lyketsos CG, et al. Major and minor depression in Alzheimer's disease: prevalence and impact. *J Neuropsychiatry Clin Neurosci*, 9: 556–561, 1997.

36. Steele C, et al. Psychiatric symptoms and nursing home placement of patients with Alzheimer's disease. *Am J Psychiatry*, 147: 1049–1051, 1990.

37. Bassuk SS, et al. Depressive symptomatology and incident cognitive decline in an elderly community sample. *Arch Gen Psychiatry*, 55(12): 1073–1081, 1998.

38. Bremner JD, et al. Hippocampal volume reduction in major depression. *Am J Psychiatry*, 157(1): 115–118, 2000.

39. Bremner JD, et al. Reduced volume of orbitofrontal cortex in major depression. *Biol Psychiatry*, 51(4): 273–279, 2002.

40. Coffey CE. The role of structural brain imaging in ECT. *Psychopharmacol Bull*, 30(3): 477–483, 1994.

41. Sheline YI. Brain structural changes associated with depression. In: *Depression and Brain Dysfunction*, eds. F Gilliam, AM Kanner, YI Sheline. London: Taylor & Francis, pp. 85–104, 2006.

42. Öngür D, et al. Glial reduction in the subgenual prefrontal cortex in mood disorders. *Proc Natl Acad Sci USA*, 95: 13290–13295, 1998.

43. Rajkowska G, et al. Morphometric evidence for neuronal and glial prefrontal cell pathology in major depression. *Biol Psychiatry*, 45(9): 1085–1098, 1999.

44. Cotter DR, et al. Glial cell abnormalities in major psychiatric disorders: the evidence and implications. *Brain Res Bull*, 55: 585–595, 2001.

45. Cotter D, et al. Reduced glial cell density and neuronal size in the anterior cingulate cortex in major depressive disorder. *Arch Gen Psychiatry*, 58: 545–553, 2001.

46. Cotter D, et al. Reduced neuronal size and glial cell density in area 9 of the dorsolateral prefrontal cortex in subjects with major depressive disorder. *Cereb Cortex*, 12: 386–394, 2002.

Neurobiological Aspects of Depression: How Do They Affect Neurologic Disorders?

Hrvoje Hecimovic

Zagreb Epilepsy Center, Department of Neurology, University Hospital, Zagreb, Croatia

Introduction

Studies of the neurobiological basis of psychiatric disorders, particularly depression, are one of the hallmarks of the past decade. This is mostly due to the translational integration of basic science findings in the genetics and neurochemistry of brain dysfunction and development of new clinical neuroimaging protocols. This chapter will review recent advances in the field and discuss their clinical implications in regard to neurological disorders.

Depression is the most prevalent psychiatric disorder and has a complex etiology and clinical presentation. Mood disorders such as major depressive disorder (MDD) are common, severe, chronic, and often life-threatening illnesses [1]. Suicide is estimated to be the cause of death in up to approximately 15% of individuals with MDD, and a negative impact on many other systemic organ effects has been recognized. Thus, MDD is a systemic disease with deleterious effects on multiple organ systems. The costs associated with disability and premature death represent a significant economic burden, and the World Health Organization's report on the Global Burden of Disease has positioned MDD among the leading causes of disability worldwide, and one that is likely to represent an increasing problem in the coming years.

Multiple risk factors and heterogeneous etiologies contribute to depressive symptoms [2]. Researchers have tried to explain the means by which a combination of genetics and environmental factors influence its onset, development, and severity of symptoms. Recent neuroimaging studies of the human brain examined the association of depression with certain structural and functional disturbances, suggesting that a dysfunction in neural circuits is responsible for mood changes. Understanding interconnectivity of the structures, neurotransmitter pathways, and molecular mechanisms implicated in this dysfunction creates a basis for better understanding of the clinical phenotype of the disease. MDD has long been viewed mainly on a neurochemical basis, but recent studies have repeatedly associated it with regional reductions in human brain volume, as well as in the quantity or volume of glia and neurons in specific brain areas. Current research shows that MDD arises from the interaction of multiple susceptibility genes and environmental factors. Clinical symptoms are not limited only to episodic mood disturbances; rather, a whole spectrum of cognitive, sensory, motoric, autonomic, endocrine, and sleep abnormalities often coexist.

Structural imaging studies using magnetic resonance imaging (MRI) have demonstrated reduced gray matter volume primarily in the

Depression in Neurologic Disorders: Diagnosis and Management, First Edition.

Edited by Andres M. Kanner.

orbital and medial prefrontal cortex, ventral striatum, and hippocampus in depressed subjects relative to healthy control samples [3]. Complementary postmortem neuropathological studies have shown significant reductions in cortical volumes, glial cells, and neurons in the subgenual prefrontal cortex (Cg 25), orbital cortex, dorsal anterolateral prefrontal cortex, and changes in the anterior insula and in the amygdala. The marked reduction in glial cells in these regions has been associated with recent findings that glia play important roles in regulating synaptic glutamate concentration and in releasing trophic factors that are important in the development and maintenance of synaptic networks. Positron emission tomography (PET) imaging studies have revealed multiple focal or more widespread abnormalities of regional cerebral blood flow (CBF) and glucose metabolism in limbic and prefrontal cortical structures in mood disorders [4]. The majority of evidence shows that in unmedicated subjects with familial MDD, regional CBF and metabolism are increased in the amygdala, orbital cortex, and medial thalamus and decreased in the dorsomedial/dorsal anterolateral prefrontal cortex and subgenual cingulate cortex in comparison to healthy controls. Using functional imaging, researchers have suggested functional networks that include limbic–thalamic–cortical or more complex limbic–striatal–pallidal–thalamic–cortical circuits, with the amygdala, orbital, and medial prefrontal cortex and areas of the striatum and thalamus in the pathophysiology of MDD. The same circuits have been implicated in other studies with patients with primarily neurological disorders and are probably best studied in chronic epilepsy.

Severe stressors have also been associated with an increased risk for the onset of MDD in susceptible individuals.

Activation of the hypothalamic–pituitary–adrenal (HPA) axis has been the best investigated and appears to mediate many of these effects. Stress-induced neuronal atrophy is prevented by adrenalectomy and worsened by exposure to high concentrations of glucocorticoids. A significant number of patients with Cushing's syndrome, in which pituitary gland adenomas result in cortisol hypersecretion, can exhibit depressive symptoms and hippocampal volume reduction.

Following corrective surgical treatment, hippocampal volume increases roughly in proportion to the treatment-associated decrease in urinary free cortisol concentrations. Stress and glucocorticoids also reduce cellular resilience. It is plausible that chronic or recurrent stress lowers the threshold for cellular death. The exact mechanism is unclear but probably depends on the facilitation of glutamatergic signaling.

The reduction in the resilience of hippocampal neurons may also result in decreased expression of brain-derived neurotrophic factor (BDNF). BDNF and other neurotrophic factors are necessary for the survival and function of neurons, implying that a sustained reduction of these factors could affect neuronal viability. It appears that endogenous neurotrophic factors primarily act by inhibiting cell death cascade in addition to providing necessary trophic support. Evidence also suggests that the cyclic AMP response element-binding protein (CREB) cascade is upregulated by antidepressant treatment. Thus, chronic antidepressant treatment may enhance CREB phosphorylation and increase the expression of a major gene regulated by CREB, that is, the one encoding BDNF. The role of the cyclic adenosine monophosphate (cAMP)–CREB cascade and BDNF in the actions of antidepressant treatment has also been investigated by studies demonstrating that upregulation of these pathways increases performance in behavioral models of depression. Several lines of evidence support the hypothesis that chronic antidepressant treatment produces neurotrophic-like effects. Antidepressant treatment may induce greater regeneration of catecholamine axon terminals in the cerebral cortex and enhance hippocampal neurons growth and synaptic plasticity [5].

Anatomy of frontolimbic network

The majority of studies suggest that hippocampal volume loss in humans is associated with depression [3], and functional imaging studies point to dysfunction in the frontolimbic network in patients with MDD. These results are in concordance with reports from animal, lesional, and human postmortem studies. It appears that there is a direct pathway from the hippocampus to the specific structures in the mesial prefrontal cortical areas. This pathway has been used as a model to study interconnectivity between frontolimbic structures, which are supposedly associated with mood changes [6]. A detailed neuroanatomy of these structures will now be described.

Hippocampus

The hippocampus (*sea horse*, in Greek) is a structure with rich connections that plays a central role in behavioral and other studies of mood, learning, and memory. This structure also has important functions in stress response mediated via the HPA axis and in neuroplasticity.

Hippocampal afferent pathways

Hippocampal main afferents originate in the frontal lobe; Brodmann areas (BA) 12, 13, and 25; occipital lobe (BA 19); and temporal lobe (BA 20, 22, 35, 36, and 38). They provide inputs from the sensory systems by direct projections to the entorhinal cortex. This structure then projects further to the Ammon's horn or the CA1, CA2, and CA3 layers. Neurons from the frontal lobe cortex (BA 9 and 46) and parietal lobe (BA 7 and 23) project directly to the Ammon's horn. Information is then processed through a local hippocampal network from the dentate gyrus to the Ammon's horn and the subiculum. Further, visceral fibers from the basal and lateral nuclei of the amygdala project to the hippocampus via BA 28. Fibers from the anterior and midline thalamic nuclei pass through the cingulum to the entorhinal cortex, but one bundle also projects directly to the hippocampus. Projections from the supramammilary region of the hypothalamus pass through the fornix to the entorhinal area and the hippocampus proper [7, 8] (Figure 2.1).

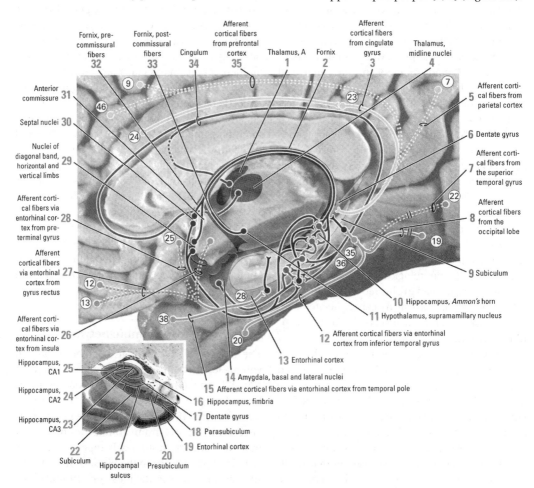

Figure 2.1 Hippocampal afferent pathways. Reproduced from Woolsey T et al. The Brain Atlas: A Visual Guide to the Human Central Nervous System, 2nd Edition. 2002, p.213.

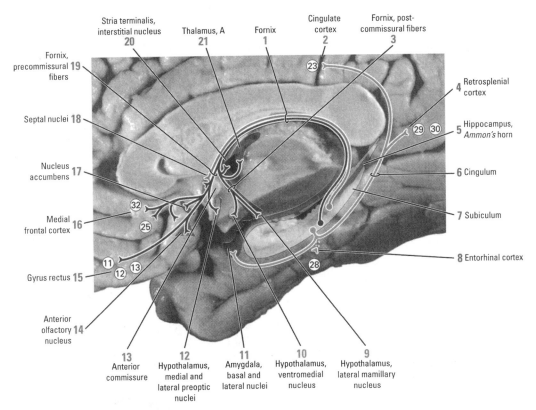

Figure 2.2 Hippocampal efferent pathways. Reproduced from Woolsey T et al. The Brain Atlas: A Visual Guide to the Human Central Nervous System, 2nd Edition. 2002, p.215.

Hippocampal efferent pathways

The majority of hippocampal efferents originate in the Ammon's horn and the subiculum. The fibers from the subiculum then form the fornix, which is divided by the anterior commissure into the precommissural and postcommisural fornix. Axons in the precommissural fornix synapse on the septal nuclei, nucleus accumbens (NAc), preoptic nucleus of the hypothalamus, and the anterior olfactory nucleus and then project to the medial frontal cortex and the gyrus rectus, including BA 11, 12, 13, 25, and 32, respectively. Postcommissural fornix fibers project to the interstitial nucleus of the stria terminalis, anterior nucleus of the thalamus, and ventromedial and lateral mammilary nuclei of the hypothalamus. Additional fibers from the subiculum synapse directly in the basal and lateral nuclei of the amygdala, entorhinal cortex, and retrosplenial cortex, and some of them pass the cingulum

and terminate in the cingulate cortex. Fibers from the Ammon's horn terminate in the septal nuclei via the precommissural fornix (Figure 2.2).

Amygdala

The amygdala (*almond*, in Greek) receives information from the sensory systems and from the visceral afferents. This structure consists of five smaller nuclei organized in three groups: the central nucleus, the cortical and medial nuclei, and the basal and lateral nuclei, incorporating various functions.

Amygdalar afferent pathways

There are five main afferent pathways in the amygdala. Projections from the cerebral cortex and temporal lobe terminate in all amygdalar nuclei: the insular fibers and the fibers from BA 20, 21, 22, and 38 project to the central nucleus; the insular fibers, the fibers from BA 20, 21, 22, 35, 36, and 38, and some subiculum efferents project to the basal and lateral nuclei. Other subiculum projections terminate in the cortical and medial nuclei of the amygdala.

Further, axons from BA 12, 13, 14, 23, 24, and 25 connect to the central nucleus, while those from BA 11, 12, and 24 project to the basal and lateral nuclei. Axons from the interstitial nucleus of the stria terminalis join the fibers from the ventromedial nucleus of the hypothalamus and lateral hypothalamic area and terminate in the central, medial, and cortical nuclei of the amygdala. Fibers from the olfactory bulb terminate in the medial and cortical amygdalar nuclei (Figure 2.3).

Amygdalar efferent pathways

The five amygdalar nuclei project diffusely using four groups of axons. The central nucleus of the amygdala projects to the substantia innominata, nuclei of the diagonal gyrus, lateral hypothalamic area, interstitial nucleus of stria terminalis, and septal nuclei (Figure 2.4). Axons from the central nucleus also course in the medial forebrain bundle to reach their targets in the brain stem. In the midbrain, the fibers terminate in the parafascicular nucleus, ventral tegmental area, pars compacta of the substantia nigra, perpendicular nucleus, periaqueductal gray matter, and the dorsal raphé nuclei. In the pons and medulla, the

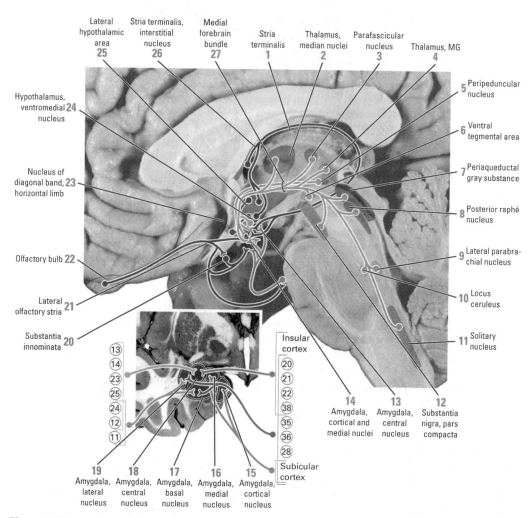

Figure 2.3 Amygdalar afferent pathways. Reproduced from Woolsey T et al. The Brain Atlas: A Visual Guide to the Human Central Nervous System, 2nd Edition. 2002, p.217.

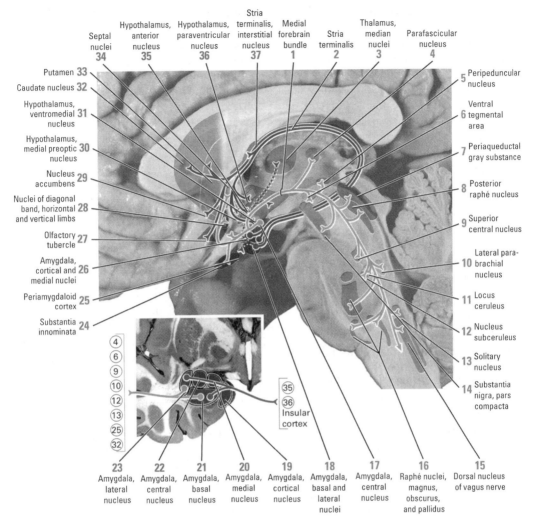

Figure 2.4 Amygdalar efferent pathways. Reproduced from Woolsey T et al. The Brain Atlas: A Visual Guide to the Human Central Nervous System, 2nd Edition. 2002, p.219.

projections end in the superior central nucleus, lateral parabrachial nucleus, locus coeruleus (LC), nucleus subcoeruleus, raphé nuclei magnus, pallidus and obscurus, nucleus of the solitary tract, and dorsal nucleus of the vagal nerve.

Amygdalar efferents from the basal, lateral, medial, and cortical nuclei pass through the stria terminalis to innervate the interstitial nucleus of the stria terminalis and the paraventricular, anterior, ventromedial, and preoptic nuclei of the hypothalamus. Fibers from the basal and lateral nuclei that link with the stria terminalis also innervate the caudate nucleus and putamen, the

NAc, and the olfactory tubercle of the telencephalon. Further, some axons connect directly through the temporal lobe to the septal nuclei and the nucleus of the diagonal gyrus.

Prefrontal cortex

Neuroanatomical, histological, and pharmacological studies suggest that the cortical afferents originating in the hippocampus and amygdala are primarily projected to the specific structures of the orbital and medial prefrontal cortex, both in humans and in monkeys [6]. Extensive research using various staining techniques and injections of specific tracers showed that there are more than 20 architectonic areas that can be differentiated within the orbital and medial cortex. Some studies suggest that these areas can be grouped into two interactive "networks." The orbital network receives sensory inputs, including smell, taste, visceral afferents, somatic afferents, and vision, and appears to be particularly related to food and eating. In contrast, the medial network supplies the major cortical efferents to the visceromotor structures in the hypothalamus and periaqueductal gray. These networks have distinct connections with limbic structures, striatum, and the mediodorsal thalamus. It also appears that rich interconnections between the two networks support information exchange from viscerosensory to visceromotor systems and vice versa.

Neurotransmitters in neurobiology of depression

Although studies show that neurotransmitters play a major role in neurobiology of mood disorders, it is unclear whether they present a primary modulating pathway or final common pathway. Major neurotransmitters described in this modulatory pathway are serotonin, norepinephrine, dopamine, and γ-aminobutyric acid.

Role of serotonin in neurobiology of depression

The majority of dorsal raphé neurons synthesize serotonin. This secretion is regulated via the 5-HT_{1A} autoreceptors located on the cell bodies. The raphé nuclei are localized along the midline of the brain stem, and the dorsal raphé nucleus lies in the ventral quadrant of the periaqueductal grey. The rostral group of nuclei includes the caudal linear, median raphé, and dorsal raphé nucleus with efferent projections directed rostrally. The caudal group, which includes the raphé magnus, raphé obscurus, raphé pallidus nuclei, and a cluster of neurons in the lateral reticular formation of the myelencephalon, projects mainly to the caudal brain stem.

The 5-HT receptors are the most diverse of the monoamine receptors. Their projections reach distant brain areas. The serotoninergic system also modulates other transmitter systems with its widespread connections. The main role of the central 5-HT system is to regulate the behavioral inhibitory system and it is implicated in the regulation of food intake, circadian rhythms, mood, anxiety, sleep, aggression, and impulsivity. Serotonergic dysfunction has been proposed in a number of neuropsychiatric disorders [9].

The 5-HT receptors have been identified and classified on the basis of structural similarity and subdivided into seven families. Each receptor has a specific localization and distinct effector pathways. The $5\text{-HT}_{1,2,4-7}$ receptor families are members of the G protein-coupled receptor superfamily. The 5-HT_3 receptor differs and belongs to the gated ionophore receptor superfamily. The largest family of the 5-HT receptors is the 5-HT_1, with five 5-HT receptor subtypes. The 5-HT_{1A} receptors act as somatodendritic autoreceptors in the raphé nuclei and postsynaptically in the hippocampus, septum, and amygdala, where they initiate neuronal inhibition. They are also located on the astrocytes in the frontal and limbic cortex [10]. A knockout transgenic mouse that lacks the 5-HT_{1A} receptors has an increased sensitivity to anxiety caused by an increased serotonergic tone due to the failed negative feedback at the 5-HT_{1A} autoreceptor [11].

Release of the 5-HT in the synaptic cleft is followed by inactivation, and then it is transported back into the presynaptic terminal by the serotonin transporter (5-HTT). It can be either degraded by monoamino oxidase (MAO) to 5-hydroxyindoleacetic acid (5-HIAA) or repackaged into secretory vesicles via the 5-HTT.

Human 5-HTT exhibits voltage dependence and may alter excitability of the neurons. Decreased brain and platelet 5-HTT binding is a frequent observation in depression. Tricyclic antidepressants (TCAs) and selective serotonin reuptake inhibitors (SSRIs) also bind to the 5-HTT. It appears that most antidepressants used in clinical practice are potent 5-HTT antagonists. Animal and human studies have investigated the contribution of the serotonergic system in the neurobiology of temporal lobe epilepsy (TLE). Genetic epilepsy-prone rats have reduced hippocampal 5-HT receptor density, and an impairment of serotonergic activity may enhance seizure severity. Serotonin-induced anticonvulsant effect was mostly mediated by hippocampal 5-HT_{1A} receptors. Human studies have demonstrated decreased 5-HT_{1A} receptor binding in the ictal onset and ictal spreading temporal lobe regions, midbrain raphé, and thalamus in mesial and neocortical TLE.

Decreased availability of the 5-HT_{1A} receptors highly correlates with the degree of epileptogenicity of cortical areas. The 5-HT transporter is a transmembrane protein responsible for reuptake of 5-HT from the synaptic cleft. The 5-HTT is encoded by a single copy gene (SLC6A4) that contains two common polymorphisms: a 44 base pair (bp) insertion/deletion in the promoter region (5-HTT gene-linked polymorphic region, 5-HTTLPR) and a 17 bp variable number of tandem repeats in the second intron (VNTR-2). It was demonstrated that long (L) and short (S) variants of the 5-HTTLPR differentially modulate transcription of the 5-HTT gene, with the L variant being more efficient in a recessive manner. Similarly, 12-repeat allele of the VNTR-2 intron was shown to have stronger enhancer-like properties than shorter alleles. The 5-HTT genetic variations have been found to affect basal cerebral metabolic activity in limbic structures in normal populations and were observed to be associated with depression, schizophrenia, and suicidal behavior.

Role of norepinephrine in neurobiology of depression

Norepinephrine (NE) is the principal sympathetic neurotransmitter in the periphery, with abundant connections throughout the brain and the entire cortex. Cell bodies of NE are found in the LC of the dorsal pons. Many structures participate in mediation of stress responses and autonomic functions, such as the paraventricular nucleus, lateral hypothalamus, and preoptic area, and project their fibers toward the LC, adding further support for the role of the NE system in stress and arousal. Main LC efferents are cortical terminal fibers primarily ending in the layers I, IV, and V, suggesting a role of NE in modulating intracortical and thalamocortical transmission. These findings indicate that projections to the thalamus might have a role in coordinating activity related to levels of arousal, along with a role in sensory and motor gating. Projections to the thalamus are important in learning and memory, and hypothalamic fibers

have a role in neuroendocrine effects related to the state of arousal.

The NE receptors consist of α and β classes. The α receptor has two subclasses, the α_1 and α_2, which are as distinct as the α and β classes. Several investigations using α_{2A}- and α_{2C}-adrenergic receptor knockout mice suggest that the α_{2A}-adrenergic receptor is "stress protective" and that the α_{2C}-adrenergic receptor mediates stress susceptibility. All NE receptors belong to the G protein-linked receptor superfamily and thus mediate slower neuromodulatory postsynaptic responses.

In depressed patients, studies have suggested NE system dysfunction [12]. Evidence shows that prolonged exposure to stress decreases α_{2A}-receptor density, specifically in the amygdala and hippocampus. Further, LC, which is the main NE-containing nucleus in the brain, showed increased density of the α_2 adrenergic receptors in suicide victims with a history of major depression. The results also showed increased activity of tyrosine hydroxylase in the LC in addition to decreased density of the NE transporter. The majority of these effects are reproduced by NE depletion in the brain and to some extent reversed by antidepressant administration.

Role of dopamine in neurobiology of depression

Another neurotransmitter, dopamine (DA), is transported into storage vesicles in both DA- and NE-producing neurons via amine-specific transporters. NE-specific neurons, however, contain dopamine β-hydroxylase within the vesicles that rapidly transforms DA to NE via hydroxylation of the β-carbon. After NE is released into the synaptic cleft following vesicle fusion, it is rapidly returned to the synaptic terminals via the NE transporter. These specific carriers are located on the outer membrane of the synaptic terminals. The NE transporter is inhibited by many classes of antidepressants that acutely increase synaptic NE concentration. L-DOPA has been shown to relieve mood symptoms in patients with Parkinson's disease. DA reuptake inhibitors such as bupropion have been studied as antidepressants. The potential role of dopamine in the neurobiology of depression is further supported by regional specificity of dopaminergic projections from the ventral tegmental area to the prefrontal cortex, striatum, and anterior cingulate. However, no study has clearly shown whether dopaminergic stimulation alone can alleviate depressive symptoms [13].

Role of γ-aminobutyric acid in neurobiology of depression

Early evidence show that a γ-aminobutyric acid (GABA) deficit in central neurons may result in depressive symptoms. Lower plasma GABA levels and a decreased quantity of $GABA_B$-binding sites were found in the brains of patients with and without depression who completed suicide. Some investigators suggest that GABA has an inhibitory effect on the biogenic amine neurotransmitters and that this inhibition may be implicated in the local network via interneurons. It has also been suggested that GABA deficit in mood disorders is complementary to the hypothesis of alterations in NE and 5-HT function in mood disorders.

Models of neurobiology of depression

Monoaminergic theory

This brain system has received the greatest attention in neurobiological studies of MDD. Effective antidepressant drugs achieve their primary biochemical effects by regulating synaptic concentrations of serotonin and NE. It was shown that treatment with antihypertensives, such as reserpine, which deplete these monoamines, can precipitate depressive episodes in susceptible individuals. Thus, the "monoaminergic hypothesis" of depression suggests that depression is caused by decreased monoamine function. Two structurally unrelated compounds that were developed primarily for nonpsychiatric conditions, iproniazid and imipramine, had potent antidepressant effects in humans and were shown to enhance central serotonin or noradrenaline transmission.

Signaling pathways form specific networks that modulate signals generated by neurotransmitter and neuropeptide systems [14]. A major intracellular pathway that mediates effects of several classes of antidepressants is the cAMP cascade, which is regulated by both 5-HT and NE [15].

Receptor activation leads to the generation of the cAMP via the stimulation of adenylyl cyclase by the G protein subtype Gsα. The generation of the cAMP then results in activation of cAMP-dependent protein kinase (PKA), and one of its substrates is the transcription factor CREB. This protein in its phosphorylated form regulates transcriptional activity. Overexpression of CREB in the hippocampus results in an antidepressant effect and suggests that CREB may serve as a potential molecular target for therapeutic agents [16]. Chronically administered antidepressants have also been shown to upregulate the CREB in the hippocampus. This effect has been reproduced in human postmortem tissues and linked to antidepressant-like responses in animal models. Current antidepressant agents offer a better therapeutic response; however, they are still designed to increase monoamine transmission, either by inhibiting neuronal reuptake (SSRI) or by inhibiting degradation (MAO inhibitors). Although these monoamine-based agents are potent antidepressants, the cause of depression is not a simple deficiency of central monoamines. MAO inhibitors and SSRIs produce immediate increases in monoamine transmission, whereas their mood-enhancing properties require days to weeks of continuous treatment. Interestingly, experimental depletion of monoamines can produce a mild reduction in mood in unmedicated depressed patients, but such manipulations do not alter mood in healthy controls. It is now thought that acute increases in the amount of synaptic monoamines induced by antidepressants produce secondary neuroplastic changes that involve transcriptional and translational changes and mediate molecular and cellular plasticity. Thus, while monoamine-based antidepressants remain the first line of therapy for depression, their long therapeutic delays and low remission rates have encouraged the search for more effective agents. The serotonin receptors involved in the action of SSRIs remain largely unknown, although selective agonists of the serotonin 5-HT4 receptor produce rapid antidepressant effects in rodents (in a couple of days).

Experiments on mice deficient in P-glycoprotein, a molecule in the blood–brain barrier that transports specific molecules back into the bloodstream, have shown that several antidepressants are substrates for P-glycoprotein. Human polymorphisms in the gene encoding P-glycoprotein significantly alter antidepressant efficacy in depressed individuals, suggesting the value of pharmacogenetic testing when selecting antidepressant agents.

Theory of the HPA axis dysfunction

The HPA axis is important in understanding the neurobiology of depression. There are specific brain structures that control the activity of the HPA axis, including the hippocampus (with an inhibitory effect on hypothalamic neurons) and the amygdala (with a direct excitatory influence). Glucocorticoids from the circulation exert powerful feedback on the HPA axis and, under physiological conditions, appear to enhance hippocampal inhibition of the HPA activity and probably hippocampal function in general.

It has been well documented that neurons from the paraventricular nucleus of the hypothalamus secrete corticotrophin-releasing factor (CRF), which stimulates the synthesis and release of adrenocorticotropin (ACTH) from the anterior part of the pituitary gland. ACTH stimulates the synthesis and release of glucocorticoids from the adrenal cortex. Prolonged increased concentration of glucocorticoids, for example during severe stress, is harmful and can damage hippocampal neurons, possibly by a reduction of dendritic branching and loss of dendritic spines included in glutamatergic synaptic inputs. Clinical studies show that excessive activation of the HPA axis is observed in almost half of individuals with depression, and this effect is partially reversed by antidepressant treatment.

Recent reports also suggested hypersecretion of the CRF in some depressed patients, which was also reversed with antidepressant treatment. CRF is a major neuropeptide mediator of stress responses in the central nervous system (CNS) and is expressed in the paraventricular nucleus of the hypothalamus to coordinate the release of ACTH from the anterior pituitary. CRF levels are increased in the cerebrospinal fluid in suicide victims and in persons with depression. Two CRF receptors, CRF_1 and CRF_2, are abundant in the brain, and there is a hypothesis that both are involved in response to stress.

Central administration of the CRF_1 antisense oligodeoxynucleotides resulted in anxiolytic effects against both the CRF concentration and psychological stressors. There were also observations of a downregulation in the CRF receptor number in the frontal cortex of depressed patients compared to controls. Further, chronic administration of CRF to normal volunteers resulted in HPA axis alterations indistinguishable from those of patients with major depression.

Neurotrophic theory

The neurotrophic hypothesis of depression summarizes the research on neurotrophic factors and their role in the neurobiology of depression and its treatment [17]. Previous studies described the role of neurotrophic factors in the regulation of neuronal growth and differentiation during development; however, more recent studies have suggested their importance in plasticity and survival of adult neurons and glia. BDNF is a member of the nerve growth factor family, and it has been shown to increase synaptic strength, survival, and growth of mature neurons through activation of a transmembrane receptor that contains intrinsic tyrosine kinase B activity (TrkB).

In animals, stress decreases levels of BDNF expression in the dentate gyrus and pyramidal cell layer of the hippocampus. This reduction appears to be mediated by glucocorticoid action and by increases in serotonergic transmission. Chronic, but not acute, administration of antidepressant drugs or chronic electroconvulsive treatment increased BDNF expression and prevented a stress-induced decrease in BDNF levels. Some groups [18] found in postmortem studies increased BDNF expression in the dentate gyrus, hilus, and supragranular regions in subjects treated with antidepressant medications compared with untreated subjects. Induction of the BDNF by antidepressants is at least partly mediated via the CREB.

It has been suggested that chronic antidepressant treatment upregulates the cAMP cascade in the hippocampus and cerebral cortex, increases levels of cAMP-dependent PKA, and enhances expression of the CREB [16]. These observations indicate that agents that activate this pathway could potentially be useful in treatment of depression. cAMP-specific phosphodiesterase

(phosphodiesterase type 4 inhibitor, PDE4) is responsible for the breakdown of cAMP, and phosphodiesterase inhibitors were shown to prevent cAMP degradation. The proposal that phosphodiesterase inhibitors can theoretically reduce symptoms of depression generated another strategy for antidepressant drug development.

A large body of evidence from preclinical studies shows that several forms of stress reduce BDNF-mediated signaling in the hippocampus, which is reversed with chronic treatment with antidepressants. Similar changes have been observed in the postmortem human hippocampus of the people who were depressed as well as in the concentrations of serum BDNF. It has been suggested that there are complex interactions between the BDNF polymorphism, a polymorphism in the serotonin transporter gene, and stressful life events. A marked cellular effect of some antidepressant treatments is the induction of adult hippocampal neurogenesis. Moreover, treatment with antidepressants, possibly through the actions of CREB or other transcriptional regulators, is shown to increases the amount of several growth factors in the hippocampus that influence neurogenesis. These include BDNF as well as vascular endothelial growth factor, which have antidepressant and proneurogenic properties in rodents. The mechanisms by which new neurons may restore mood are still uncertain. Activity-dependent increases in neurogenesis may enhance activity propagation through the hippocampus and allow hippocampal networks to adapt. Promoting depressive symptoms in response to stress may differ between different neural circuits and be distinct from the changes that underlie depression in the absence of external stress. It is also plausible that the neuroplastic events required for antidepressant efficacy may function through separate but parallel circuits and common final pathways.

Neuroimmune theory

Cytokines are humoral mediators with a role in innate and adaptive immunity. Recent studies provided mostly indirect evidence that cytokines may also act as mood modulators [19]. Both peripherally and centrally synthesized cytokines can activate cytokine receptors within the CNS. Low doses of interleukin (IL)-1 produce social

withdrawal and decreased exploratory and sexual behavior in some animals. This is mediated by the release of proinflammatory cytokines such as interferon-α (IFN-α), tumor necrosis factor-α (TNF-α), IL-6, and IL-1β, which activate the HPA axis and central monoamine systems. Clinical studies show that approximately a third of the patients treated with recombinant IFNs develop depression as a side effect of treatment. Thus, immune activation may occur in a group of depressed subjects. Some authors have suggested that this result is linked with coexisting autoimmune conditions such as rheumatoid arthritis, in which broader system inflammation increases the risk of producing depressive mood change. Some preclinical studies also indicate that blocking proinflammatory cytokine-mediated signaling can produce antidepressant effects. Mice with targeted deletions of the gene encoding IL-6 or those encoding the TNF-α receptors show antidepressant-like behavioral phenotypes, and a centrally administered antagonist of the IL-1β receptor reversed the behavioral effects of chronic stress. In future studies, support for this hypothesis will focus on determination of largely unknown neural pathways involved in the behavioral effects of cytokines to delineate the intercellular interactions between brain macrophages, glia, and neurons within this circuitry. This is a promising field that will increase our understanding of the mechanistic interaction between the immune system, synaptic plasticity, and antidepressants, and may lead to the ultimate development of a novel spectrum of therapeutics for severe mood disorders.

Regulation of synaptic plasticity by TNF-α and IL-1

Increased levels of TNF-α have been observed in several neuropathological states associated with learning and memory deficits. The pathophysiological levels of TNF-α have been shown to inhibit long-term potentiation (LTP) in the CA1 region as well as in the dentate gyrus of the rat hippocampus. LTP produces a long-lasting increase in synaptic efficacy and is an important underlying mechanism of learning and memory formation. It has also been shown that the TNF receptor knockout mice demonstrate impaired long-term depression (LTD) in the CA1 region of the hip-

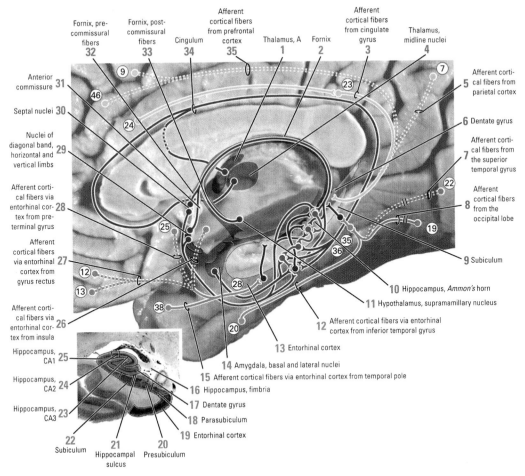

Figure 2.1 Hippocampal afferent pathways. Reproduced from Woolsey T et al. The Brain Atlas: A Visual Guide to the Human Central Nervous System, 2nd Edition. 2002, p.213.

Labels (clockwise from top left):

- 32 — Fornix, pre-commissural fibers
- 33 — Fornix, post-commissural fibers
- 34 — Cingulum
- 35 — Afferent cortical fibers from prefrontal cortex
- 1 — Thalamus, A
- 2 — Fornix
- 3 — Afferent cortical fibers from cingulate gyrus
- 4 — Thalamus, midline nuclei
- 31 — Anterior commissure
- 30 — Septal nuclei
- 29 — Nuclei of diagonal band, horizontal and vertical limbs
- 28 — Afferent cortical fibers via entorhinal cortex from pre-terminal gyrus
- 27 — Afferent cortical fibers via entorhinal cortex from gyrus rectus
- 26 — Afferent cortical fibers via entorhinal cortex from insula
- 25 — Hippocampus, CA1
- 24 — Hippocampus, CA2
- 23 — Hippocampus, CA3
- 22 — Subiculum
- 21 — Hippocampal sulcus
- 20 — Presubiculum
- 5 — Afferent cortical fibers from parietal cortex
- 6 — Dentate gyrus
- 7 — Afferent cortical fibers from the superior temporal gyrus
- 8 — Afferent cortical fibers from the occipital lobe
- 9 — Subiculum
- 10 — Hippocampus, *Ammon's* horn
- 11 — Hypothalamus, supramamillary nucleus
- 12 — Afferent cortical fibers via entorhinal cortex from inferior temporal gyrus
- 13 — Entorhinal cortex
- 14 — Amygdala, basal and lateral nuclei
- 15 — Afferent cortical fibers via entorhinal cortex from temporal pole
- 16 — Hippocampus, fimbria
- 17 — Dentate gyrus
- 18 — Parasubiculum
- 19 — Entorhinal cortex

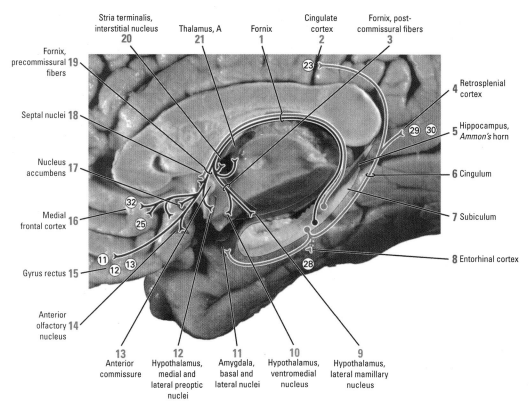

Figure 2.2 Hippocampal efferent pathways. Reproduced from Woolsey T et al. The Brain Atlas: A Visual Guide to the Human Central Nervous System, 2nd Edition. 2002, p.215.

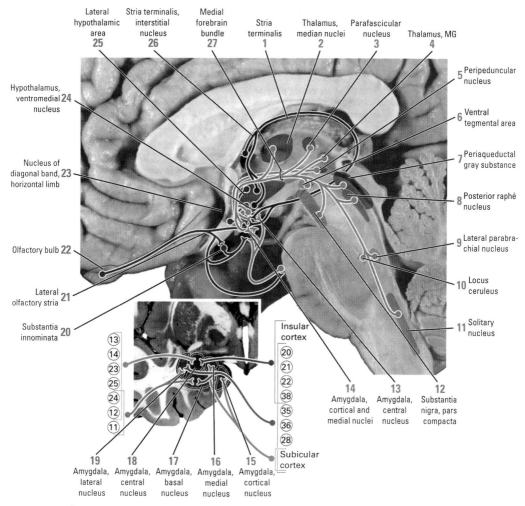

Lateral hypothalamic area **25**
Stria terminalis, interstitial nucleus **26**
Medial forebrain bundle **27**
Stria terminalis **1**
Thalamus, median nuclei **2**
Parafascicular nucleus **3**
Thalamus, MG **4**

Hypothalamus, ventromedial **24** nucleus

Nucleus of diagonal band, **23** horizontal limb

Olfactory bulb **22**

Lateral **21** olfactory stria

Substantia **20** innominata

5 Peripeduncular nucleus

6 Ventral tegmental area

7 Periaqueductal gray substance

8 Posterior raphé nucleus

9 Lateral parabrachial nucleus

10 Locus ceruleus

11 Solitary nucleus

Insular cortex

⑬ ⑭ ㉓ ㉕ ㉔ ⑫ ⑪

⑳ ㉑ ㉒ ㊳ ㉟ ㊱ ㉘

Subicular cortex

14 Amygdala, cortical and medial nuclei
13 Amygdala, central nucleus
12 Substantia nigra, pars compacta

19 Amygdala, lateral nucleus
18 Amygdala, central nucleus
17 Amygdala, basal nucleus
16 Amygdala, medial nucleus
15 Amygdala, cortical nucleus

Figure 2.3 Amygdalar afferent pathways. Reproduced from Woolsey T et al. The Brain Atlas: A Visual Guide to the Human Central Nervous System, 2nd Edition. 2002, p.217.

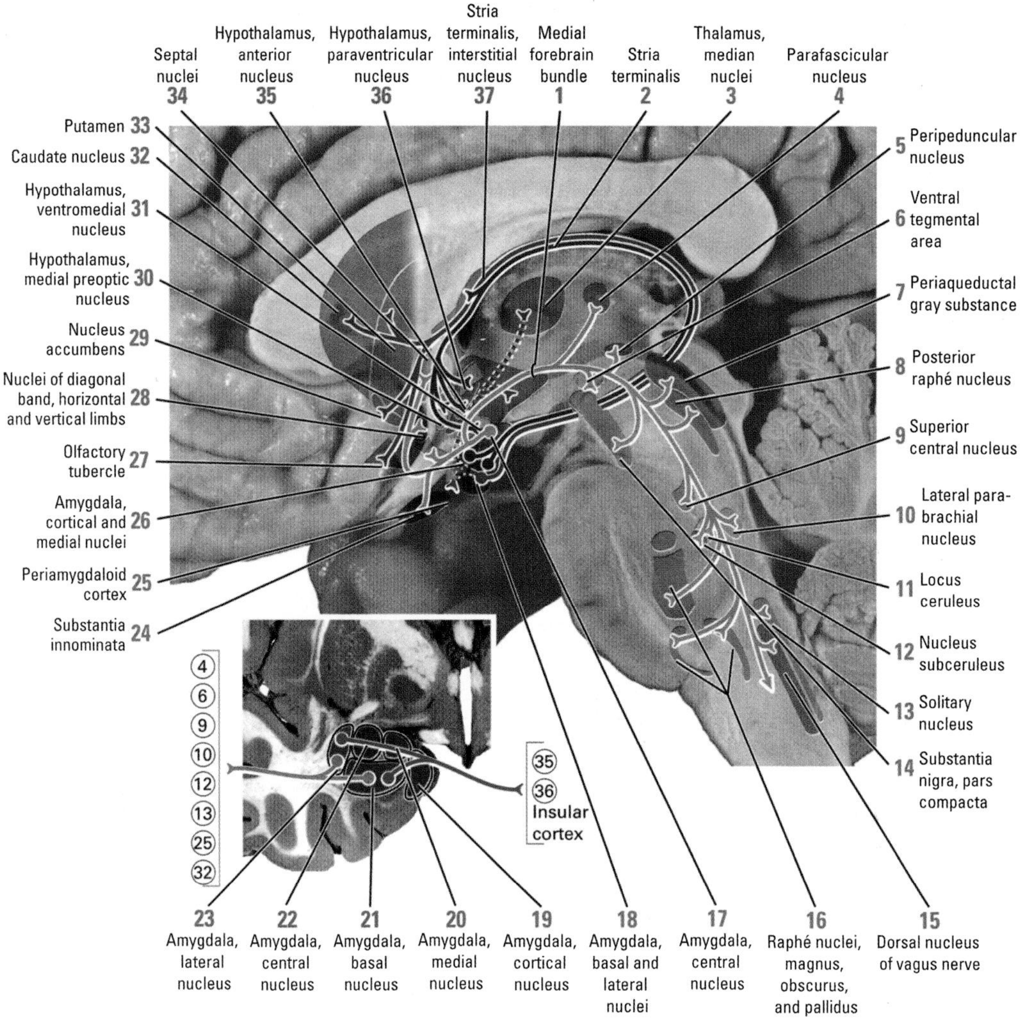

Septal nuclei 34
Hypothalamus, anterior nucleus 35
Hypothalamus, paraventricular nucleus 36
Stria terminalis, interstitial nucleus 37
Medial forebrain bundle 1
Stria terminalis 2
Thalamus, median nuclei 3
Parafascicular nucleus 4
Putamen 33
Caudate nucleus 32
Hypothalamus, ventromedial 31 nucleus
Hypothalamus, medial preoptic 30 nucleus
Nucleus accumbens 29
Nuclei of diagonal band, horizontal 28 and vertical limbs
Olfactory tubercle 27
Amygdala, cortical and 26 medial nuclei
Periamygdaloid cortex 25
Substantia innominata 24
5 Peripeduncular nucleus
Ventral 6 tegmental area
7 Periaqueductal gray substance
8 Posterior raphé nucleus
9 Superior central nucleus
Lateral para- 10 brachial nucleus
11 Locus ceruleus
12 Nucleus subceruleus
13 Solitary nucleus
14 Substantia nigra, pars compacta
4
6
9
10
12
13
25
32
35
36
Insular cortex
23 Amygdala, lateral nucleus
22 Amygdala, central nucleus
21 Amygdala, basal nucleus
20 Amygdala, medial nucleus
19 Amygdala, cortical nucleus
18 Amygdala, basal and lateral nuclei
17 Amygdala, central nucleus
16 Raphé nuclei, magnus, obscurus, and pallidus
15 Dorsal nucleus of vagus nerve

Figure 2.4 Amygdalar efferent pathways. Reproduced from Woolsey T et al. The Brain Atlas: A Visual Guide to the Human Central Nervous System, 2nd Edition. 2002, p.219.

pocampus. TNF-α knockout mice showed improved performance on spatial memory and learning tasks, and TNF-α overexpressing mice were significantly impaired on spatial learning and memory tasks. These findings of the TNF-α effects on synaptic plasticity appear to have important behavioral correlates *in vivo*. Although more recent studies of the role of TNF-α in regulating synaptic plasticity appear more conflicting, it is plausible that there is a fine balance between pathophysiological and physiological levels of TNF-α. Under pathophysiological conditions, when central TNF-α levels are elevated, LTP is likely to be inhibited, while under physiological conditions, low levels of TNF-α serve as modulators of homeostatic synaptic plasticity. Some studies suggest that TNF-α has deleterious effects on synaptic plasticity; however, recent evidence shows that physiologically low levels of TNF-α may be important in brain development as well as in "synaptic scaling." Independent of the important role of TNF-α in homeostatic scaling, this effect of TNF-α on Ca^{2+} homeostasis may also have implications for neuronal toxicity, especially when extracellular levels of TNF-α are high, as seen in a number of neuropathological conditions.

Recent evidence suggests that IL-1 may modulate synaptic plasticity and behavioral systems. It has been suggested that pathophysiological levels of IL-1 can have negative effects on hippocampal-dependent memory and learning processes, while stress-induced inhibition of hippocampus-dependent conditioning can be reversed by the IL-1RA, an IL-1 receptor antagonist. In accordance with these behavioral effects, IL-1 was found to impair LTP in the hippocampus.

It has been shown that administration of IL-1RA in rats impairs memory in the water maze and passive avoidance paradigms, both of which are associated with hippocampal functioning. Similarly, mice with a targeted deletion of IL-1R1 display severely impaired hippocampal-dependent memory, diminished short-term plasticity, and exhibit no LTP, both *in vivo* and *in vitro*. Other studies showed that the physiological levels of IL-1 are needed for memory formation, and a slight increase in the brain IL-1 levels can even improve memory. However, any significant divergence from the physiological range, either by excess elevation in IL-1 levels induced by exogenously administered IL-1 or enhanced endogenous release of IL-1 or by blockade of IL-1 signaling, results in impaired memory. Interestingly, mice with a deletion of the IL-1 receptor or with restricted overexpression of IL-1 antagonist did not display stress-induced behavioral or neuroendocrine changes. Further support for the role of immune system activation in the pathogenesis of depressive disorders comes from studies noting that the antidepressants desipramine and fluoxetine reduce the inflammatory reaction in ovalbumin-sensitized rats in the lipopolysaccharide (LPS) animal model of autoimmunity.

Involvement of cytokines in the pathogenesis of depression

Considering the evidence supporting the role of proinflammatory cytokines in the regulation of synaptic plasticity and new data suggesting that synaptic plasticity is impaired in mood disorders, it is conceivable that activation of the immune system network may be related to some aspects of the complex pathophysiology of depressive disorders. Hyperactivation of the immune system results in increased TH1 cytokines. Several animal studies have shown that administration of cytokines such as IL-1 or activation of macrophages and other inflammatory immune cells by systemic LPS treatment provokes "sickness behavior" symptoms. Motivation and some cognitive functions also appear to be affected. Mice lacking the enzyme required to synthesize IL-1 have reduced "sickness behavior" and lower expression of neurotoxic antinflammatory mediator genes in the brain after peripheral endotoxin injection. In addition, deletion of either TNF-α receptor 1 (TNFR1) or TNF-α receptor 2 (TNFR2) genes results in antidepressant-like effects.

The incidence of depressive disorders associated with cytokine therapy is highly variable, ranging from 0% to 40% in different studies. The explanations for these variations are probably related to the specific disease being treated, the cytokine type and dose being used, and the outcome measures and psychiatric history. In most cases, these depressive symptoms are treated effectively with antidepressants. In healthy human volunteers, depression, anxiety, and memory impairment are associated with immune activation by the bacterial endotoxin LPS and are correlated with serum IL-1 and TNF-α levels induced by that treatment.

Earlier findings in animal studies showing that cytokines may play a modulatory role in the development of depression-like behaviors have partially been correlated in clinical studies. Immunotherapy with IL-2 or IFN-α is often associated with marked cognitive disturbances, and neurovegetative symptoms such as fatigue, sleep disturbances, irritability, appetite suppression, and depressed mood correlate with elevated serum levels of IFN-α, IL-6, IL-8, and IL-10.

Cytokines are potential therapeutic modulators in mood disorders

Stress is a common risk factor for the development of MDD. It is plausible that most initial episodes of MDD are preceded by an identifiable stressor. In line with this hypothesis is the notion that stress may provide a link between MDD and inflammation. Existing preclinical and clinical evidence indicates that acute and chronic stress elevates levels of proinflammatory cytokines, such as IL-1 and TNF-α, and activates their signaling pathways in the periphery and in the CNS. Additional data to support the concept of cytokine hypothesis are provided by clinical studies of patients with MDD who present with a significant rise in serum levels of proinflammatory cytokines, such as TNF-α, IL-1 IL-6, IL-12, IL-6R, IL-2, IL-2R, IL-1RA, and IFN-α. It is interesting that some other severe psychiatric disorders such as bipolar disorder and schizophrenia have also been associated with increased inflammatory response and elevated levels of proinflammatory cytokines. It has been shown that some patients with MDD have an imbalance between pro- and anti-inflammatory cytokines, which can be attenuated following treatment with the antidepressants such as fluoxetine, sertraline, or paroxetine. Other recent studies indicate that MDD patients with abnormal allelic variants of the genes for IL-1 and TNF-α and higher levels of TNF-α showed a reduced responsiveness to antidepressant treatment. Several studies also indicate a potential modulatory response following excitotoxicity and microglial activation in the etiology of MDD. Activation of the immune system has been

observed in patients with MDD, resulting in increased levels of circulating proinflammatory cytokines. There are different modulatory pathways governing how proinflammatory cytokines can contribute to glutamate neurotoxicity: directly, via activation of the kynurenine pathway in microglia and increased production of quinolinic acid and glutamate release, and indirectly, via decreasing glial glutamate transporter activity leading to reduced glutamate removal from the extracellular space and by inducing long-term activation of microglia to release TNF-α and IL-1 in a positive feedback manner. Antidepressants have been shown to inhibit INF-α-induced microglia production of IL-6 and nitric oxide, suggesting that inhibiting brain inflammation may represent a novel mechanism of action of antidepressants. Inflammation-mediated imbalance of glutamatergic neurotransmission appears to be similarly implicated in other psychiatric disease, suggesting that immune-mediated glutamatergic disbalance may have a role in the pathophysiology of psychiatric illnesses, including MDD, that are associated with significant cognitive impairments.

There have been some indications that antidepressant drugs may induce changes in TNF-α expression and function in the brain. Treatment with the TCA desipramine depletes neuron-localized TNF-α mRNA and proteins in certain brain regions that may regulate mood expression. Administration of desipramine and amitriptyline, as well as the SSRI zimelidine, decreased TNF-α levels and facilitated NE release. Facilitation of noradrenergic neurotransmission induced by decreased levels of TNF-α in the brain is important to the efficacy of desipramine. This effect appears to be shared by other types of antidepressant drugs. Administration of amitriptyline or zimelidine transformed TNF-α regulation of NE release to facilitation, an effect that occurs in association with α2-adrenergic receptor activation. This field of evidence is growing rapidly and shows that some antidepressants regulate TNF-α levels in the brain and possibly modulate noradrenergic and to some extent serotonergic and dopaminergic neurotransmission. Thus, early evidence shows a regulatory role of TNF-α-induced modulation of synaptic plasticity in the mechanism of antidepressant action.

Antidepressants can inhibit the production and release of proinflammatory cytokines and stimulate the production of anti-inflammatory cytokines, suggesting that reductions in inflammation may contribute to treatment response. This indicates that inhibiting proinflammatory cytokine signaling is a potential strategy for treating depressive disorders, especially in patients with increased inflammatory activity before therapy who are less likely to respond to conventional agents. Cytokine antagonists appear to have antidepressant-like effects, even in the absence of an immune challenge. In humans, administration of the TNF-α blockers has been found to attenuate the depressive symptoms that accompany immune system activation. Thus, it is possible that anticytokine actions may represent a novel therapeutic target in the treatment of depressive disorders in the future. It is also possible that anti-inflammatory cytokines such as IL-4 and IL-10 may also be useful in such therapies.

Neural networks of mood dysfunction

Several brain regions and circuits have been shown to regulate emotions, reward, and executive function, and dysfunctional changes within these highly interconnected limbic regions have been implicated in depression and antidepressant actions [20]. A large amount of the evidence from human postmortem and neuroimaging brain studies of depressed patients shows reductions in gray matter volume and glial density, particularly in the prefrontal cortex and the hippocampus, which are regions thought to mediate the cognitive and emotional aspects of depression, such as feelings of worthlessness and guilt. In contrast to structural studies, experiments investigating brain function, such as functional magnetic resonance imaging (fMRI) or PET, show that activity of the amygdala and subgenual cingulate (Cg25) cortex is strongly correlated with dysphoric emotions. Neuronal activity within these regions is increased by transient sadness in healthy volunteers and is chronically increased in depressed individuals. This activity does return to normal levels with successful antidepressant treatment. Reflecting the structural nature of depression, deep brain stimulation applied to the white matter tracts surrounding Cg25 produced a sustained reversal of depressive symptoms in a small cohort of treatment-resistant patients [21]. Deep brain stimulation, achieved through the stereotactic surgical placement of stimulating electrodes, has also provided a significant improvement in clinical ratings when applied to the NAc, a striatal subregion that is important for reward and for hedonic deficits in depression. These networks are modulated by various monoamine projections from midbrain and brain stem nuclei (dopamine from the ventral tegmental area, serotonin from the dorsal raphé nuclei, and noradrenaline from the LC). Some recent studies have also hypothesized the role of some hypothalamic nuclei in mediating neurovegetative signs of depression. Despite the significant body of evidence describing neural circuits that may mediate symptoms of depression, we are still far from understanding them even in normal individuals. Combining these data with risk factors for depression, the genotype and phenotype of depressed individuals will be even more relevant in future studies [22].

Structural MRI studies

The majority of research in MRI evaluations of depressed subjects suggests structural brain abnormalities. Most studies of patients with MDD showed reduced hippocampal volumes, which is associated with early age of onset, number of previous episodes, or longer duration of untreated depression. However, a significant minority of similar studies failed to determine any association between volume reductions and clinical phenotype of MDD. Reports of hippocampal volume change in bipolar disorder have also been contradictory. There have been reports of increased, decreased, or no change in the hippocampal volume. None of the studies showed any definite changes in the total intracranial volume between patients with depression and healthy subjects.

Volume reduction in MDD was further reported in the prefrontal cortex, primarily in the anterior cingulate and gyrus rectus. Inconsistent results were found regarding amygdala volumes. Studies showed either a reduction in the left amygdala volume, asymmetry of the structure, an increase in bilateral amygdala volume after the first episode of MDD, or a reduction in the bilateral core nuclei [23]. Another approach of some groups was to measure the hippocampus–amygdala complex as a single structure, but these studies found no changes in its volume in comparison with healthy controls. Volume examination of the basal ganglia found decreased left caudate or putamen or no change in the volume. Most studies that assessed white matter changes in people with MDD found an increase in the white matter hyperintensities either periventricularly or more frontally [24]. This is an interesting new avenue of approach that may significantly contribute to the understanding of neural pathways.

Functional positron emission tomography studies

Functional neuroimaging studies should be viewed as complementary to the existing biochemical and structural evidence. A potential advantage of these studies is that they can help improve patient selection for drug therapy or other therapies such as cognitive–behavioral therapy. These studies may also improve treatment monitoring for patients with psychiatric illnesses.

More of these studies were done using PET to measure brain glucose metabolism and blood flow changes. Multiple groups proposed a model of limbic-cortical dysfunction, suggesting that hypometabolism in the prefrontal areas, mesial prefrontal cortex, anterior cingulate, and striatum [25] and an increase in the amygdala glucose metabolism are responsible for symptoms of apathy, attention deficits, executive function impairments, and psychomotor slowing, which are typical for patients with depression [26]. Observed hypermetabolism in other regions, such as in the hypothalamus, insula, and brain stem appears to be responsible for symptoms of disturbed sleep, appetite, and libido. There is no consensus concerning a relationship between blood flow changes and glucose metabolism abnormalities in depressed patients compared to the severity of the disease as measured by scales such as the Beck Depression Inventory or the Hamilton Depression Rating Scale.

More recent data from PET studies using radiolabeled isotopes suggest more specific pathways of neurotransmission [27]. The majority of these studies examined abnormalities in the ligands binding in unipolar and bipolar disorder. Although these data indicated specific areas of dysfunction and some evidence related them to specific clinical symptoms or antidepressant treatment, the common conclusion is still hypothetical [28]. Various other neuroimaging modalities focused on brain white matter changes and more detailed analysis of the pathways involved in psychiatric diseases also promise new insights.

The described model of frontolimbic dysfunction subserves specific but related functions such as mood, cognition, emotions, and circadian rhythm. There is still a need for larger longitudinal studies in selected populations of patients with mood dysfunction. This way, clinicians can better select patients for appropriate therapies, monitor their treatments, and aim for better outcomes.

Conclusion

Our understanding of the neurobiology of depression has evolved substantially, from early speculations about an excess of black bile to theories that focus on chemical imbalances. Most recent hypotheses include gene–environment interactions in conjunction with endocrine, immunological and metabolic mediators, and the current knowledge of cellular, molecular, and epigenetic forms of plasticity (Table 2.1). However, major gaps in the explanation of depression and its treatment still exist. Novel insights into pharmacogenetics and immunomodulatory pathways may bring new ideas and direct future therapies. We should also better understand the biological basis of the efficacy of deep brain stimulation in depression and the therapeutic possibilities of viral-mediated gene delivery, which has been applied successfully in other neuropsychiatric disorders. Finally, depression that occurs as a comorbid condition primarily to neurological diseases, which are described in other chapters, may have different characteristics. Exploring these differences will help us better understand the neurobiology of both disorders [29]. Depressive disorder is complex in its nature, and only multidisciplinary approaches can provide new insights into the neurobiological bases of depression.

Table 2.1 Neurobiology of depression

	Neurochemical Transporters	Neuromodulators	Neural circuit	Major Depression Phenotype
Genotype ⇕ Environment (stressful life events) ⇔	Serotonin (5-HT$_{1A}$, 5-HTT) Norepinephrine (catecholamine depletion) Dopamine (dopamine depletion) GABA (GABA depletion) ⇔	Monoamines (cAMP cascade, CREB) HPA axis dysfun ction (↑CRF) Neurotrophic response (↓BDNF, ↓CREB) Neuroimmune response (↑cytokines, ↑IL-I, ↑TNF-α) ⇔	Hippocampus (↓volume) Amygdala (↓ volume, ↑CBF, ↑FDG uptake) PFC (↓volume, ↓ FDG uptake in Cg 25) Hypothalamus (↓activity) Basal ganglia (↓ volume of caudate and putamen) ⇔	Impaired learning Impaired memory Psychomotor change Increased stress sensitivity Anhedonia Disturbed sleep Autonomic dysfunction Endocrine dysfunction

PEARLS TO TAKE HOME

- Genetics, psychosocial maturation, and stressful events have a cumulative impact on major depressive disorder.
- Gene–environment interactions seem to be a major predictor of a person's risk for major depressive disorder.
- Structural and functional brain abnormalities in patients with major depressive disorder may be associated with abnormal function of the HPA axis, low levels of BDNF, and imbalance of neurotransmitters.
- Current options for antidepressant treatment are limited by the delayed onset of action, lack of efficacy, and adverse outcomes.
- Some chronic neurological disorders have increased prevalence of depression.

Acknowledgment

This work was funded by the Epilepsy Foundation grant to HH.

References

1. Krishnan V, Nestler EJ. The molecular neurobiology of depression. *Nature*, 455(7215): 894–902, 2008.
2. aan het Rot M, Mathew SJ, Charney DS. Neurobiological mechanisms in major depressive disorder. *CMAJ*, 180(3): 305–313, 2009.
3. Sheline YI, Sanghavi M, Mintun MA, et al. Depression duration but not age predicts hippocampal volume loss in medically healthy women with recurrent major depression. *J Neurosci*, 19(12): 5034–5043, 1999.
4. Drevets WC. Neuroimaging and neuropathological studies of depression: implications for the cognitive-emotional features of mood

disorders. *Curr Opin Neurobiol*, 11(2): 240–249, 2001.

5. Hado-Vieira R, Salvadore G, Luckenbaugh DA, et al. Rapid onset of antidepressant action: a new paradigm in the research and treatment of major depressive disorder. *J Clin Psychiatry*, 69(6): 946–958, 2008.

6. Price JL. Prefrontal cortical networks related to visceral function and mood. *Ann N Y Acad Sci*, 877: 383–396, 1999.

7. Woolsey T, Hanaway J, Gado M. *The Brain Atlas: A Visual Guide to the Human Central Nervous System*, 2nd ed. Hoboken, NJ: John Wiley & Sons, Inc., 2003.

8. Duvernoy HM. *The Human Hippocampus: Functional Anatomy, Vascularization and Serial Sections with MRI*. Berlin, Germany: Springer-Verlag, 1998.

9. Delgado PL, Price LH, Miller HL, et al. Serotonin and the neurobiology of depression. Effects of tryptophan depletion in drug-free depressed patients. *Arch Gen Psychiatry*, 51(11): 865–874, 1994.

10. Azmitia EC, Gannon PJ, Kheck NM, et al. Cellular localization of the 5-HT1A receptor in primate brain neurons and glial cells. *Neuropsychopharmacology*, 14(1): 35–46, 1996.

11. Gross C, Zhuang X, Stark K, et al. Serotonin1A receptor acts during development to establish normal anxiety-like behaviour in the adult. *Nature*, 416(6879): 396–400, 2002.

12. Wong ML, Kling MA, Munson PJ, et al. Pronounced and sustained central hypernoradrenergic function in major depression with melancholic features: relation to hypercortisolism and corticotropin-releasing hormone. *Proc Natl Acad Sci USA*, 97(1): 325–330, 2000.

13. Lambert G, Johansson M, Agren H, et al. Reduced brain norepinephrine and dopamine release in treatment-refractory depressive illness: evidence in support of the catecholamine hypothesis of mood disorders. *Arch Gen Psychiatry*, 57(8): 787–793, 2000.

14. Nestler EJ, Barrot M, DiLeone RJ, et al. Neurobiology of depression. *Neuron*, 34(1): 13–25, 2002.

15. Coyle JT, Duman RS. Finding the intracellular signaling pathways affected by mood disorder treatments. *Neuron*, 38(2): 157–160, 2003.

16. Chen AC, Shirayama Y, Shin KH, et al. Expression of the cAMP response element binding protein (CREB) in hippocampus produces an antidepressant effect. *Biol Psychiatry*, 49(9): 753–762, 2001.

17. Shirayama Y, Chen AC, Nakagawa S, et al. Brain-derived neurotrophic factor produces antidepressant effects in behavioral models of depression. *J Neurosci*, 22(8): 3251–3261, 2002.

18. Chen B, Dowlatshahi D, MacQueen GM, et al. Increased hippocampal BDNF immunoreactivity in subjects treated with antidepressant medication. *Biol Psychiatry*, 50(4): 260–265, 2001.

19. Khairova RA, Hado-Vieira R, Du J, et al. A potential role for pro-inflammatory cytokines in regulating synaptic plasticity in major depressive disorder. *Int J Neuropsychopharmacol*, 12(4): 561–578, 2009.

20. Hecimovic H, Gilliam F. Neurobiology of depression and new opportunities for treatment. In: *Depression and Brain Dysfunction*, eds. F Gilliam, AM Kanner, YI Sheline. New York: Taylor & Francis Group, 2005.

21. Mayberg HS, Lozano AM, Voon V, et al. Deep brain stimulation for treatment-resistant depression. *Neuron*, 45(5): 651–660, 2005.

22. Gilliam F, Santos J, Vahle V, et al. Depression in epilepsy: ignoring clinical expression of neuronal network dysfunction? *Epilepsia*, 45, Suppl. 2: 28–33, 2004.

23. Sheline YI, Gado MH, Price JL. Amygdala core nuclei volumes are decreased in recurrent major depression. *Neuroreport*, 9(9): 2023–2028, 1998.

24. Taylor WD, Steffens DC, MacFall JR, et al. White matter hyperintensity progression and late-life depression outcomes. *Arch Gen Psychiatry*, 60(11): 1090–1096, 2003.

25. Meyer JH, Kruger S, Wilson AA, et al. Lower dopamine transporter binding potential in striatum during depression. *Neuroreport*, 12(18): 4121–4125, 2001.

26. Drevets WC, Price JL, Simpson JR Jr., et al. Subgenual prefrontal cortex abnormalities in mood disorders. *Nature*, 386(6627): 824–827, 1997.

27. Drevets WC, Frank E, Price JC, et al. PET imaging of serotonin 1A receptor binding

in depression. *Biol Psychiatry*, 46(10): 1375–1387, 1999.

28. Hecimovic H, Goldstein JD, Sheline YI, et al. Mechanisms of depression in epilepsy from a clinical perspective. *Epilepsy Behav*, 4, Suppl. 3: S25–S30, 2003.

29. Gilliam F, Hecimovic H, Sheline Y. Psychiatric comorbidity, health, and function in epilepsy. *Epilepsy Behav*, 4, Suppl. 4: S26–S30, 2003.

Idiopathic Depressive Disorders: Basic Principles

John J. Barry
Department of Psychiatry, Stanford School of Medicine, Palo Alto, CA, USA

Clinical manifestations of idiopathic depressive disorders

Mood disorders have become an increased concern among health-care professionals. It has been estimated that 26% of women and 12% of men will experience a depressive disorder in their lifetime [1, 2]. In fact, depression ranks fourth in the list of the most important medical issues worldwide [2]. There is also speculation that prevalence of the disorder is rising, especially in the young. Depression associated with bipolar disorder is also increasingly being recognized and may now account for up to 50% of depressive episodes in patients [1].

In order to fully appreciate the overlap between the clinical appearances of depression as it presents in patients with a primary central nervous system (CNS) disorder, it is imperative to understand the features of an idiopathic depressive disorder. The purpose of this chapter will be to review the primary manifestations of mood disorders not associated with or secondary to a comorbid neurologic disorder as they present in the general population. Definitions of the two major categories of mood disorders will be outlined as defined by the *Diagnostic and Statistical Manual of Mental Disorders*, Fourth Edition (DSM-IV). This review will be followed by a discussion of comorbidity issues, that is, depressive disorders associated with another psychiatric or medical illness. Since the co-occurrence of anxiety disorders and depression is particularly problematic, it will be a major focus of the discussion. The natural history of a treated mood disorder will follow, along with treatment issues, focusing on a definition of "effective treatment" of an idiopathic mood disorder.

Mood disorders: general issues

Given the aforementioned rates of mood disorders in the general population, it is surprising that the recognition of clinical depression is seriously neglected. It has been estimated that the presence of an idiopathic depressive disorder is missed in over two-thirds of patients [3–5]. The same issue can certainly be noted in depression coupled with a CNS disorder [6].

The economic burden of mood disorders is severe. It has been noted that by 2020, depression will be the second leading cause of disability behind only cardiovascular disease [7]. In underdeveloped countries, it will be the leading cause of disability. The economic costs are also astounding. Counting absenteeism and decreased productivity, depression may cause upwards of $44 billion per year in the United States [8]. This represents an excess of $31 billion compared with workers without depression [9]. It has also been estimated that 72% of those with depressive disorders are included in the work force [10].

Depression in Neurologic Disorders: Diagnosis and Management, First Edition.
Edited by Andres M. Kanner.
© 2012 Blackwell Publishing Ltd. Published 2012 by Blackwell Publishing Ltd.

Quality of life is impacted as well. People with idiopathic depressive disorders have a precipitous decrease in their quality of life equal to that seen in medical conditions such as arthritis and kidney disease [11]. Finally, morbidity and mortality of many medical illnesses are significantly affected by depressive illness, and a prevalent and significant bidirectionality also exists [12–15]

Definition of mood disorders

According to the DSM-IV-TR (fourth edition, text revision), mood disorders are grouped into "mood episodes" and "mood disorders" [16]. It must be understood that these are phenomenological descriptions that categorize disease based on symptomatology, not biology. Thus, there may be many diseases that in themselves are discrete biological entities but manifest with an associated depression. In addition, depression may have many subtypes that are in themselves unique; however, at present, the state of the art is not sensitive enough to discriminate between them. This may be true for depression associated with grief, bipolar disorder, psychotic depression, and certainly depression associated with CNS disorders and the iatrogenic depressive disorders associated with their treatment. The appearance of the disorder may be generally the same, but important differences exist that may extend to treatment as well [17].

Mood episodes are characterized into those that are major depressive or those associated with bipolar disease with manic, mixed, or hypomanic states [16]. Mood disorders can be bifurcated into two major categories: unipolar and bipolar affective disorders (BADs). In addition, mood disorders can be grouped into those appearing as a consequence of a general medical condition or a substance-induced mood dysfunction [16].

Unipolar depressive disorders can be further broken down into major depressive disorders (MDDs), dysthymic disorders, and depressive disorders not otherwise specified. MDD is a severe mood disorder defined as a symptom complex lasting for at least 2 weeks and displaying at least five of the features listed in Table 3.1 [16]. Dysthymic disorder is more persistent than MDD but milder in intensity, as defined in Table 3.2 [16]. As will be discussed later, residual depressive symptoms may be present after the treatment of a mood disorder and may result in a persistent decline in quality of life [18]. In addition, the diagnosis of MDD may be associated with qualifiers, including MDD with psychotic features, melancholia, catatonia, atypical features, or postpartum

Table 3.1 Symptoms of a major depressive episode [16]

- Five or more of the symptoms listed below occurring during a 2-week period or more and must include the presence of depressed mood or loss of interest:
  - Problems with appetite and associated weight loss or gain
  - Psychomotor agitation or retardation
  - Loss of interest and drive
  - Difficulty concentrating and making decisions
  - Worthlessness, guilt, frustration
  - Repeated thoughts of death or suicide
  - Sleep disturbance

Table 3.2 Symptoms of a dysthymic disorder [16]

- For at least 2 years for more days than not—depressed mood

- While depressed, at least two of the following symptoms were found without reprieve for not more than 2 months at a time:
  - Fatigue
  - Increased or decreased appetite
  - Sleep dysfunction
  - Low self-esteem
  - Difficulty with concentration or decisions
  - Hopelessness

- Caveats—no episode of MDD occurred at the onset of the illness and the symptoms cannot be explained as those associated with a psychotic disorder or a manic or substance abuse disorder and the symptoms are serious enough to cause psychological consequences.

onset. Each categorical grouping may have specific treatment implications.

Bipolar disorder presents as a fluctuating chronic disease that consists of episodes of elevated mood lasting for greater than 1 week and associated with at least three of the following symptoms: racing thoughts, decreased need for sleep, pressured speech, distractibility, and increased goal-directed activity, which may include agitation, intrusiveness, grandiosity, and impulsive pleasure-seeking activity. Psychosis may be a part of the illness in more severe episodes. One type of mood cycle will often be followed by another featuring the opposite mood polarity, for example, mania then depression. An increased suicide risk of up to 19% [19] is also present. Mixed episodes that combine depressive and manic symptoms during the same episode may also take place. In 15% of patients, "rapid cycling" takes place, with four or more cycles per year. As alluded to earlier, the depressive phase noted during a BAD cycle appears to be a distinct entity from that seen with an MDD. It may have its own characteristics, course, and treatment response, with antidepressants actually inducing mania (classified as a substance-induced mood disorder) [20]. These facts are important when reviewing mood symptoms in patients with mood disorders since increased rates of BAD may be seen with neurologic disorders such a epilepsy [14] and multiple sclerosis [21].

Comorbidity of mood disorders with medical illnesses

Depression can be both a cause and a consequence of medical illness and is a common comorbid phenomenon. Its presence is more the rule than the exception. For example, depression appears to increase the risk of coronary heart disease and is a major factor in mortality from myocardial infarction. Reasons for this association are many and include physiological factors, for example, increased hypothylamic–pituitary–adrenal axis hyperactivity with cortisol elevation, platelet activation and hypercoagulability, and elevated levels of pro-inflammatory cytokines accelerating atherosclerosis [15]. Cancer, HIV/AIDS, and neurologic disorders that are the subject of this book also provide examples of this fact. In addition, several authors have commented on the bidirectionality of depression in neurologic disorders such as epilepsy where depression may have a causal effect of the development of a somatic illness [12–14].

Comorbidity of mood disorders and other psychiatric illnesses

The National Comorbidity Survey noted that 79% of lifetime-to-date psychiatric disorders are observed to be comorbid with other psychiatric disorders [22]. Probably the most frequent and important comorbidity of lifelong depression is the presence of an anxiety disorder. Just as in depression, anxiety disorders can be subdivided into several different categories. They include Generalized Anxiety Disorder (GAD), Panic Disorder, Posttraumatic Stress Disorder (PTSD), Phobias, Obsessive Compulsive Disorder, and Acute Stress Disorder [16]. The overall incidence of a comorbidity of an anxiety and depressive disorder has been quoted in one review at 40% to 75% [23]. Kessler et al. [22] noted that 51% of patients experiencing a major depressive episode also had a concomitant anxiety disorder. In another review, 48.6% of adolescences and young adults with an MDD manifested symptoms consistent with an anxiety disorder as well [24].

The presence of comorbid depression and anxiety is a harbinger of a more treatment-refractory course of illness. It is also associated with more severe symptoms, poorer outcomes, increased suicidality, and expanded medical utilization [25–27]. In patients with anxiety and depressive disorders, depression may begin earlier and have a worse course [28]. Comorbid depression and anxiety appears to affect longevity of symptoms. For example, after 32 months, 41% of a comorbid group retained symptoms, in contrast to 4.7% of people in the general population who had either a persistent depressive or anxiety disorder initially [29]. Patients with panic disorder and depression have a 15-fold increased incidence of suicidal ideation [30, 31]. Treatment intervention will also be affected.

The comorbidity of depression and anxiety is seen in a variety of settings. A high comorbidity has been found in adolescence, which is also associated with more severe symptoms [32]. This association is also noted in people with chronic diseases such as cancer [33], migraine [34], irritable bowel syndrome [35], and epilepsy [36]. In a review by Katon et al. evaluating only randomized controlled studies of >100 patients, the severity of physical symptoms was as strongly correlated with anxiety and depression as it was with physiological measures [26]. The diseases evaluated were diabetes, coronary heart disease, pulmonary disease, asthma, congestive heart disease, osteoarthritis, and rheumatoid arthritis.

A review of the neurobiological aspects of depressive and anxiety disorders helps explain the high comorbid occurrence of these conditions. The neurobiological aspects of depressive disorders have been reviewed in a previous section of this book (see Chapter 2). Overlapping neuroanatomical pathways of both depressive and anxiety disorders may explain the clinical features noted above [28]. For example, the ventral prefrontal cortex appears to function as an executive area in emotional disorders and chemically, structurally, and functionally shows abnormalities in both of these disorders [28]. The amygdyla also functions abnormally in these disorders, and the hippocampus may be damaged in untreated long-term depression. Reduced hippocampal volume may also be a vulnerability factor for the development of PTSD with trauma [28]. The fact that antidepressants are effective for both anxiety and depressive disorders implies a common neurocircuitry and common operant neurotransmitter systems. It appears that the stimulation of neurogenesis may be a common pathway for the treatment of both disorders, and there may be common genetic pathways here as well [28]. It has been observed that anxiety and depression may be manifestations of a single illness [37]. However, different types of environmental risks seem to cause GAD and MDD. For example, loss and humiliation may result in MDD, while danger may be associated more with GAD. Common effective treatments argue for extensive overlap of physiological causes; however, there are differences. For example, benzodiazapines work well for anxiety but do not resolve depressive symptoms [28]. Others have reviewed several models to explain this phenomena [23].

Identification of a mood disorder using psychometric tools

In psychiatry, the gold standard for the measurement of the presence of a mood disorder is the Structured Clinical Interview for DSM-IV Axis I Disorders (SCID). Every other test measuring or following the progress of the treatment of depression is based on a comparison with the SCID. These tests include both self-rating and self-assessment scales.

The most commonly used self-rating scales for the evaluation of general psychiatric communities are the Beck Depression Inventory (BDI) and the Center for Epidemiological Studies Depression Scale (CES-D). Both of these psychometric tools have been validated in screening for depression in epilepsy patients. Other measures in common use in psychiatry include the Hospital Anxiety and Depression Scale (HADS) and, for geriatric patients, the Geriatric Depression Scale (GDS). Interviewer-administered devices include the Hamilton Rating Scale for Depression (HAM-D) and the Montgomery–Åsberg Depression Rating Scale (MADRS), among others. For further details on these instruments please refer to Yonkers and Samson [38].

A word of caution regarding overreliance on psychometric tools is indicated. Patients may complain of depression that compromises their quality of life regardless of the results of a psychometric test. Items on some psychometric tests ask for "changes" in mood, and patients who have had a lengthy episode of depression will answer these questions negatively, causing a spuriously low score. Treatment may thus be necessary regardless of the test score.

Treatment issues

Natural history of an idiopathic depressive disorder

Depression is an episodic disorder that tends to have a relapsing and remitting course. With the index episode of depression, the expected response (greater than 50% resolution of symptoms) to an antidepressant drug (AD) is in the realm of 50–65% [18, 39, 40]. However, residual symptoms frequently remain. Subsyndromal depression results from and may be the cause of relapse. This is a critical factor in the treatment of this disorder. Compared to patients who have made a complete recovery, it is estimated that there is a five times greater incidence of relapse in patients with residual symptoms [18, 41]. Clearly, depression is "dimensional not categorical" [18].

Undertreatment of MDD is frequent. Katon noted that of the 55% of patients identified with an MDD in a primary care clinic, only 11% were appropriately treated [42].

Interventions

Evaluation The psychometric tools mentioned earlier are utilized with particular attention to the presence of suicidal ideation and anxiety, as noted previously. Bipolar disorder should also be evaluated. The Mood Disorder Questionnaire (MDQ) is a reasonable screening instrument. It is a 13-item self-rating questionnaire, in which the score can range from 0 to 13. A score of >6 is a cut-off point suggestive of a Bipolar Spectrum Disorder.

Two other features of the patient's history should alert the physician to the presence of BAD: a family history of BAD and a history of an induction of mood elation with the use of ADs. Evaluation is critical because treatment of a bipolar depression is different from that of a unipolar mood disorder. The rest of this chapter concerns unipolar depression [43].

Other causes of a depressive disorder should be assessed, including medical and iatrogenic causes. If treatment is necessary, options are discussed with the patient, including psychotherapy, which may be individual, couples, or group therapy. Individual therapy may include cognitive–behavior therapy (CBT) or interpersonal therapies.

Nonpharmacological treatment There appears to be clinical efficacy for nonpharmacological interventions, especially those consisting of CBT and interpersonal therapies [44, 45]. Pharmacotherapy was compared with nonpharmacological interventions in the National Institute of Mental Health (NIMH) Collaborative Research Program for Depression, and equal efficacy was found with several important caveats [45]. First, it appears that medication provides more effectiveness for patients with a more severe depression. Second, combination psychotherapy and medication provide a synergistic effect. This was confirmed in a study evaluating the antidepressant nefazodone and cognitive–behavioral analysis system (CBAS) intervention. The combination group had an 85% response rate, compared with 55% for the medication group and 46% for the CBAS group [46]. CBT has also been shown to be useful for residual depressive symptoms, resulting in fewer relapses [43, 47].

Pharmacological therapy Before beginning an antidepressant, a detailed history is imperative, as it may help to guide antidepressant treatment. For example, an AD that worked in the past can be considered as a first option. Also, drug interactions must be reviewed, and a family history of response to one antidepressant may indirectly reveal a genetic factor influencing the patient's possible AD response. A personal history of prior depressive episodes, onset and course of the depression, plus a history of childhood neglect and abuse may also provide a clue to a possible poor response to ADs [48–50].

Pharmacological intervention requires appropriate recognition and adequate treatment. Treatment algorithms have been developed to maximize efficacy. Today, clinicians have access to several families of AD. These include tricyclic antidepressants (TCAs), monoamine oxidase inhibitors (MAOI), selective serotonin reuptake inhibitors (SSRIs), and serotonin and norepinephrine reuptake inhibitors (SNRIs). A detailed review of each family and their pharmacologic effects can be found in Chapter 8.

Studies performed to evaluate treatment as usual compared with a standardized approach have documented the superiority of a guidelines approach [51–55]. As previously stated, patients are frequently underdosed, receive inadequate follow-up, and stop their medications early. Thus, there appears to be a significant gap between what is felt to be best practice and what is actually delivered [56]. It is the author's experience that patients will often report efficacy of treatment, but when measured by a standardized measure (e.g., BDI), high levels of depression remain. An algorithm often helps to ensure improved patient satisfaction over treatment as usual [57]. This observation was proven by the Texas Medication Algorithm Project [58, 59]. In that study, 60% of the patients had a medical illness.

The response rate after an initial pharmacological intervention was discussed earlier. In general, unless other information is gleaned from the patient's personal or family history, a serotonin reuptake inhibitor (fluoxetine, paroxetine, sertraline, citalopram, escitalopram) provides the practitioner with a useful first-line intervention with maximum efficacy and minimum side effects. However, some authors postulate the superiority of antidepressants with more complex neurotransmitter activity [14, 60]. In addition, targeting specific prominent symptoms associated with the mood disorder may also affect the treatment approach. For example, patients with prominent pain complaints may be given an SNRI such as venlafaxine or duloxetine, while those with melancholic features may respond better to an SNRI, mirtazepine, or a TCA. Patients with atypical features may be more preferably treated with an MAOI or SSRI. Cost may also be a factor. Generic SSRIs are the least expensive, while brand-name SNRIs are more expensive [43, 61].

SNRIs such as venlafaxine may have distinct advantages. SNRIs have more complex and widespread neurotransmitter effects by acting on serotonin, norepinephrine, and, in higher dosages, dopamine. This may result in higher remission rates than seen with SSRIs [14, 60] and faster onset of action than a medication such as fluoxetine [60]. Conversely, they are more difficult to use, more expensive, and may result in increases in blood pressure with increasing dosages [62]. In addition to the ADs cited above, there are other psychotropic drugs compounds, particularly those used for augmentation strategies of the antidepressant effect. These include mood-stabilizing agents (e.g., lithium, lamotrigine), atypical antipsychotics (quetiapine and aripiprazole, for example), and CNS stimulants (methylphenidate) [43].

Acute, continuation, and maintenance phases of treatment

When an effective dose of an AD is reached, it generally takes from 6 to 12 weeks until remission. During this interval, the patient should be watched for increasing suicidal ideation, especially when energy returns before the depression lifts. The next phase of treatment consists of a continuation phase lasting from 4 to 9 months. This period consolidates treatment and is a time of potential relapse. Maintenance therapy is reserved for patients with repeated episodes of depression, for whom the probability of relapse may reach 85%. In addition, a history of severe depression, especially with suicidal ideation, continued residual depressive complaints, or psychotic features may catalyze the treating physician to continue maintenance treatment indefinitely [43, 63].

Given the necessity to treat depression adequately, it is important to watch for the patient developing tolerance to the AD and a return of symptoms. This may occur in 9–33% of patients [64]. In addition, when titrating off of an AD, patients need to be warned of drug withdrawal, which may involve symptoms such as agitation, vivid dream activity, nausea, dizziness, and neurologic complaints [14, 62].

Treatment-resistant depression

As noted previously, the goal of depression treatment is the complete resolution of symptoms, that is, remission. One area of interest in the treatment of idiopathic depressive disorders is what to do when there is a lack of response to an initial trial of an AD. This situation was evaluated in the Sequenced Treatment Alternatives to Relieve Depression (STAR*D) investigation. This study involved 3671 patients who manifested symptoms of an MDD and were treated with AD in an algorithmic fashion. Interestingly, two-thirds of the group had a recurrent depressive disorder, the same number had a concurrent medical illness, and 44.6% had a concurrent anxiety disorder [65]. All patients were started on citalopram. It is important to note that the mean dosage was 48.3 mg/day for a time to remission of 6.7 weeks [66]. Both of these facts are important since much of the literature in the treatment of CNS disorders shows studies using less mean AD dosing [8]. Another important factor in the study is the recommended frequency of visits, a suggestion that may need to be transferred to patients treated for comorbid mood and neurologic disorders. Of the 1721 patients in the study without suicidal ideation, 7% developed emergent suicidal ideation, which resolved in two-thirds of those patients by the end of the study. It is unclear whether this was due to the medication [43, 67].

With nonresponse to an initial intervention, a series of switch and augmentation strategies were used. Full descriptions are supplied elsewhere [43]. The remission rate for the first intervention of citalopram was 36.8%, with the next step accruing another 30.6%, step three with 13.7%, and the final step with 13.0%. The overall cumulative remission rate was 67%, but only 43% sustained remission over time [43]. Thus, alternatives are needed. Other augmentation strategies that have shown efficacy are again described elsewhere [43, 68, 69].

Alternative interventions

The most effective intervention in the treatment of severe acute resistant depression is electroconvulsive therapy (ECT), especially when it is associated with a high suicidal risk [70]. A description of its usage can be found in References [70, 71]. In general, unilateral electrode placement is utilized to minimize memory impairment from the procedure but may not be as effective as bilateral treatment. Sessions are decreased in frequency after an initial response. Relapse is frequent after ECT treatment if effective AD therapy is not given, and thus ECT itself may be used as a long-term strategy for the treatment of a severe refractory disorder [43].

Other nonpharmacological interventions include vagus nerve stimulation. Initially used for people with epilepsy and refractory seizures, vagus nerve stimulation was evaluated by Rush et al. for refractory MDD and depression associated with BAD. A 40% response rate was found [72, 73]. This resulted in a sham-controlled study, which after 10 weeks showed nonstatistically significant response on the HAM-D; however, a secondary measure, the Inventory of Depressive Symptomatology Self-Report, a response rate of 17.0% for the active group and 7.3% for the control group was found, which was statistically significant [74]. In a 1-year evaluation of treated patients compared with a treatment-as-usual group, response for the active group was 27% versus 13% for the treatment-as-usual group. These results led to an approval for the device in those patients with an MDD who have failed four or more adequate AD treatments [43, 75].

Another possibly useful intervention for resistant MDD is repetitive transcranial magnetic stimulation (rTMS). In a recent sham-controlled randomized study by George et al., left prefrontal TMS for moderate resistant MDD was found to be efficacious. In the active TMS group, 14.1% remitted, while only 5.1% responded in the sham treatment group. In the open-label follow-up, 30.2% of the remaining patients responded [76]. In 2008, the Food and Drug Administration (FDA) approved the intervention for the treatment of resistant depression.

Finally, deep brain stimulation is being developed as a possible intervention for people with a severely refractory depressive disorder. This was investigated in six patients by Mayberg et al., with four patients responding to treatment and three in full remission. The discussion of this intervention is beyond the scope of this chapter [77].

Special circumstances

As mentioned previously, comorbid depression and anxiety is a frequent occurrence. Treatment of both disorders is imperative and often requires the use of an anxiolytic and an AD. Medications such as TCA, SSRIs, venlafaxine, and mirtazepine are useful interventions. A specific anxiolytic can be used initially and titrated off as the AD shows increasing activity [78–80]. In addition, CBT treatment has also shown efficacy for comorbid symptoms [81].

Depression seen in the context of a BAD requires different therapeutic intervention than in the context of a unipolar MDD. The first line of treatment is a mood stabilizer and not an antidepressant, which may catalyze a cycle shift, that is, induce a manic episode and possible cycle acceleration [82]. These issues are discussed in an update from the Texas Implementation of Medication Algorithm [83]. Further discussion of these issues can be found in Reference [43].

Two other special situations are important to mention regarding the treatment of an idiopathic depressive disorder. The presence of psychotic features in the context of a depressive disorder also requires a different interventional approach and heightens the possibility of suicide [2]. In addition to an AD, an antipsychotic agent is required for effective treatment, with ECT the treatment of choice [43, 84]. Finally, geriatric patients also present a special situation. It is important to remember that depression is seen in nearly 6.5% of elderly individuals and accounts for 18% of suicides in the normal population [85].

Metabolic changes and drug–drug interactions must be taken into consideration, and ADs with anticholinergic properties (e.g., TCAs) should be avoided.

Conclusion

This chapter aimed to review the phenomenology of depressive disorders as seen in patients with idiopathic mood dysfunction. The natural course of the disorder was reviewed in addition to treatment issues, both with and without pharmacological intervention. With this information, it is hoped that the overlap of depression seen in the general population can be adequately compared to the appearance and treatment issues of depression comorbid with a CNS disorder. Differences and similarities can then be better clarified, resulting in an improved understanding of the disorder in general.

💡 PEARLS TO TAKE HOME

1. It is imperative to understand the features of an idiopathic depressive disorder to recognize and treat depression as it appears in CNS diseases.
2. Recognition of mood disorders in the general population is missed in over two-thirds of patients, resulting in an astounding economic burden.
3. Comorbidity of mood disorders and other psychiatric illnesses is frequent. Anxiety and mood disorders appear together in 40–75% of patients and may be a harbinger of a possibly more serious course with treatment resistance.
4. The neurobiology of both mood and anxiety disorders overlaps significantly.
5. Identification of mood disorders has been aided by the use of easy-to-use psychometric screens.
6. Nonpharmacological and pharmacological interventions may be synergistic when used in combination.
7. Consensus guidelines have been developed using information gleaned from several algorithm studies.

8. Other special interventions include electroconvulsive treatment, transcranial magnetic stimulation, vagus nerve stimulation, and deep brain stimulation.
9. Different treatment modalities need to be considered for patients with a depression associated with a BAD and a depressive disorder with psychotic features.

References

1. Akiskal H. Mood disorders. In: *Comprehensive Textbook of Psychiatry*, eds. B Sadock and V Sadock. New York: Lippincott Williams & Williams, pp. 1559–1575, 2005.
2. Barry JJ. The recognition and management of mood disorders as a comorbidity of epilepsy. *Epilepsia*, 44, Suppl. 4: 30–40, 2003.
3. Coyle J, et al. Non-detection of depression by primary care physicians reconsidered. *Gen Hosp Psychiatry*, 17: 3–12, 1995.
4. Hirschfeld RM, et al. The National Depressive and Manic-Depressive Association consensus statement on the undertreatment of depression. *JAMA*, 277: 333–340, 1997.
5. Hermann BP, et al. Psychiatric comorbidity in chronic epilepsy: identification, consequences, and treatment of major depression. *Epilepsia*, 41, Suppl. 2: S31–S41, 2000.
6. Ettinger AB, et al. Symptoms of depression and anxiety in pediatric epilepsy patients. *Epilepsia*, 39(6): 595–599, 1998.
7. Glass RM. Awareness about depression: important for all physicians. *JAMA*, 289: 3169–3173, 2003.
8. Barry JJ, Jones JE. What is effective treatment of depression in people with epilepsy. *Epilepsy Behav*, 6(4): 520–528, 2005.
9. Stewart WF, et al. Cost of lost productive work time among US workers with depression. *JAMA*, 289: 3135–3144, 2003.
10. Davidson JRT, Meltzer-Brody SE. The underrecognition and undertreatment of depression: what is the breath and depth of the problem. *J Clin Psychiatry*, 60, Suppl. 7: 4–9, 1999.
11. Spitzer RL, et al. Health-related quality of life in primary care patients with mental disorders:

results from PRIME-MD 1000 Study. *JAMA*, 274: 1511–1517, 1995.

12. Kanner AM. Depression in epilepsy: prevalence, clinical semiology, pathogenic mechanisms, and treatment. *Biol Psychiatry*, 54(3): 388–398, 2003.

13. Kanner AM. Depression and the risk of neurological disorders. *Lancet*, 366(9492): 1147–1148, 2005.

14. Barry J, et al. Affective disorders in epilepsy. In: *Psychiatric Issues in Epilepsy: A Practical Guide to Diagnosis and Treatment*, eds. AB Ettinger and AM Kanner. Philadelphia, PA: Lippincott Williams & Williams, pp. 203–247, 2007.

15. Evans DL, Charney D. Mood disorders and medical illness: a major public health problem. *Biol Psychiatry*, 3: 177–180, 2003.

16. Association AP. *Diagnostic and Statistical Manual of Mental Disorders*, 4th ed. Washington, DC: American Psychiatric Press, 1994.

17. Higgins ES, George MS. *The Neuroscience of Clinical Psychiatry*, New York: Lippincott Williams& Wilkins, 2007.pp. 227–237.

18. Judd LL, et al. Major depressive disorder: prospective study of residual subthreshold depressive symptoms as predictor of rapid relapse. *J Affect Disord*, 50: 97–108, 1998.

19. American Psychiatric Association. Practice guidelines for the treatment of patients with bipolar disorder. *Am J Psychiatry*, 151, Suppl. 12: 1–36, 1994.

20. Schatzberg AF. Bipolar disorder: recent issues in diagnosis and classification. *J Clin Psychiatry*, 59, Suppl. 6: 5–10, 1998.

21. Kanner AM, Barry JJ. Is the psychopathology of epilepsy different from that of nonepileptic patients? *Epilepsy Behav*, 2: 170–186, 2001.

22. Kessler RC, et al. Lifetime and 12-month prevalence of DSM-III-R psychiatric disorders in the United States—results from the national comorbidity survey. *Arch Gen Psychiatry*, 51: 8–19, 1994.

23. Shankman SA, Klein DN. The relation between depression and anxiety: an evaluation of the tripartite, approach-withdrawal and valence-arousal models. *Clin Psychol Rev*, 23: 605–637, 2003.

24. Wittchen HU, et al. Prevalence of mental disorders and psychological impairments in adolescents and young adults. *Psychol Med*, 28: 109–126, 1998.

25. van Balkom AJLM, et al. Comorbid depression, but not comorbid anxiety disorders, predicts poor outcome in anxiety disorders. *Depress Anxiety*, 25: 408–415, 2008.

26. Katon WJ, et al. The association of depression and anxiety with medical symptom burden in patients with chronic medical illness. *Gen Hosp Psychiatry*, 29: 147–155, 2007.

27. Brown LA, et al. The impact of panic-agoraphobic comorbidity on suicidality in hospitalized patients with major depression. *Depress Anxiety*, 27: 310–315, 2010.

28. Keller MB. Untangling depression and anxiety: clinical challenges. *J Clin Psychiatry*, 66(11): 1478–1487, 2005.

29. Young AS, et al. Persistent depression and anxiety in the United States: prevalence and quality of care. *Psychiatr Serv*, 59(12): 1391–1398, 2008.

30. Goodwin R, et al. Panic and suicidal ideation in primary care. *Depress Anxiety*, 14: 244–246, 2001.

31. Fawcett J, et al. Time-related predictors of suicide in major depression disorder. *Am J Psychiatry*, 147: 1189–1194, 1990.

32. O'Neil KA, et al. Comorbid depressive disorders in anxiety-disordered youth: demographic, clinical, and family characteristics. *Child Psychiatry Hum Dev*, 41(3): 330–341, 2010.

33. Brown LF, et al. The association of depression and anxiety with health-related quality of life in cancer patients with depression and/or anxiety. *Psychooncology*, 19(7): 734–741, 2010.

34. Tietjen GE, et al. Depression and anxiety: effect on the migraine-obesity relationship. *Headache*, 47(6): 876–877, 2007.

35. Hillila MT, et al. Comorbidity and use of health-care services among irritable bowel syndrome sufferers. *Scand J Gastroenterol*, 42(7): 799–806, 2007.

36. Jones JE, et al. Rates and risk factors for suicide, suicidal ideation, and suicide attempts in chronic epilepsy. *Epilepsy Behav*, 4, Suppl. 3: S31–S38, 2003.

37. Maj M. "Psychiatric comorbidity": an artefact of current diagnostic systems? *Br J Psychiary*, 186: 182–184, 2005.

38. Yonkers KA, Samson J. Mood disorder measures. In: *Handbook of Psychiatric Measures*, ed. AJ Rush, et al. Washington, DC: American Psychiatric Association, pp. 515–549, 2005.

39. Greden JF. Unmet need: what justifies the search for a new antidepressant? *J Clin Psychiatry*, 63, Suppl. 2: 3–7, 2002.

40. Kennedy SH, et al. *Treating Depression Effectively*, New York: Martin Dunitz, 2004.

41. Paykel ES, et al. Residual symptoms after partial remission: an important outcome in depression. *Psychol Med*, 25: 1171–1180, 1995.

42. Katon WJ. Clinical and health services relationships between major depression, depressive symptoms, and general medical illness. *Biol Psychiatry*, 54: 216–226, 2003.

43. Barry JJ, et al. Consensus statement: the evaluation and treatment of people with epilepsy and affective disorders. *Epilepsy Behav*, 13: S1–S29, 2008.

44. Agras WS. Behavioral therapy. In: *Comprehensive Textbook of Psychiatry/VI*, ed. BJ Sadock. Baltimore, MD: Williams & Wilkins, 1995.

45. Hollon SD, et al. Psychotherapy and medication in the treatment of adult and geriatric depression: which monotherapy or combined treatment? *J Clin Psychiatry*, 66(4): 455–468, 2005.

46. Keller MB, et al. A comparison of nefazodone, the cognitive behavioral-analysis system of psychotherapy, and their combination for the treatment of chronic depression. *N Engl J Med*, 342: 1462–1470, 2000.

47. Fava GA, et al. Six-year outcome for cognitive behavioral treatment of residual symptoms in major depression. *Am J Psychiatry*, 155: 1462–1470, 1998.

48. Hermann BP, Wyler AR. Depression, locus of control, and the effects of epilepsy surgery. *Epilepsia*, 30(3): 332–338, 1989.

49. Hermann BP, et al. Learned helplessness, attributional style, and depression in epilepsy. Bozeman Epilepsy Surgery Consortium. *Epilepsia*, 37(7): 680–686, 1996.

50. Boland RJ, Keller MB. Treatment of depression. In: *Textbook of Psychopharmacology*, eds. AF Schatzberg and DB Nemeroff. Washington, DC: American Psychiatric Press, pp. 547–565, 2004.

51. Trivedi MH, Kleiber BA. Using treatment algorithms for the effective management of treatment-resistant depression. *J Clin Psychiatry*, 62, Suppl. 18: 25–29, 2001.

52. Trivedi MH, et al. Use of treatment algorithms for depression. *J Clin Psychiatry*, 67(9): 1458–1465, 2006.

53. Katon WJ, et al. Collaborative management to achieve treatment guidelines: impact of depression in primary care. *JAMA*, 273: 1026–1031, 1995.

54. Katon WJ, et al. Stepped collaborative care for primary care patients with persistent symptoms of depression: a randomized trial. *Arch Gen Psychiatry*, 56: 1109–1115, 1999.

55. Katon WJ, et al. The pathways study: a randomized trial of collaborative care in patients with diabetes and depression. *Arch Gen Psychiatry*, 61: 1042–1049, 2004.

56. Trivedi M, et al. Maximizing the adequacy of medication treatment in controlled trials and clinical practice: STAR*D measurement-based care. *Neuropsychopharmacology*, 32: 2479–2489, 2007.

57. Trivedi M. Use of decision support tools for treatment algorithms. *CNS Spectr*, 12(8): 9–16, 2007.

58. Trivedi MH, et al. Clinical results for patients with major depressive disorder in the Texas Medication Algorithm Project. *Arch Gen Psychiatry*, 61(7): 669–680, 2004.

59. Trivedi MH. Remission of depression and the Texas Medication Algorithm Project. *Manag Care Interface*, Suppl. B: 9–13, 2003.

60. Thase ME, et al. Remission rates during treatment with venlafaxine or selective serotonin reuptake inhibitors. *Br J Psychiatry*, 178: 234–241, 2001.

61. Abramowicz M. Drugs for psychiatric disorders. *Treat Guidel Med Lett*, 4(46): 35–46, 2006.

62. Bezchlibnyk-Butler KZ, et al. Antidepressants. In: *Clinical Handbook of Psychotropic Drugs*, eds. KZ Bezchlibnyk-Butler and JJ Jeffries. Ashland, OH: Hogrefe & Huber Publishers, 2007.Antidepressants; Ashland, OH

63. Charney DS, et al. Treatment of depression. In: *Textbook of Psychopharmacology*, eds. AF Schatzberg and CB Nemeroff. Washington, DC: American Psychiatric Press, pp. 705–731, 1998.

64. Sharma V. Loss of response to antidepressants and subsequent refractoriness: diagnostic issues in a retrospective case series. *J Affect Disord*, 64: 99–106, 2001.

65. Sackeim H, et al. Acute and longer-term outcomes in depressed outpatients requiring one or several treatment steps: a STAR*D report. *Am J Psychiatry*, 163: 1905–1917, 2006.

66. Trivedi MH, et al. Evaluation of outcomes with citalopram for depression using measurement-based care in STAR*D: implications for clinical practice. *Am J Psychiatry*, 163(1): 28–40, 2006.

67. Zisook S, et al. Clinical correlates of the worsening or emergence of suicidal ideation during SSRI treatment of depression: an examination of citalopram in the STAR*D study. *J Affect Disord*, 117(1–2): 63–73, 2009.

68. DeBattista C, et al. Gonadal and adrenal steroids in the treatment of major depression. *Depress Mind Body*, 2(3): 94–98, 2006.

69. DeBattista C. Augmentation and combination strategies for depression. *J Psychopharmacol*, 20: 11–18, 2006.

70. Figiel GS, et al. Electroconvulsive therapy. In: *Textbook of Psychopharmacology*, eds. AF Schatzberg and CB Nemeroff. Washington, DC: American Psychiatric Press, pp. 523–545, 1998.

71. American Psychiatric Association *The Practice of Electroconvulsive Therapy: Recommendations for Treatment, Training, and Privileging (A Task Force Report of the American Psychiatric Association)*, 2nd ed. Washington, DC: American Psychiatric Association, 2001.

72. Rush JA, et al. Vagus nerve stimulation for treatment-resistant depression: a multicenter study. *Biol Psychiatry*, 47: 276–286, 2000.

73. Nahas Z, et al. Two-year outcome of vagus nerve stimulation (VNS) for treatment of major depressive episodes. *J Clin Psychiatry*, 66: 1097–1104, 2005.

74. Rush AJ, et al. Vagus nerve stimulation for treatment-resistant depression: a randomized, controlled acute phase trial. *Biol Psychiatry*, 58(5): 347–354, 2005.

75. George MS, et al. A one-year comparison of vagus nerve stimulation with treatment as usual for treatment-resistant depression. *Biol Psychiatry*, 58(5): 364–373, 2005.

76. George MS, et al. Daily left prefrontal transcranial magnetic stimulation therapy for major depressive disorder—a sham-controlled randomized trial. *Arch Gen Psychiatry*, 67(5): 507–516, 2010.

77. Mayberg HS, et al. Deep brain stimulation for treatment resistant depression. *Neuron*, 45: 651–660, 2005.

78. Pollack MH, Marzol PC. Pharmacotherapeutic options in the treatment of comorbid depression and anxiety. *CNS Spectr*, 5(12): 23–30, 2000.

79. Pollack MH, et al. Combined paroxetine and clonazepam treatment strategies compared to paroxetine monotherapy for panic disorder. *J Psychopharmacol*, 17(3): 276–282, 2003.

80. Gorman JM, Papp LA. Efficacy of venlafaxine in mixed depression-anxiety states. *Depress Anxiety*, 12, Suppl. 1: 77–80, 2000.

81. Allen LB, et al. Cognitive-behavioral therapy (CBT) for panic disorder: relationship of anxiety and depression comorbidity with treatment outcome. *J Psychopathol Behav Assess*, 32: 185–192, 2010.

82. Manji HK, et al. The cellular neurobiology of depression. *Nat Med*, 7: 541–547, 2001.

83. Suppes T, et al. The Texas implementation of medication algorithms: update to the algorithms for treatment of bipolar 1 disorders. *J Clin Psychiatry*, 66: 870–886, 2005.

84. Schatzberg AF, et al. Augmentation strategies for treatment-resistant disorders. In: *Manual of Clinical Psychopharmacology*. Washington, DC: American Psychiatric Press, pp. 437–480, 2003.

85. Crystal S, et al. Diagnosis and treatment of depression in the elderly Medicare population: predictors, disparities, and trends. *J Am Geriatr Soc*, 51(12): 1718–1728, 2003.

Screening Instruments for Depression in Neurologic Disorders: Their Application in the Clinic and in Research

Andres M. Kanner[1] and Angela Strobel Parsons[2]
[1]Departments of Neurological Sciences and Psychiatry, Rush Medical College at Rush University; Laboratory of EEG and Video-EEG-Telemetry; Section of Epilepsy and Rush Epilepsy Center, Rush University Medical Center, Chicago, IL, USA
[2]Chicago College of Osteopathic Medicine, Midwestern University, Downers Grove, IL, USA

Introduction

Neurologic disorders, including epilepsy, stroke, dementias, Parkinson's disease (PD), essential tremor, Huntington's disease (HD), migraines, and multiple sclerosis (MS), are often associated with psychiatric comorbidities, of which depressive disorders (DDs) are the most frequent [1]. In most cases, it is assumed that DDs are a complication of the fundamental neurologic disorder. Yet, the relationship between neurologic disorders and DDs is complex. Indeed, several studies published in recent years have identified the existence of a bidirectional relationship between DDs and stroke [2–4], epilepsy [5–7], dementia [8–10], and PD [11, 12]. This bidirectional relationship suggests not only that patients with these conditions are at a greater risk of developing a DD, but also that patients with a DD are at an increased risk for developing one of these neurologic disorders (this bidirectional relation is discussed in great detail in the respective chapter of the book).

Comorbid DDs have been found to have a negative impact on the quality of life of these patients,

their suicidal risk, and worsen the course and response to treatment of the neurologic disorders. Thus, early identification and treatment of DDs is of the essence; yet, more often than not, DDs remain unrecognized and untreated. Screening instruments may provide an initial solution to this serious problem. These consist of self-reporting instruments or questionnaires administered by an examiner. The former type has the advantage of allowing patients to complete the instruments while waiting to be seen by their physician, whereas in the latter, the examiner must be trained in their administration.

Among the screening instruments developed for the identification of primary DDs, the Beck Depression Inventory (BDI) [13], the Hospital Anxiety and Depression Scale (HADS) [14], the Zung Scale (ZS) [15], the Geriatric Depression Scale (GDS) [16], and the Center for Epidemiological Studies Depression Scale (CES-D) [17] are the most frequently used, while the Hamilton Depression Rating Scale (HAM-D) [18] is an examiner-rating scale with wider exposure. All of these instruments investigate the presence of symptoms for the previous 2 weeks and yield a severity score.

Depression in Neurologic Disorders: Diagnosis and Management, First Edition.
Edited by Andres M. Kanner.
© 2012 Blackwell Publishing Ltd. Published 2012 by Blackwell Publishing Ltd.

While the advantage of screening instruments in clinical practice is well recognized, the following caveats need to be taken into consideration:

1. The clinical manifestations of a comorbid DD may differ from those of a primary DD (e.g., epilepsy, some cases of stroke, PD, and dementia) [19]. In such cases, the use of screening instruments not validated for specific neurologic conditions may yield false-positive or negative findings.
2. Somatic and cognitive symptoms (e.g., fatigue, headache, slow thinking, poor concentration) are commonly included in these screening instruments as symptoms of depression but can often be the expression of a neurologic symptom or adverse events of medication used for the treatment of the neurologic condition. If the symptoms result from the underlying neurologic disorder, they can lead to high total scores that may falsely suggest a depressive episode. For example, one of the frequently used screening instruments for primary DD, the Patient Health Questionnaire-9, has five of its nine items devoted to investigating somatic and cognitive symptoms [20]. Accordingly, this instrument should not be used in patients with neurologic disorders.
3. Patients may be limited in their ability to reliably complete self-report screening instruments due to cognitive deficits from the underlying neurologic disorder. In fact, most of these self-report screening instruments have been validated in people with normal intelligence; thus, their use in cognitively impaired patients is likely to yield false-positive or false-negative findings.
4. Anxiety disorders are a very frequent comorbid condition of DDs in patients with and without neurologic disorders. Thus, when screening for DDs, it is worth including a screening instrument for anxiety disorder. The Patient Health Questionnaire–Generalized Anxiety Disorder-7 (GAD-7) is a seven-item, self-rating scale that investigates symptoms of anxiety in the last 2 weeks [21]. Each item is scored in a Likert scale ranging from 0 to 3 (0 = absent, 3 = most or all of the time); a

score of >10 is suggestive of a generalized anxiety disorder. The absence of any somatic or cognitive items is also an advantage of this instrument. An alternative is the HADS. Neither of these two instruments have been validated in patients with neurologic disorders, however [14].

5. It should be emphasized that screening instruments do not establish a psychiatric diagnosis. They are indicative of psychiatric symptoms occurring in the previous 2 or 4 weeks, and suggest the possibility of a psychiatric disorder. However, it is important to confirm the psychiatric diagnosis using formal psychiatric evaluations or examiner-administered structured interviews that can yield diagnoses of psychiatric disorders according to the *Diagnostic and Statistical Manual of Mental Disorders* (fourth edition and beyond, e.g., DSM-IV-TR [fourth edition, text revision]) [22] or of those presenting as atypical forms of DD, a frequent occurrence in neurologic disorders.

This chapter reviews the screening instruments commonly used in five neurologic disorders (epilepsy, MS, stroke, dementia, and PD) and comments on their advantages and limitations.

Depression in epilepsy

Depressive disorders occur in patients with epilepsy with a higher prevalence than in matched healthy controls [23], ranging from 3% to 9% in patients with controlled epilepsy to 20% to 55% in patients with recurrent seizures [24–26]. The Canadian Community Health Survey (CCHS 1.2) was used to investigate the prevalence of psychiatric comorbidity in persons with epilepsy compared with those without epilepsy [26]. In a sample of 36,984 subjects, 0.6% was identified with epilepsy, 17.4% of which had a lifetime prevalence of major DDs, compared with 10.7% in the general population. Patients with epilepsy were found to have a lifetime prevalence of mood disorders of 24.4% versus 13.2% in the general population. Suicidal ideation is twice as high in patients with epilepsy.

Depressive disorders in epilepsy can often be identical to primary DDs. Yet, in a significant percentage of patients, they have an atypical clinical presentation that does not meet any DSM diagnostic criterion [24]. Mendez et al. found that 50% of depressive episodes in patients with epilepsy had to be classified as atypical depression [27]. The atypical forms of DD very often present as clusters of symptoms of irritability, anxiety, depression, and neurovegetative symptoms [28–30], which have a chronic course and can be interrupted by recurrent symptom-free periods lasting days to weeks and mimicking a dysthymic disorder. Thus, the term *dysthymic-like disorder of epilepsy* was suggested and identified in 69 (70%) patients in one study [28]. These DDs were milder in severity than a major depressive episode but caused a significant disruption in daily activities, quality of life, and social relations. "Interictal dysphoric disorder" (IDD) is another term used to describe the atypical manifestations of DDs. Blumer and Altshuler identified eight affective-somatoform symptoms as the core of the IDD [29]: irritability, depressive moods, anergia, insomnia, pains, anxiety, phobic fears, and euphoric moods. In their opinion, the presence of three affective-somatoform symptoms was sufficient to be associated with significant disability. Nearly one-third to one-half of patients with epilepsy seeking medical care present a clinical picture compatible with an IDD of sufficient degree to warrant pharmacological treatment. IDD tends to develop 2 years or more after the onset of epilepsy.

Symptoms or episodes of depression can be identified prior to the onset of seizures (preictal period) as an expression of the actual seizures (ictal symptoms) or following seizures (postictal period, which may extend up to 120 hours after a seizure) [31–35]. More commonly, depressive episodes occur independently of seizures (interictal symptoms or episodes). Little data exist regarding peri-ictal symptoms, which are often unrecognized by clinicians. Furthermore, the vast majority of screening instruments have only been used in the identification of interictal depressive symptoms and episodes.

Screening instruments

Among the available screening instruments developed for patients with primary DDs, only two have been validated in patients with epilepsy: the Beck Depression Inventory-II (BDI-II) [12] and the CES-D [17]. One self-rating instrument, the Neurological Disorders Depression Inventory for Epilepsy (NDDI-E), was developed to identify major depressive episodes specifically in people with epilepsy [36]. Another self-rating instrument, the Interictal Dysphoric Disorder Inventory (IDDI), was developed to identify IDD [37]. Finally, one questionnaire, The Rush Postictal Psychiatric Symptoms Questionnaire, was developed to identify postictal psychiatric symptoms [35].

The NDDI-E. This six-item self-report screening instrument investigates the presence of six symptoms of depression during the previous 2 weeks. Each symptom is scored on a Likert scale (1 = not present, 4 = all or most of the time). A score of >15 is suggestive of a major depressive episode, with a sensitivity of 81% and a specificity of 90%. This instrument is devoid of any item that identifies somatic or cognitive symptoms that are common in depressive episodes but can often be the expression of toxicity to antiepileptic drugs or cognitive disturbances associated with the seizure disorder or the underlying neurologic disorder. This is one of the advantages of the instrument since it minimizes the risk of false-positive high total scores resulting from the presence of adverse events associated with antiepileptic drugs or of cognitive disturbances related to the underlying seizure disorder. This instrument has been used with increasing frequency in the United States; it has already been validated and translated into Portuguese [38] and is being validated and translated into Spanish, French, Arabic, Hebrew, German, Hindi, and Japanese.

The BDI-II and CES-D. These are both self-rating screening instruments used to identify symptoms of depression occurring in the last 2 weeks [12, 17]. Jones et al. found the mean sensitivities for these instruments to be 93% and 80%, respectively, in people with epilepsy [39]. The CES-D was used in a study comparing the prevalence of depressive symptomatology among patients with epilepsy, asthma, and healthy controls; patients with epilepsy experienced symptoms of depression with a significantly greater frequency (36.5%) and severity than people with asthma (27.8%) and healthy controls (11.8%) [40].

The IDDI. This is a 38-item self-report questionnaire specifically developed to identify IDD and its eight cardinal symptoms during the last 12 months. The initial 32 items investigate these symptoms' presence, frequency, severity, and global impairment. The time course of these symptoms and their relation with epileptic seizures and therapy are investigated with six items included in the appendix of the instrument. A diagnosis of IDD is defined by the presence of at least three symptoms of at least "moderate" or "severe" severity and causing "moderate" or "severe" distress. Apart from the diagnosis, this instrument yields separate scores for individual symptoms and degree of severity defined by frequency and impairment scores. Mula and Trimble [37] compared the sensitivity and specificity of the IDDI between 117 patients with epilepsy (E) and 112 patients with migraine (M) and did not find any group difference in IDD prevalence (E = 17%; M = 18.7%) and IDDI total scores (E = 4.1 ± 2.0 vs. M = 3.8 ± 2.0).

The Rush Postictal Psychiatric Symptoms Questionnaire. This is the only screening instrument developed to identify postictal psychiatric symptoms [35]. It is a 42-item questionnaire administered by the health-care professional to identify 26 psychiatric and five cognitive postictal symptoms, of which nine are symptoms of depression. Each question inquires about the frequency of symptoms during the postictal period, defined as the 72 hours following a seizure. For each symptom, there are questions related to its occurrence during the *interictal* period as well. For symptoms identified during both interictal and postictal periods, there is a follow-up question to compare severity between the two periods. This questionnaire generates descriptive data but does not yield a severity score. For example, in one study of 100 consecutive patients with treatment-resistant epilepsy, 43% endorsed postictal symptoms of depression with a median duration of 24 hours [35].

Depression in MS

Depression symptoms have been identified in approximately 80% of patients with MS [41–43], while a lifetime prevalence of major DDs has been found in 22.8% of MS patients compared

with 16% in the general population [44, 45]. Patients with MS have also been shown to have a higher prevalence of depression than patients with other chronic medical illnesses. Depression in MS may be indistinguishable from primary mood disorders. A cautionary note is in order because symptoms of MS (cognitive, somatic, and neurovegetative) can often be confused with symptoms of a DD.

Screening instruments

MS is one of the neurologic disorders that shares common somatic and cognitive symptoms with DDs. Thus, clinicians must keep this in mind when using screening instruments for DDs. In one study, for example, the exclusion of confounding symptoms of fatigue and cognitive symptoms resulted in a decrease in overall prevalence rates of depression in both patients with MS (from 15.7% to 6.8%) and patients with no MS (from 7.4% to 3.2%) [46]. Conversely, another study found that successful treatment of depression led to improved scores when all 21 items of the BDI-II were included; however, only 12 of 17 items of the HAM-D, including somatic symptoms, showed improvement [47].

The BDI has been shown to be a good screening instrument for depression in MS [48]. One study found that BDI cut-off scores yielded a sensitivity of 71% and a specificity of 79% for major depression [49].

The CES-D has also been found to be a good screening instrument in population-based studies of patients with MS [50–52]. Chwastiak et al. found that 41.8% of 739 patients were experiencing symptoms of depression (CES-D score ≥16); the scores of 29.1% of the subjects ranged between moderate and severe (score ≥21) [51]. Of note, patients with advanced MS were much more likely to experience depressive symptoms than subjects with minimal disease.

Abbreviated screening instruments are also effective. The Beck Depression Inventory-Fast Screen (BDI-FS) discriminated patients with MS undergoing treatment for DD from untreated patients with MS [53]. Likewise, the sensitivity and specificity of the two-question instrument Patient Health Questionnaire-2 (PHQ2) was investigated in a study of 260 patients with MS (the first question inquires about the presence of depressed mood and the second about the ina-

Table 4.1 Diagnostic accuracy of Simple (PHQ2) screening items for MS [54]]

Screening item	Sensitivity% (95% CI)	Specificity% (95% CI)	PPV% (95% CI)	NPV% (95% CI)
No. 1 only	75 (62–84)	94 (89–97)	73 (61–83)	91 (86–95)
No. 2 only	75 (62–84)	94 (89–97)	81 (68–89)	91 (86–95)
Nos. 1 and 2	51 (38–63)	98 (94–99)	90 (74–97)	85 (80–89)
No. 1 or 2	99 (91–100)	87 (81–91)	72 (61–80)	99 (96–100)

PPV, positive predictive value; NPV, negative predictive value.

bility to experience pleasure). Sixty-seven patients (26%) met diagnostic criteria of major depression with the major depression module of the Structured Clinical Interview for the DSM (SCID) [54]. The two questions of the PHQ2 identified 99% (95% confidence interval [CI]: 91–100%) of cases (see Table 4.1).

Depression in stroke

The occurrence of a DD after a stroke is commonly referred to as poststroke depression (PSD). Its prevalence has been estimated to range between 30% and 72%, depending on the setting where patients were studied (e.g., population based, hospital, rehab facility) and the instruments used to identify the DD. In a study conducted in four communities, the pooled prevalence of all types of PSD was 31.8% (30% to 44%). The occurrence of PSD peaks between the third and sixth month after the stroke [55]. Symptoms of major depression can persist for a long time: major depression was found to last for approximately 1 year (27%) and minor depression for more than 2 years (20%) [56–58].

As in the case of epilepsy, a bidirectional relationship between stroke and DD has been previously identified [2–4, 59, 60]. In addition, the occurrence of PSD negatively affects the recovery of cognitive function and the ability to perform activities of daily living and increases the mortality risk of these patients [61].

PSD can present as a major depressive episode and/or minor depression, with the caveat that psychomotor retardation may be more frequently identified than in primary DD. For example, slowness and psychomotor retardation were found as a differentiating symptom in PSD, while anhedonia and concentration difficulty were found in patients with primary DD [62]. Furthermore, PSD can worsen the severity of

neurovegetative symptoms and fatigue. In one study, reduced sleep, level of energy, and libido were significantly more frequent in depressed than nondepressed patients with stroke at initial evaluation and at 3, 6, 12, and 24 months [57]. Vascular depression refers to a form of PSD identified in older patients (after the age of 65) with a history of bilateral overt or silent strokes or subcortical bilateral white matter ischemic disease. However, clinical manifestations of PSD are most often similar to primary late-onset depression.

Screening instruments

As with other neurologic disorders, the most frequently used self-rating scales in studies of PSD include the BDI [13], the HADS [14], the ZS [15], the GDS [16], and the CES-D [17], while the HAM-D [18] is one of the most frequently used examiner rating scales. Aben et al. found that the sensitivity of the BDI and HADS ranged between 80% and 90%, while their specificity was 60% in a study of 202 consecutive patients. The HAM-D yielded a sensitivity of 78.1% and a specificity of 74.6% [63]. The GDS and ZS had the highest sensitivity and the ZS had the highest positive predictive value (PPV) (93%) in a study of 40 elderly patients with stroke, of whom 17 were found to be depressed [64]. O'Rourke et al. found the HADS to be inadequate in identifying anxiety or PSD 6 months after a stroke in a study of 105 consecutive patients [65].

Healey et al. studied the sensitivity and specificity of several screening instruments in 49 elderly patients with stroke (mean age: 78.8 ± 6.9 years) [66]. The instruments included the Brief Assessment Schedule Depression Cards (BASDEC) and the BDI-FS. Using cut-off scores of ≥7, the BASDEC yielded a sensitivity of 100% and a specificity of 95% for major depression, whereas the BDI-FS (cut-off scores ≥4) had a sensitivity of 71% and a specificity of 74%. When patients with minor depression were included in analyses, the sensitivity for the BASDEC decreased to 69% while the specificity remained high (97%), and the sensitivity of the BDI-FS decreased to 62% while the specificity remained almost unchanged (78%).

A single-item screening tool for depression was conducted for 122 consecutive patients at Yale admitted with an acute stroke who did not have communication or severe cognitive problems and who were still in the hospital in the second week poststroke [67]. This instrument was derived from the Yale–Brown Obsessive Compulsive Scale (YBOCS). The Montgomery–Åsberg Depression Rating Scale (MADRS) was used as a comparator. At week 2, it had a sensitivity of 86% (57/66), a specificity of 84% (46/55), a PPV of 86% (57/66), and a negative predictive value (NPV) of 84% (46/55), with an overall efficiency of 85% (103/121). At month 3, it had a sensitivity of 95% (52/55), a specificity of 89% (32/36), a PPV of 93% (52/56), and a NPV of 91% (32/35), with an overall efficiency of 92% (84/91).

Gainotti et al. developed the Poststroke Depression Scale (PSDS) [68], an instrument with 10 items that include guilt feelings, depressed mood, neurovegetative symptoms, thoughts of death or suicide, apathy and loss of interest, hyperemotionalism, anxiety, catastrophic reactions, anhedonia, and diurnal mood variations. The investigators administered the PSDS and the HAM-D to 124 patients with stroke, 45 of whom met *Diagnostic and Statistical Manual of Mental Disorders*, Third Edition, Revised (DSM-III-R) criteria of major depression and 47 of minor depression. Scores were compared with those obtained on the same scales from 17 psychiatric patients also diagnosed with major depression on the basis of DSM-III-R diagnostic criteria. The investigators suggested that the PSDS demonstrated a continuum between major and minor forms of PSD. They concluded that in patients with stroke, a DSM-III-based diagnosis of major PSD could be in part inflated by symptoms that are typical of major depression (such as apathy and neurovegetative symptoms) in a patient free from brain damage but that could be due to the brain lesion in a stroke patient.

Aphasia often makes it difficult for clinicians to identify PSD and use screening instruments [69]. Depressed mood in patients with aphasia was detected using the Stroke Aphasic Depression Questionnaire (SADQ) [70]. In this study, 70 discharged patients with stroke were evaluated using the SADQ, the HADS, and the Wakefield Depression Inventory. The SADQ was also administered to 17 patients with aphasia on two occasions at a 4-week interval. The SADQ scores were significantly related to other measures of depression ($r = 0.22$–0.52, $p < 0.05$). A shortened 10-item version showed higher validity ($r = 0.32$–0.67, $p < 0.01$). Test–retest analysis also indicated that the SADQ is reliable over a 4-week interval ($r = 0.72$, $p < 0.001$). Sackley et al. found that the SADQ yielded a sensitivity of 77% and a specificity of 78% in a study of 88 patients with stroke [71]. Bennett et al. compared the Stroke Aphasic Depression Questionnaire Hospital Version (SADQ-H), Signs of Depression Scale (SODS), Visual Analogue Mood Scale (VAMS) and Visual Analogue Self-Esteem Scale (VASES) in screening for mood problems after stroke [72]. The SADQ-H, Stroke Aphasic Depression Questionnaire Hospital, 10-item version (SADQ-H10), and SODS were all appropriate for screening for depression after stroke but not for screening for anxiety. The authors recommended the SADQ-H10 for screening purposes and the VAMS and VASES for assessing severity.

Depression in dementia

The prevalence of DDs in patients with dementia has been estimated to range between 30% and 50% [73, 74]. One study evaluating the presence of depression across the life span revealed that up to 50% of patients with Alzheimer's disease or PD develop a DD, compared to 12% of patients seen in primary care settings. The existence of a bidirectional relationship has also been suggested by several authors since as many as two-thirds of patients with dementia exhibit symptoms of depression or depressive episodes up to 3 years before the onset of cognitive deficits [75]. One study showed that in patients with dementia, 10.6% suffer from major depression and 29.8% from minor depression [76].

Screening instruments

Various screening instruments are currently in use to determine the severity of depression in patients with dementia. A study by Canuto et al. evaluated the French version of the Health of the Nation Outcome Scale (HoNOS) 65+ compared to the Mini-Mental State Examination, GDS, Brief Psychiatric Rating Scale, the Katz Index of Independence in Activities of Daily Living, and the Global Assessment of Functioning scale [77]. The HoNOS consists of 13 items: behavioral disturbance, nonaccidental self-injury, problem drinking or drug use, cognitive problems, problems related to physical illness or disability, problems associated with hallucinations and/or delusions, problems with depressive symptoms, other mental and behavioral symptoms, problems with relationships, problems with activities of daily living, problems with living conditions, and problems with activities, plus drug management. The HoNOS 65+ provided a sensitivity of 95% and a specificity of 88%. The study indicated that the HoNOS 65+ scale is useful to evaluate depression in patients with dementia.

The Cornell Scale for Depression and Dementia (CSDD) was found to be equally valuable in patients with and without dementia [78, 79]. The CSDD contains questions relating to mood symptoms, behavioral disturbance, physical signs, cyclic functions, and ideational disturbance [79]. The study included 145 patients: 73 with depression only, 36 with depression and dementia, and 36 in the control group (11 with dementia). The CSDD has the best sensitivity (93%) and specificity (97%), indicating its use in patients with dementia and depression. In addition, the study showed the decreased validity of the 15-item Geriatric Depression Scale (GDS-15) when applied to cognitively impaired elderly patients. The only disadvantage of using the CSDD is the need for a reliable informant, which is not always possible when dealing with cognitively impaired patients.

The HAM-D has also been shown to be a reliable instrument to identify DD in patients with Alzheimer's disease [80]. The most important symptom was shown to be a depressed underlying mood.

Depression in PD

Major depression in PD has been identified in 5–25% of patients and minor depression in 25–50% [81–84]. In one population-based study of 245 patients with PD, 45.5% reported a mild form of depression [83], while in another community population sample, 19.6% met criteria for moderate to severe depression [81]. Recognition of nonmotor symptoms of PD is low in a neurologic setting, with a diagnostic accuracy for the treating neurologists of 35% for depression, 42% for anxiety, 25% for fatigue, and 60% for sleep disturbance [85].

As in epilepsy and stroke, depression can have a negative impact on quality of life in patients with PD [86–90]. Depression was the most significant predictor variable of poor health-related quality of life in a multicenter study conducted by the Global Parkinson's Disease Survey Steering Committee that included 2020 patients with PD and 687 caregivers across six countries [88]. Only 1% of patients reported feeling depressed, while 50% were considered to be experiencing symptoms of depression based on the study criteria (BDI score >10). In fact, DD has been found to be the variable most closely related to poor quality of life, while the stage and duration of PD and cognitive impairment had a lesser impact [90]. In a study by Ravina et al., a total of 114 (27.6%) of 413 patients were identified with a DD during a mean follow-up period of 14.6 months [87]. Forty percent of these subjects were neither treated with antidepressants nor referred for further psychiatric evaluation. Depression significantly predicted impairment in activities of daily living and increased the need for PD-specific symptomatic therapy (hazard ratio = 1.86; 95% CI 1.29, 2.68).

A bidirectional relationship between PD and depression has been suggested in two population-based studies [11, 12]. The first study included a cohort of age-matched individuals with and without depression [11]. Among the 1358 subjects with depression, 19 developed PD, and among the 67,570 subjects without depression, 259 developed PD. People with depression were three times more likely to develop PD than people without depression in multivariable analysis (hazard ratio of 3.13 [95% CI: 1.95–5.01]). The second study investigated whether depression preceded the onset of PD in an age-matched population [12]. Among patients who developed PD, 9.2% had a history of depression compared with 4.0% of the control population, yielding an odds ratio for a depression history of 2.4 (95% CI: 2.1–2.7).

One study found that the severity of depressive symptoms in patients with PD and patients with primary DD was comparable [91]. Yet, compared with primary DDs, which most often begin in the fourth decade of life, DDs in patients with PD usually begin late in life. Dysphoric symptoms, including irritability, pessimism, and sadness, are more frequent in patients with PD, whereas feelings of failure, guilt, and self-blame are less frequent in PD than in primary DDs. Patients with PD are less likely to commit suicide even though they have higher prevalence of suicidal ideation. Anxiety symptoms have been found in two-thirds of patients with PD with depressive symptoms; conversely, 97% of patients with PD with an anxiety disorder have been found to exhibit depressive symptoms.

Screening instruments

BDI, HADS, GDS, and the MADRS are often used as screening instruments for depression in patients with PD [92–94]. As with epilepsy, MS, and stroke, the presence of somatic symptoms resulting from PD may be a potential problem resulting in a false-positive diagnosis of depression. One group of investigators found a high sensitivity and low specificity at cut-off scores of 8/9 with the BDI, while scores of 16/17 or higher yielded a low sensitivity and high specificity [93]. Similar findings showed that the BDI and MADRS show similar accuracy within the receiver operating characteristic (ROC) curves (84.3% for MADRS and 79.7% for BDI) [92]. The same study showed that lower cut-off scores (11/12) of the HAM-D and MADRS (14/15) yielded maximal sensitivity, but at the expense of a low specificity, while maximum discrimination between depressed and nondepressed patients with PD was reached at cut-off scores of 13/14 and 14/15, respectively [92]. Other investigators compared the GDS to the HAM-D against the Structured Clinical Interview for Axis I DSM IV Disorders (SCID). An ROC curve established points of maximum specificity/sensitivity for the GDS at a cutoff of 9/10 (sensitivity = 0.809, specificity = 0.837,

PPV = 0.584, NPV = 0.939) and for the HDRS at a cutoff of 12/13 (sensitivity 0.810, specificity = 0.821, PPV = 0.580, NPV = 0.934) [94].

Mondolo et al. investigated the validity of the HADS and GDS in patients with PD [95]. A high specificity and PPV were reached at a cut-off score of 12/13 for the GDS and at a cut-off score of 11/12 for the HADS. Serrano-Duenas and Soledad Serrano compared a six-item version of the Hamilton Depression Rating Scale (HAM-D6) against the original 21-item tool (HAM-D21) using the DSM-IV criteria for major depression. They found that the HAM-D6 is probably as good as the 21-item scale [96].

Conclusion

Depressive disorders are a common comorbidity in neurologic disorders with significant negative impacts on the course of the disorder, quality of life, and response to treatment. Despite their relatively high prevalence, these disorders often go unrecognized and untreated. This problem may be mitigated with the judicious use of screening instruments. While it may be theoretically ideal to have specific screening instruments for depression validated for each neurologic disorder, the available instruments appear to yield acceptable sensitivities and specificities. Nevertheless, some neurological conditions feature special complications, such as cognitive impairment or language disorder, that may necessitate modification of tools in order to allow accurate completion. Ultimately, detection of depression mandates a full clinical assessment and appropriate treatment and aftercare to improve patient outcomes.

⚲ PEARLS TO TAKE HOME

- The clinical manifestations of comorbid DDs may differ from those of primary DDs (e.g., epilepsy, some cases of stroke, PD, and dementia).
- Neurologic disorders and DDs share common symptoms (somatic and cognitive symptoms presenting as fatigue, headache, slow thinking, and poor concentration) that are often included in screening instruments as symptoms of depression but can often be

the expression of a neurologic symptom or adverse event of medication used for the treatment of the neurologic condition. In cases of the latter, high scores of screening instruments may yield false-positive diagnoses of DDs.

- Screening instruments alone do not establish a psychiatric diagnosis of DD; rather, they are indicative of psychiatric symptoms occurring in the previous 2 or 4 weeks, and may suggest the possibility of a DD that needs to be confirmed with a formal psychiatric evaluation.
- Screening instruments developed for primary DDs have been found to be very useful in epilepsy, stroke, PD, dementia, and MS.
- Screening instruments have been developed specifically to identify major depressive episodes in patients with epilepsy and to identify PSD.
- Given the high comorbidity of DDs and anxiety disorders, screening for anxiety symptoms should always be conducted as well.

References

1. Kanner AM. Depression and the risk of neurological disorders. *Lancet*, 366(9492): 1147–1148, 2005.
2. May M, McCarron P, Stansfeld S, et al. Does psychological distress predict the risk of ischemic stroke and transient ischemic attack? The Caerphilly Study. *Stroke*, 33: 7–12, 2002.
3. Larson SL, Owens PL, Ford D, et al. Depressive disorder, dysthymia, and risk of stroke. Thirteen-year follow-up from the Baltimore Epidemiological Catchment Area Study. *Stroke*, 32: 1979–1983, 2001.
4. Jonas BS, Mussolino ME. Symptoms of depression as a prospective risk factor for stroke. *Psychosom Med*, 62: 463–471, 2000.
5. Forsgren L, Nystrom L. An incident case referent study of epileptic seizures in adults. *Epilepsy Res*, 6: 66–81, 1990.
6. Hesdorffer DC, Hauser WA, Annegers JF, et al. Major depression is a risk factor for seizures in older adults. *Ann Neurol*, 47: 246–249, 2000.
7. Hesdorffer DC, Hauser WA, Olafsson E, et al. Depression and suicidal attempt as risk factor for incidental unprovoked seizures. *Ann Neurol*, 59(1): 35–41, 2006.
8. Modrego PJ, Ferrandez J. Depression in patients with mild cognitive impairment increases the risk of developing dementia of Alzheimer type: a prospective cohort study. *Arch Neurol*, 61: 1290–1293, 2004.
9. Kessing LV, Andersen PK. Does the risk of developing dementia increase with the number of episodes in patients with depressive disorder and in patients with bipolar disorder? *J Neurol Neurosurg Psychiatry*, 75: 1662–1666, 2004.
10. Dal Forno G, Palermo MT, Donohue JE, et al. Depressive symptoms, sex, and risk for Alzheimer's disease. *Ann Neurol*, 57(3): 381–387, 2005.
11. Leentgens AFG, Van Der Akker M, Metsemakers JFM, et al. Higher incidence of depression preceding the onset of Parkinson's disease: a register study. *Mov Disord*, 18: 414–418, 2003.
12. Nilsson FM, Kessing LV, Bowlig TG. Increased risk of developing Parkinson's disease for patients with major affective disorder: a register study. *Acta Psychiatr Scand*, 104: 380–386, 2001.
13. Beck AT, Steer RA, Garbing MG. Psychometric properties of the Beck Depression Inventory: twenty five years of evaluation. *Clin Psychol Rev*, 8: 77–100, 1988.
14. Zigmond AS, Snaith RP. The hospital anxiety and depression scale. *Acta Psychiatr Scand*, 67: 361–370, 1983.
15. Zung WW. A self-rating depression scale. *Arch Gen Psychiatry*, 12: 63–70, 1965.
16. Yesavage JA, Brink TL, Rose TL. Development and validation of the Geriatric Depression Screening Scale. A preliminary report. *J Psychiatr Res*, 17: 37–49, 1982.
17. Van Dam NT, Earleywine M. Validation of the Center for Epidemiologic Studies Depression Scale-Revised (CESD-R): pragmatic depression assessment in the general population. *Psychiatry Res*, 186(1): 128–132, 2011.

18. Hamilton M. A rating scale for depression. *J Neurol Neurosurg Psychiatry*, 23: 56–62, 1960.

19. Kanner AM. Depression in epilepsy: prevalence, clinical semiology, pathogenic mechanisms and treatment. *Biol Psychiatry*, 54: 388–398, 2003.

20. Gilbody S, Richards D, Barkham M. Diagnosing depression in primary care using self-completed instruments: UK validation of PHQ-9 and CORE-OM. *Br J Gen Pract*, 57(541): 650–652, 2007.

21. Kroenke K, Spitzer RL, Williams JB, et al. Anxiety disorders in primary care: prevalence, impairment, comorbidity, and detection. *Ann Intern Med*, 146: 317–325, 2007.

22. American Psychiatric Association. *DSM-IV-TR*. Washington, DC: APA Press, 2004.

23. Kanner AM, Balabanov A. Depression in epilepsy: how closely related are these two disorders? *Neurology*, 58, Suppl. 5: S27–S39, 2002.

24. Jacoby A, Baker GA, Steen N, et al. The clinical course of epilepsy and its psychosocial correlates: findings from a UK community study. *Epilepsia*, 37(2): 148–161, 1996.

25. O'Donoghue MF, Goodridge DM, Redhead K, et al. Assessing the psychosocial consequences of epilepsy: a community-based study. *Br J Gen Pract*, 49(440): 211–214, 1999.

26. Tellez-Zenteno JSF, Patten SB, Wiebe S. Psychiatric comorbidity in epilepsy: a population-based analysis. *Epilepsia*, 48: 2336–2344, 2007.

27. Mendez MF, Cummings J, Benson D, et al. Depression in epilepsy. Significance and phenomenology. *Arch Neurol*, 43: 766–770, 1986.

28. Kanner AM, Kozak AM, Frey M. The use of sertraline in patients with epilepsy: is it safe? *Epilepsy Behav*, 1(2): 100–105, 2000.

29. Blumer D, Altshuler LL. Affective disorders. In: *Epilepsy: A Comprehensive Textbook*, Vol. II, eds. J Engel and TA Pedley. Philadelphia: Lippincott-Raven, pp. 2083–2099, 1998.

30. Kraepelin E. *Psychiatrie*, Vol. 3. Leipzig, Germany: Johann Ambrosius Barth, 1923.

31. Blanchet P, Frommer GP. Mood change preceding epileptic seizures. *J Nerv Ment Dis*, 174: 471–476, 1986.

32. Williams D. The structure of emotions reflected in epileptic experiences. *Brain*, 79: 29–67, 1956.

33. Weil A. Depressive reactions associated with temporal lobe uncinate seizures. *J Nerv Ment Dis*, 121: 505–510, 1955.

34. Daly D. Ictal affect. *Am J Psychiatry*, 115: 97–108, 1958.

35. Kanner AM, Soto A, Gross-Kanner H. Prevalence and clinical characteristics of postictal psychiatric symptoms in partial epilepsy. *Neurology*, 62: 708–713, 2004.

36. Gilliam FG, Barry JJ, Meador KJ, et al. Rapid detection of major depression in epilepsy: a multicenter study. *Lancet Neurol*, 5(5): 399–405, 2006.

37. Mula M, Trimble MR. What do we know about mood disorders in epilepsy? In: *Psychiatric Controversies in Epilepsy*, eds. AM Kanner and S Schachter. London: Academic Press, pp. 49–66, 2008.

38. de Oliveira GN, Kummer A, Salgado JV, et al. Brazilian version of the Neurological Disorders Depression Inventory for Epilepsy (NDDI-E). *Epilepsy Behav*, 19(3): 328–331, 2010.

39. Jones JE, Herman BP, Woodard JL, et al. Screening for major depression in epilepsy with common self-report depression inventories. *Epilepsia*, 46(5): 731–735, 2005.

40. Ettinger A, Reed M, Cramer J; Epilepsy Impact Project Group. Depression and comorbidity in community-based patients with epilepsy or asthma. *Neurology*, 63(6): 1008–1014, 2004.

41. Feinstein A. Multiple sclerosis and depression. In: *The Clinical Neuropsychiatry of Multiple Sclerosis*. Cambridge, UK: Cambridge University Press, pp. 26–50, 1999.

42. Minden SL, Orav JO, Reich P. Depression in multiple sclerosis. *Gen Hosp Psychiatry*, 9: 426–434, 1987.

43. Patten SB, Metz LM, Reimer MA. Biopsychosocial correlates of lifetime major depression in a multiple sclerosis population. *Mult Scler*, 6(2): 115–120, 2000.

44. Kessler RC, McGonagle KA, Zhao S, et al. Lifetime and 12-month prevalence of DSM-III-R psychiatric disorders in the United

States: results from the National Comorbidity Study. *Arch Gen Psychiatry*, 51: 8–19, 1994.

45. Patten SB, Beck CA, Williams JV, et al. Major depression in multiple sclerosis: a population-based perspective. *Neurology*, 61(11): 1524–1527, 2003.

46. Krupp LB, Alvarez LA, LaRocca NG, et al. Fatigue in multiple sclerosis. *Arch Neurol*, 45: 435–437, 1988.

47. Mohr DC, Hart SL, Goldberg A. Effects of treatment for depression on fatigue in multiple sclerosis. *Psychosom Med*, 65(4): 542–547, 2003.

48. Aikens JE, Reinecke MA, Pliskin NH, et al. Assessing depressive symptoms in multiple sclerosis: is it necessary to omit items from the original Beck Depression Inventory? *J Behav Med*, 22: 127–142, 1999.

49. Moran PJ, Mohr DC. The validity of Beck Depression Inventory and Hamilton Rating Scale for Depression items in the assessment of depression among patients with multiple sclerosis. *J Behav Med*, 28(1): 35–41, 2005.

50. Sullivan MJ, Weinshenker B, Mikail S, et al. Screening for major depression in the early stages of multiple sclerosis. *Can J Neurol Sci*, 22(3): 228–231, 1995.

51. Chwastiak L, Ehde DM, Gibbons LE, et al. Depressive symptoms and severity of illness in multiple sclerosis: epidemiologic study of a large community sample. *Am J Psychiatry*, 161(8): 1504, 2004.

52. Patten SB, Lavorato DH, Metz LM. Clinical correlates of CES-D depressive symptom ratings in an MS population. *Gen Hosp Psychiatry*, 27(6): 439–445, 2005.

53. Benedict RH, Fishman I, McClellan MM, et al. Validity of the Beck Depression Inventory-Fast Screen in multiple sclerosis. *Mult Scler*, 9(4): 393–396, 2003.

54. Mohr DC, Hart SL, Julian L. Screening for depression among patients with multiple sclerosis: two questions may be enough. *Mult Scler*, 13: 215–219, 2007.

55. Robinson RG. Poststroke depression: prevalence, diagnosis, treatment and disease progression. *Biol Psychiatry*, 54: 376–387, 2003.

56. Eastwood MR, Rifat SL, Nobbs H, et al. Mood disorder following cerebrovascular accident. *Br J Psychiatry*, 154: 195–200, 1989.

57. Fedoroff JP, Starkstein SE, Parikh RM, et al. Are depressive symptoms non-specific in patients with acute stroke? *Am J Psychiatry*, 148: 1172–1176, 1991.

58. Burvill PW, Johnson GA, Jamrozik KD, et al. Prevalence of depression after stroke: the Perth Community Stroke Study. *Br J Psychiatry*, 166: 320–327, 1995.

59. Colantonio A, Kasi SV, Ostfeld AM. Depressive symptoms and other psychosocial factors as predictors of stroke in the elderly. *Am J Epidemiol*, 136: 884–894, 1992.

60. Everson SA, Roberts RE, Goldberg DE, et al. Depressive symptoms and increased risk of stroke mortality over a 29-year period. *Arch Intern Med*, 158: 1133–1138, 1998.

61. Parikh RM, Robinson RG, Lipsey JR, et al. The impact of post-stroke depression on recovery in activities of daily living over two year follow-up. *Arch Neurol*, 47: 785–789, 1990.

62. Lipsey JR, Robinson RG, Pearlson GD, et al. Nortriptyline treatment of post-stroke depression. A double-blind study. *Lancet*, 1(8372): 297–300, 1984.

63. Aben I, Verhey F, Lousberg R, et al. Validity of the Beck Depression Inventory, hospital anxiety and depression scale, SCL-90, and Hamilton depression rating scale as screening instruments for depression in stroke patients. *Psychosomatics*, 43(5): 386–393, 2002.

64. Johnson G, Burvill PW, Anderson CS, et al. Screening instruments for depression and anxiety following stroke: experience in the Perth community stroke study. *Acta Psychiatr Scand*, 91(4): 252–257, 1995.

65. O'Rourke S, MacHale S, Signorini D, et al. Detecting psychiatric morbidity after stroke: comparison of the GHQ and the HAD Scale. *Stroke*, 29(5): 980–985, 1998.

66. Healey AK, Kneebone II, Carroll M, et al. A preliminary investigation of the reliability and validity of the Brief Assessment Schedule Depression Cards and the Beck Depression Inventory-Fast Screen to screen for depression in older stroke survivors. *Int J Geriatr Psychiatry*, 23(5): 531–536, 2008.

67. Watkins CL, Lightbody CE, Sutton CJ, et al. Evaluation of a single-item screening tool for depression after stroke: a cohort study. *Clin Rehabil*, 21: 846–852, 2007.

68. Gainotti G, Azzoni A, Razzano C, et al. The Post-Stroke Depression Rating Scale: a test specifically devised to investigate affective disorders of stroke patients. *J Clin Exp Neuropsychol*, 19(3): 340–356, 1997.

69. Townend E, Brady M, McLaughlan K. A systematic evaluation of the adaptation of depression diagnostic methods for stroke survivors who have aphasia. *Stroke*, 11: 3076–3083, 2007.

70. Sutcliffe LM, Lincoln NB. The assessment of depression in aphasic stroke patients: the development of the Stroke Aphasic Depression Questionnaire. *Clin Rehabil*, 12(6): 506–513, 1998.

71. Sackley CM, Hoppitt TJ, Cardoso K. An investigation into the utility of the Stroke Aphasic Depression Questionnaire (SADQ) in care home settings. *Clin Rehabil*, 20(7): 598–602, 2006.

72. Bennett HE, Thomas SA, Austen R, et al. Validation of screening measures for assessing mood in stroke patients. *Br J Clin Psychol*, 45(Pt 3): 367–376, 2006.

73. Lykestsos CG. The interface between depression and dementia: where are we with this important frontier? *Am J Geriatr Psychiatry*, 18(2): 95, 2010.

74. Korczyn AD, Halperin I. Depression and dementia. *J Neurol Sci*, 283: 139–142, 2009.

75. Jorm AF. Is depression a risk factor for dementia or cognitive decline? *Gerontology*, 46: 219–227, 2000.

76. Lamberty GJ, Bielauskas LA. Distinguishing between depression and dementia in the elderly: a review of neuropsychological findings. *Arch Clin Neuropsychol*, 8: 149–170, 1993.

77. Canuto A, Rudhard-Thomazic V, Herrmann FR, et al. Assessing depression outcome in patients with moderate dementia: sensitivity of the HoNOS65+ scale. *J Neurol Sci*, 283: 69–72, 2009.

78. Korner A, Lauritzen L, Abelskov K, et al. The Geriatric Depression Scale and the Cornell Scale for Depression in Dementia. A validity study. *Nord J Psychiatry*, 60: 360–364, 2006.

79. Alexopoulos GS. *The Cornell Scale for Depression in Dementia: Administration & Scoring Guidelines*, New York: Weill Medical College of Cornell University, 2002.

80. Naarding P, Leentjens AFG, van Kooten F, et al. Disease-specific properties of the Hamilton rating scale for depression in patients with stroke, Alzheimer's dementia, and Parkinson's disease. *J Neuropsychiatry Clin Neurosci*, 14: 329–334, 2002.

81. Tandberg E, Larsen JP, Aarsland D, et al. The occurrence of depression in Parkinson's disease—a community-based study. *Arch Neurol*, 53: 175–179, 1996.

82. Schrag A, Jahanshahi M, Quinn NP. What contributes to depression in Parkinson's disease? *Psychol Med*, 31: 65–73, 2001.

83. Gotham AM, Brown RG, Marsden CD. Depression in Parkinson's disease: a quantitative and qualitative analysis. *J Neurol Neurosurg Psychiatry*, 49: 381–389, 1986.

84. Cummings JL. Depression and Parkinson's disease: a review. *Am J Psychiatry*, 149: 443–454, 1992.

85. Shulman LM, Taback RL, Rabinstein AA, et al. Non-recognition of depression and other non-motor symptoms in Parkinson's disease. *Parkinsonism Relat Disord*, 8: 193–197, 2002.

86. Starkstein SE, Mayberg HS, Leiguarda R, et al. A prospective longitudinal study of depression, cognitive decline, and physical impairments in patients with Parkinson's disease. *J Neurol Neurosurg Psychiatry*, 55: 377–382, 1992.

87. Ravina B, Camicioli R, Como PG, et al. The impact of depressive symptoms in early Parkinson disease. *Neurology*, 69(4): E2–E3, 2007.

88. The Global Parkinson's Disease Survey Steering Committee. Factors impacting on quality of life in Parkinson's disease: results from an international survey. *Mov Disord*, 17: 60–67, 2002.

89. Kuopio AM, Marttila RJ, Helenius H, et al. The quality of life in Parkinson's disease. *Mov Disord*, 15: 216–213, 2000.

90. Schrag A, Jahanshahi M, Quinn N. What contributes to quality of life in patients with Parkinson's disease? *J Neurol Neurosurg Psychiatry*, 69: 308–312, 2000.

91. Merschdorf U, Berg D, Csoti I, et al. Psychopathological symptoms of depression in Parkinson's disease compared to major depression. *Psychopathology*, 36: 221–225, 2003.

92. Leentjens AF, Verhey FR, Lousberg R, et al. The validity of the Hamilton and Montgomery-Asberg depression rating scales as screening and diagnostic tools for depression in Parkinson's disease. *Int J Geriatr Psychiatry*, 15: 644–649, 2000.

93. Leentjens AF, Verhey FR, Luijckx GJ, et al. The validity of the Beck Depression Inventory as a screening and diagnostic instrument for depression in patients with Parkinson's disease. *Mov Disord*, 15(6): 1221–1224, 2000.

94. Silberman CD, Laks J, Capitão CF, et al. Recognizing depression in patients with Parkinson's disease: accuracy and specificity of two depression rating scale. *Arq Neuropsiquiatr*, 64(2B): 407–411, 2006.

95. Mondolo F, Jahanshahi M, Granà A, et al. Evaluation of anxiety in Parkinson's disease with some commonly used rating scales. *Neurol Sci*, 28(5): 270–275, 2007.

96. Serrano-Duenas M, Soledad Serrano M. Concurrent validation of the 21-item and 6-item Hamilton Depression Rating Scale versus the DSM-IV diagnostic criteria to assess depression in patients with Parkinson's disease: an exploratory analysis. *Parkinsonism Relat Disord*, 14: 233–238, 2008.

Suicidality in Neurologic Diseases

Yukari Tadokoro[1] and Andres M. Kanner[2]
[1]Department of Neuropsychiatry, School of Medicine, Aichi Medical University, Aichi-ken, Japan
[2]Departments of Neurological Sciences and Psychiatry, Rush Medical College at Rush University; Laboratory of EEG and Video-EEG-Telemetry; Section of Epilepsy and Rush Epilepsy Center, Rush University Medical Center, Chicago, IL, USA

Introduction

Suicide is defined as death caused by self-directed injurious behavior with an intent to die [1]. Suicidality encompasses suicidal ideation, which may be passive (e.g., "it would be OK if I do not wake up tomorrow") or active (e.g., developing a plan to commit suicide); suicidal behavior (e.g., "suicide attempts"); and completed suicide [2].

A history of suicidal attempt is the strongest predictor of completed suicide [1, 3]. The terminology describing suicidal attempts has varied. Canetto et al. proposed the terms "fatal suicidal behavior" and "nonfatal suicidal behavior" for suicidal acts that do and do not result in death, respectively [4]. For "nonfatal suicidal behavior," the term "attempted suicide" is commonly used in the United States.

In 2007, suicide was the eleventh leading cause of death for all ages, accounting for 34,598 deaths, or 1.4% of all fatalities registered in the United States, while the age-adjusted death rate for suicide was 11.3 deaths per 100,000, an increase of 3.7 percent from the 2006 rate. Since 2000, the age-adjusted death rate for suicide has increased by 8.6% [5].

There are no official national statistics for suicidal ideation and attempted suicide. Nevertheless, it is generally estimated that there are 25 attempts for every completed suicide [6]. A recent study by the Substance Abuse and Mental Health Services Administration (SAMHSA) reported that nearly 8.3 million adults (age 18 and older) in the United States had serious thoughts of suicide in the year 2008. The study also showed that 2.3 million adults made suicide plans, and 1.1 million adults had actually attempted suicide [7]. Several factors have been reported to contribute to suicidal behavior in general, including demographic, psychiatric, biological, medical, social, and environmental factors. Certain life events may also serve as participating issues for suicidal behavior [4, 8–10].

Demographic factors

Age is an important demographic marker of suicide risk. Although suicide rates tend to increase with age, the absolute number of cases is greater among those under 45 as compared with those over 45 years of age. Gender, ethnicity, and culture are also important factors in the epidemiology of suicide. Males are approximately 4 times more likely to die from suicide than females, while females are 3 times more likely to report attempted suicide.

Psychiatric and psychological factors

A previous suicide attempt is one of the most powerful predictors of subsequent completed suicide. About 1% of individuals who attempt suicide die within 1 year, and 10–20% will successfully commit suicide within 10 years [11]; however, the majority of individuals who commit suicide have had no previous suicide attempt. Some of the psychiatric and psychological factors associated with suicide include, in particular, clinical depression with feelings of hopelessness and/or helplessness, schizophrenia, history of or current alcohol and/or substance abuse, impulsive or aggressive tendencies, and a family history of psychiatric disorders.

Genetic factors

A family history of suicide is a recognized marker for increased risk of suicide, and there is a possibility of genetic traits leading some people to suicidal behavior.

Social and environmental factors

A number of social and environmental factors have been identified as associated with suicidal behavior. These include easy access to lethal weapons such as firearms in the home, which are used in more than half of suicides in the United States. The stigma attached to mental health can cause an unwillingness to seek help, which may result in suicidal behavior. The economic impact on suicidality is also considered to be significant, and several studies have shown increased rates of suicide during times of economic recession and high unemployment. Suicidal behavior may be associated with a history of family violence or maltreatment in childhood, including physical and sexual abuse. Relational, social, or financial losses can be devastating and predispose vulnerable people to suicidal behavior. Sexual orientation may also have an association with suicidality in young adults. Finally, in some cultures, religious beliefs are associated with suicidal behavior, as suicide may be viewed as a noble means of death.

Physical illness and suicidality

Physical illness has been identified as a risk factor for suicide, but only when associated with comorbid psychiatric illness. In a review of the literature, Mackenzie and Popkin found a higher prevalence of physical illness in people who committed suicide than in the general population, but suicide in physically ill people who did not suffer from a psychiatric disorder was rare [12]. Comorbid psychiatric disorders, in particular depressive and anxiety disorders, are not rare in people with physical illnesses [13], but more often than not they remain underdiagnosed and undertreated. While several studies have found a depressive disorder to be the most frequent risk factor of suicidal behavior, one study found a significant association between medical condition and suicidality, which persisted after adjusting for depressive illness and alcohol use [2].

Neurologic disease and suicidality

Results reported in some previous investigations of suicidal behavior in patients with neurologic diseases are uncertain and inconsistent due to methodological problems [14]. Nonetheless, the risk of suicide is known to be increased in patients with a variety of neurologic diseases.

Relationship of suicidality with common neurologic diseases

Stroke

In patients with stroke, the risk of suicide is increased, though it appears to vary according to age at the time of stroke, physical disability, comorbid psychiatric problems (mainly depression), and a history of prior stroke [15]. Kishi et al. found that suicidal ideation in patients with acute stroke was strongly associated with a previous history of stroke, but not related to the severity of physical impairment in the acute phase [16]. Most of their patients with suicidal ideation met the diagnostic criteria for major depression, while younger age, poor social support, impaired cognitive function, and sensory deficit were related to suicidal ideation as well.

Longitudinal studies conducted in Denmark also revealed that patients with stroke, especially in the younger age group, had a significantly increased risk of suicide [17, 18]. Teasdale and Engberg reported that the Standardized Mortality Rate (SMR) for patients suffering a stroke before the age of 50 was 2.85 [18]. The duration of hospitalization appeared to be negatively associated with suicide risk, as the SMR was highest for patients hospitalized for less than 1 month;

furthermore, survival analysis suggested that suicide risk was greatest within the first 5 years after a stroke.

On the other hand, some researchers have reported on delayed suicidal plans, which are strongly related to the existence of depressive disorders, especially major depression, and a prior history of stroke [19, 20]. Kishi et al. reported that patients with delayed suicidal plans had significantly more posterior lesions and a tendency to be more impaired in their social functioning and activities of daily life than patients with early plans [19]. It was also suggested that early suicidal plans might be mediated by neurobiological determinants, especially serotonergic dysfunction, whereas their development might be triggered by a psychological mechanism associated with greater physical impairment and poor social support.

One report noted that one in three patients with stroke were using antidepressants at the time the stroke occurred [21]. Forsstrom et al. also found that prestroke depression was associated with significantly shorter survival after stroke [22]. The age- and gender-adjusted hazard of suicide after stroke was higher in individuals with prestroke depression than in those without lifetime depression (adjusted hazard ratio = 2.16). About 70% of suicide victims had a history of prestroke depression, compared to 30% of those with no depression or poststroke depression.

Parkinson's disease

Although Parkinson's disease (PD) diagnosis is based on motor signs [23], and disabilities due to motor impairments dominate the clinical manifestations of the disease [24], nonmotor symptoms, mainly depression and even psychoses, have been recently recognized as significant factors of disability impacting quality of life at all stages [23–26]. Many patients were found to first suffer from depressive episodes before their first motor symptomatology. The prevalence rate of depression in PD has been reported to range from 4% to 90%, which may be attributed to the significant symptom overlap between depression and PD, such as reduced energy, psychomotor retardation, mental slowing, difficulties with concentration, and insomnia, among others [24, 25].

The combination of severe physical disabilities and depression in this generally older-aged population may cause concerns that patients with PD are at high risk for suicidal behavior [15]. However, most investigations have reported no or only a modest increase in such risk. Suicide attempts and completed suicide appear to be uncommon despite the elevated prevalence of suicidal ideation in patients with PD, and the suicide risk for patients with PD has been found to be similar to that in the general population [27–29]. Nevertheless, the general consensus appears to be that coexisting psychiatric problems have significant impact on suicidality in PD, as comorbid psychiatric symptoms, more so than PD-related disease variables, were found to be associated with suicidal behavior [28–30].

An investigation of the psychopathological features of depression in PD as compared to primary depression revealed that a history of suicide attempts was significantly more common in patients without PD with major depression than in patients with PD with depression (42% vs. 4%), while both groups experienced suicidal ideation at the same rate (76%) [31]. Depression is one of the leading causes of suicide, and it remains unclear why an increased rate of depression is not accompanied by a markedly increased risk of suicide in patients with PD. Slaughter et al. speculated that striatal dysfunction in PD may preferentially predispose the patient to mesial and ventrolateral frontal dysfunction, resulting in an apathetic depression, while leaving orbitofrontal function relatively intact [26]. They also noted that the risk of suicide may be influenced by the relative proportion of serotonin deficit to norepinephrine and dopamine levels.

Patients with PD with suicidal ideation were reported to be younger and have an earlier onset of disease [29]. The rate of suicide among married patients with PD was higher than that among single, divorced, or widowed patients with PD, which is contrary to epidemiologic observations of suicide in the general population [15]. It is noteworthy that some reports found suicide to be one of the important causes of mortality in patients with deep brain stimulation for PD [32].

Huntington's disease

Psychiatric symptoms are often the first clinical manifestation of Huntington's disease (HD), even though research and clinical emphases seem to have been placed on motor and cognitive aspects of the disease. Paulsen et al. found that 98% of their patients with HD experienced psychiatric symptoms [33] and suggested that depression, apathy, aggression, and disinhibition are common among these patients [34]. The rate of suicide in HD ranges from 0.5% to 12.7% [35]. Most investigations found a high frequency of suicide in HD families, though some noted that suicide was a rare feature of the disease [36, 37]. In his original paper, George Huntington himself mentioned "a tendency to insanity and suicide" [38] as one of the marked peculiarities of HD [39].

A study of individuals registered in the Huntington Study Groups database reported elevated rates of suicidal ideation among individuals at risk for and diagnosed with HD [33]. Those results suggest two "critical periods" of increased risk of suicide in HD during the course of the disease: with the appearance of soft signs of HD before the neurological diagnosis has been established and during the initial progression of the disease, including functional decline, after diagnosis. Studies examining information from the National Huntington Disease Research Roster (NHDRR) revealed that the frequency of suicide was higher not only in patients with HD, but also in their relatives, including those with no risk, as compared with the general U.S. population [36], and that suicide occurred more frequently in the early stage of the disease [38, 40]. The prevalence of suicide was found to be four times higher in individuals at risk for HD than in those diagnosed with HD [38]. Among at-risk individuals, one-third of the suicides occurred before the age of 30 and 40% before the age of 40 [41].

Predictive testing for HD has been available since the mid-1980s, and its implementation may play a role in suicidal behavior among individuals at risk. Nevertheless, the overall impression among tested individuals, in both decreased- and increased-risk groups, was that being informed of their genetic status with respect to the possibility of development of the disease was beneficial to them [42]. In a worldwide survey of catastrophic events (i.e., suicides, suicide attempts, and psychiatric hospitalizations) following testing for HD, only 0.97% of the participants reported to have had one of those events after receiving their test results. Of those,

84.1% were found to have an increased risk, which represented 2% of the cohort, whereas only 0.3% of those with a decreased risk experienced catastrophic events [42].

Epilepsy

As early as 1941, Prudhomme suggested that suicide occurred more frequently among patients with epilepsy than in the general population. However, many investigations have been encumbered by methodological problems [43]; thus, the reported rates of suicide among patients with epilepsy vary considerably. In a review of 21 studies, Jones et al. found that 11.5% of all deaths in people with epilepsy were caused by suicide [44], whereas Bell et al. found a rate under 5% compared with 1.4% in the general population [43].

Suicidal ideation and behavior appears to be relatively common among individuals with epilepsy, with increasing relative risk (RR) attributable to psychiatric comorbidity, particularly affective disorders [44–46]. Furthermore, the relationship between epilepsy and suicidal ideation behavior is complex and multifactorial. In a population-based Danish study, people with epilepsy had a twofold higher risk of committing suicide in the absence of any psychosocial problem; this risk increased by 32-fold in the presence of a mood disorder and by 12-fold in the presence of an anxiety or schizophreniform disorder [45]. The risk of suicide was greatest during the first 6 months after diagnosis of epilepsy (RR: 5.35). In another investigation of patients with chronic epilepsy, the highest risks for a suicide attempt were associated with a lifetime history of major depressive episodes (odds ratio [OR]: 5.9) and lifetime manic episodes (OR: 12.6) [44]. In addition, onset of epilepsy at a younger age [46] and family psychiatric history [47] have been reported as risk factors for suicide [46].

Suicidal ideation and behavior have been identified in the context of postictal psychiatric episodes. Kanner et al. found that 13% of patients with refractory partial epilepsy experienced habitual postictal suicidal ideation [48]. Furthermore, Kanemoto et al. reported that suicide attempts were more frequent during postictal psychosis (7%) than during either acute interictal psychosis (2%) or postictal confusion

(0%) in a study of patients with temporal lobe epilepsy (TLE) [49].

An increased suicide risk in individuals with TLE has been reported. Fukuchi et al. examined 43 cases of death in epilepsy and found that all suicides identified in the cohort were TLE cases [50]. This association, however, has not been supported by all studies.

Suicide has been also identified after epilepsy surgery. A meta-analysis investigating the occurrence of suicides in patients with epilepsy revealed a higher prevalence among patients who underwent epilepsy surgery than in the general population, regardless of whether a seizure-free state was achieved [51].

The use of antipsychotic drugs has been associated with a ten-fold higher risk of suicide [46]. Likewise, several types of antiepileptic drugs (AEDs) have also been related to psychiatric adverse events seen in clinical practice. In January 2008, the Food and Drug Administration (FDA) issued a safety warning regarding the risk of suicidality associated with AED administration. However, the validity of those results has been questioned because of several methodological problems [52]. The FDA alert was followed by several investigations on the relation between AEDs and suicidal ideation and behavior [53–55], which yielded conflicting results. Thus, the relation between AEDs and suicidality is yet to be established.

A bidirectional relationship between epilepsy and suicidality was suggested in a population-based case-control study of all newly diagnosed unprovoked seizures among Icelandic individuals [56]. The investigators found that a lifetime history of attempted suicide increased the risk for an unprovoked seizure by 3.5fold even after adjusting for age, gender, cumulative alcohol intake, and depression.

Dementia

Despite the high rates of psychiatric symptoms reported during the course of this disease [57], patients with dementia were found to die from suicide less often than expected [58]. Furthermore, a meta-analysis of suicide risk in patients with common neurologic and psychiatric disorders found that dementia had a lower than expected SMR due to suicide, which led to the speculation that impaired competence may be protective

against suicide by diminishing the ability to elaborate and carry out a suicidal plan [59].

In a review of literature on suicidal behavior in dementia, Haw et al. [60] found no good evidence that suicide risk in dementia was higher than in the general population, except for a study presented by Erlangsen et al. In that study, the authors reported that the suicide risk in hospital-diagnosed dementia was elevated, particularly in those aged 50–69 years, for whom the RR was 8.5 in males and 10.8 in females [61]. The time period shortly after diagnosis was associated with a higher suicide risk, though suicides continued to occur well after the initial diagnosis. In addition, the suicide risk in patients with dementia remained relatively high after controlling for mood disorders.

Depression is a common risk factor for both suicide and dementia. Multiple studies have reported that suicide ideation experienced by patients with dementia is strongly associated with comorbid depressive symptoms while being unrelated to the patient's awareness of memory and/or other cognitive disturbances, particularly in Alzheimer's disease (AD) [15, 62]. In the last decade, the diagnosis of dementia, particularly AD, is being made at earlier stages of the disease when the deterioration of the patient's cognitive functions is limited, which could possibly result in increased suicide risk [59]. Lim et al. described the clinical and neuropsychological course of two subjects with autopsy-proven AD [63]. Both had very mild early-stage AD at their last assessment prior to suicidal behavior and displayed the high-risk phenotype predisposing to suicidal behavior: male gender, highly educated professional, preserved insight, dysphoric symptoms that did not meet the criteria for major depression and postdated the onset of cognitive decline, and endorsement of suicidal ideation. The authors stated the need for awareness that early-stage AD might present a unique suicidal risk as compared with later stages.

Amyotrophic lateral sclerosis

Suicidal thoughts are not rare in patients with amyotrophic lateral sclerosis (ALS) given its devastating nature, the lack of effective treatment, and increasing dependence on caregivers [64]. Euthanasia and physician-assisted suicide (PAS) are not legal in most countries; therefore, suicide may be regarded as a last resort for patients with ALS. Fang et al. [64] reported an approximately sixfold higher risk of suicide among patients with ALS compared with age-, gender-, and calendar period-matched individuals in the general Swedish population (SMR: 5.8). Patients who committed suicide were diagnosed at a relatively younger age compared with those who did not. The highest RR for suicide was observed within the first year after the first hospitalization for ALS (SMR: 11.2).

In a prospective study, Albert et al. reported that 43.4% of patients with ALS who died during the follow-up period had thought about ending their lives, 18.9% expressed the wish to die, and 5.7% acted on that wish and planned their suicides with the use of sedatives [65]. All patients who acted on that wish had family support for hastening their deaths.

In the United States, PAS but not euthanasia has only been legal in the state of Oregon since November 1997 [66], and the number of PAS deaths has remained largely stable since 2003. The ratio of PAS deaths to non-PAS deaths for ALS was 269 to 10,000, whereas the same ratio for cancer was 39.9 to 10,000. In patients with ALS, psychological reasons may play a larger role in the unbearable suffering as compared with patients with cancer [67]. Physicians in Oregon who participate in PAS have indicated that loss of autonomy, decreasing ability to participate in enjoyable activities, and loss of dignity were the three most common end-of-life concerns in patients choosing that option [66]. These patients were more likely to be male, more highly educated, more hopeless, less religious, and rated a poor quality of life. However, recent studies have shown that a major depressive disorder (MDD) is frequent given the severity of the disease [68].

Multiple sclerosis

Studies on the relationship between suicide risk and multiple sclerosis (MS) have yielded inconsistent results due to different study designs and methodology problems; thus, comparisons among them are nearly impossible [14]. Nevertheless, the literature as a whole points to a higher suicidal risk in patients with MS than in the general population [15].

Stenager et al. conducted two analyses of patients with MS registered with the Danish Multiple Sclerosis Registry (DMSR), which comprised 5525 cases with onset of MS between the years 1953 and 1985 and 6088 cases diagnosed with MS within the same period [69]. The overall SMR for suicide was 1.83. Among male patients with MS with an onset at the age of 30 or younger, the SMR of suicide was 2.73, while their female counterparts had an SMR of 1.28. Among patients diagnosed after the age of 30, the SMRs in males and females were 3.12 and 2.12, respectively. Most suicides took place within 5 years of diagnosis, and the time of suicide appeared to be more temporally related to the time of diagnosis than to the age of onset. Indeed, the suicide risk was highest shortly after diagnosis, though it remained elevated many years after diagnosis [70]. In males, suicides were more frequent between the ages of 40 and 49 years by violent means; in addition, a history of previous suicidal behavior or a previous mental disorder (with depression as the most frequent condition), recent deterioration of MS, and moderate disability were the variables significantly associated with the suicidal risk [71]. In the case of females, the variables associated with suicide were less distinct [71]. Although it may be assumed that suicidal behavior is more likely to occur in patients with progressive, debilitating neurological conditions [72], that was not the case.

Not all suicides among patients with MS occur in the context of a clearly diagnosed depressive episode or disorder. However, a diagnosis of depression in patients with MS may be masked by overlapping symptoms such as fatigue, insomnia, appetite disturbance, and diminished ability to concentrate [25, 73]. Nonetheless, patients with MS are at increased risk for depressive disorders [71, 74], which increases the suicidal risk [25].

Migraine

Many migraine patients experience changes in mood or behavior as a prodromal or accompanying feature of their migraine attacks [75], and various medical and psychiatric conditions have been reported as comorbid conditions that accompany migraine [76]. However, few epidemiologic studies have investigated the association of migraine with suicidal behavior, and the relationship is unclear.

Breslau et al. [77] found an increased prevalence of suicide attempts among individuals with migraine compared to those without migraine, and also noted that suicide attempts had a stronger association with migraine with aura than without aura. Migraine with aura alone, without coexisting MDD, was found to be associated with a significantly increased risk for suicide attempts and suicidal ideation (4.3 and 2.4, respectively) [78]. Furthermore, when migraine with aura was accompanied by MDD, the odds for suicide attempts were markedly increased and greatly exceeded the risk associated with MDD alone (23.2 and 7.8, respectively). On the other hand, migraine without aura alone was not associated with a significantly increased risk of suicidal ideation or suicide attempts.

In an investigation of psychiatric comorbidity and suicidal risk among adolescents with chronic daily headaches conducted in Taiwan, Wang et al. also found that the suicidal risk in subjects with migraine was higher than in those without migraine (OR: 4.3) [79]. There was also a significant association between migraine headache and suicidal risk for subjects with migraine with aura (OR: 7.8) after controlling the data for age, gender, and major depressive and anxiety disorders, but not for migraine without aura, which implies that migraine with aura is an independent risk factor for a higher risk of suicide.

Traumatic brain injury

Traumatic brain injury (TBI) is a major public health problem. Unfortunately, few detailed studies of suicidality in TBI have been conducted. In a systematic literature search, Simpson and Tate found that some population-based studies reported a significantly higher prevalence of completed suicide, suicidal attempts, and suicidal ideation in individuals with TBI compared to the general population, even after controlling for psychiatric disorders [80]; however, these findings have not been confirmed in other studies [81, 82]. These inconsistent results appear to have primarily resulted from methodological differences and flaws associated with the studies.

Teasdale and Engberg provided the first population-based evidence of elevated suicide rates after diagnosis of TBI [83]. They examined Danish individuals with mild TBI and found that

death from suicide occurred in 0.59% of those with concussion, 0.61% of those with cranial fractures, and 0.84% of those with cerebral lesions. The median time intervals from injury to suicide ranged from 3 to 3.5 years for all diagnostic groups and did not differ significantly. Overall, compared to age- and gender-matched controls, the SMRs for suicide in those with concussion, cranial fractures, and cerebral lesions were 3.0, 2.7, and 4.1, respectively. In all groups, the ratios were higher for females than males, and lower for patients injured before the age of 21 or after the age of 60. Substance use was a significantly associated variable. Individuals who suffered from a TBI by an act of self-harm were seven times more likely to die from suicide compared to those who sustained a TBI from other causes.

In clinical interviews and a medical file review of outpatients with TBI, Simpson and Tate found that 17.4% of patients attempted suicide over a mean period of 5 years [84]. The lifetime attempt rate was 26.2%. Half of the patients made one attempt, while the remainder made two or more attempts. Neither injury severity nor the presence of premorbid suicide risk factors contributed to elevated levels of suicidality postinjury. Nearly half (48.3%) of the participants who made a postinjury attempt went on to make at least one further attempt [85].

Traumatic spinal cord injury

There is general agreement in published studies that the life expectancy for individuals with traumatic spinal cord injury (TSCI) has increased significantly since World War II [86]. However, suicide is becoming a major cause of death among patients with TSCI. Recent studies reported that death from suicide was 3.3–4.9 times more common in patients with TSCI than in the general population [87].

In a study of suicide following TSCI in the United States, DeVivo et al. reported that the SMR was highest between 1 and 5 years after injury, although it was also significantly elevated during the first postinjury year [88]. In addition, the SMR was highest for individuals aged 25–54 years old, but was also elevated for those aged less than 25 when compared with the general population. Overall, the suicide rate was higher for females and for individuals with paraplegia, in whom suicide was the leading cause of death. Yet, other studies reported greater risk of suicide for individuals with quadriplegia than for those with paraplegia [89, 90]. In addition, a survey performed in Denmark [86, 87] revealed that the frequency of suicide was higher in a group of marginally disabled individuals than in other functional groups of individuals with more severe disabilities.

In some cases, TSCI occurred as a result of a suicide attempt. Charlifue et al. reviewed the records of patients with TSCI available from the National Center for Health Statistics, and found that of those who committed suicide, 7% had sustained TSCI as a result of a suicide attempt [90]. Also, examination of a database containing details of individuals with TSCI as a result of a suicide attempt revealed that 7.3% of those reattempted suicide, though the majority did not [91].

Screening for suicidality

Identification of patients at risk for suicidal behavior is a seldom occurrence in a neurologist's practice, not because patients may not be experiencing suicidal ideation and/or the psychiatric comorbidities associated with a suicidal risk. In fact, this chapter clearly demonstrated the relatively high prevalence of psychiatric disorders that can facilitate and/or increase a suicidal risk. The use of screening instruments can provide a solution to this problem. These instruments should include scales that screen for depression, generalized anxiety disorder, and suicidal ideation and/or behavior. Two user-friendly options include the Beck Depression Inventory, Second Edition (BDI-II) [92], which, in addition to screening for depressive symptoms present in the last 2 weeks, includes one item that screens for suicidal ideation and behavior. The Generalized Anxiety Disorder-7 (GAD-7), is a seven-item self-rating instrument that screens for generalized anxiety disorder [93]. It takes 7 minutes for patients to complete these two instruments. Finally, the suicidality module of the Mini International Neuropsychiatric Inventory is a seven-item questionnaire that investigates the presence of suicidal attempts ever, and suicidal ideation and behavior in the last 4 weeks [94].

Conclusions

Suicidality is a relatively common psychiatric complication in patients suffering from most neurologic disorders. The relation between suicidality and neurologic disorders is complex and multifactorial. The relation between suicidality on the one hand and epilepsy and migraine on the other is bidirectional, which is an expression of common neurobiologic pathogenic mechanisms operant in these conditions. Screening for depressive and anxiety disorders and the use of short screening instruments of suicidal ideation and behavior can help identify patients at risk for suicidal behavior.

PEARLS TO TAKE HOME

- Suicidality is a term that encompasses suicidal ideation, suicidal behavior, and completed suicide.
- Suicidality is a relatively frequent complication of most major neurologic disorders, including stroke, epilepsy, MS, migraine, HD, ALS, and traumatic and spinal cord injury.
- The presence of comorbid psychiatric disorders, in particular MDDs, is one of the leading risk factors for suicidality in patients with neurologic disorders.
- Suicidality is less frequent in advanced stages of dementia and is not more frequent in patients with PD than in the general population.
- A bidirectional relationship exists between suicidality on the one hand and epilepsy and migraine with auras on the other. This suggests not only that patients with epilepsy and migraine are at increased risk of developing suicidal ideation and behavior, but also that patients with suicidal behavior are at increased risk of developing epilepsy and migraine.
- Identification of patients at risk for suicidal behavior should include the use of screening instruments that detect depressive and anxiety disorders, some of which include specific items of suicidal ideation and behavior.

References

1. Centers for Disease Control and Prevention. Definitions: Self-Directed Violence. http://www.cdc.gov/ViolencePrevention/suicide/definitions.html.

2. Druss B, Pincus H. Suicidal ideation and suicide attempts in general medical illnesses. *Arch Intern Med*, 160: 1522–1526, 2000.

3. Krug EG et al., eds. *World Report on Violence and Health*, Geneva, Switzerland: World Health Organization, 2002.

4. Chapter 7. Self-Directed Violence. http://www.who.int/violence_injury_prevention/violence/global_campaign/en/chap7.pdf.

5. National Vital Statistics Reports Volume 58, Number 19. http://www.cdc.gov/nchs/data/nvsr/nvsr58/nvsr58_19.pdf.

6. Goldsmith SK et al., eds. *Reducing Suicide: A National Imperative*, Washington, DC: National Academy Press, 2002.

7. Office of Applied Studies. Suicidal Thoughts and Behaviors among Adults. http://oas.samhsa.gov/2k9/165/suicide.cfm.

8. National Institute of Mental Health. Suicide in the U.S.: Statistics and Prevention. http://www.nimh.nih.gov/health/publications/suicide-in-the-us-statistics-and-prevention/index.shtml.

9. Nock MK, Borges G, Bromet EJ, Cha CB, Kessler RC, Lee S. Suicide and suicidal behavior. *Epidemiol Rev*, 30: 133–154, 2008.

10. Centers for Disease Control and Prevention. Suicide: Risk and Protective Factors. http://www.cdc.gov/ViolencePrevention/suicide/riskprotectivefactors.html.

11. Monk N. Epidemiology of suicide. *Epiedmiol Rev*, 9: 51–69, 1987.

12. Mackenzie TB, Popkin MK. Suicide in the medical patient. *Int J Psychiatry Med*, 17: 3–22, 1987.

13. Copsey Spring TR, Yanni L, Levenson JL. A shot in the dark: failing to recognize the link between physical and mental illness. *J Gen Intern Med*, 22: 677–680, 2007.

14. Stenager EN, Stenager E. Suicide and patients with neurologic diseases. Methodologic problems. *Arch Neurol*, 49: 1296–1303, 1992.

15. Arciniegas DB, Anderson CA. Suicide in neurologic illness. *Curr Treat Options Neurol*, 4: 457–468, 2002.

16. Kishi Y, Kosier JT, Robinson RG. Suicidal plans in patients with acute stroke. *J Nerv Ment Dis*, 184: 274–280, 1996.

17. Stenager EN, Madsen C, Stenager E, Boldsen J. Suicide in patients with stroke: epidemiological study. *BMJ*, 316: 1206, 1998.

18. Teasdale TW, Engberg A. Suicide after a stroke: a population study. *J Epidemiol Community Health*, 55: 863–866, 2001.

19. Kishi Y, Robinson RG, Kosier JT. Suicidal plans in patients with stroke: comparison between acute-onset and delayed-onset suicidal plans. *Int Psychogeriatr*, 8: 623–634, 1996.

20. Pohjasvaara T, Vataja R, Leppavuori A, Kaste M, Erkinjuntti T. Suicidal ideas in stroke patients 3 and 15 months after stroke. *Cerebrovasc Dis*, 12: 21–26, 2001.

21. Williams LS. Depression and stroke: cause or consequence? *Semin Neurol*, 25: 396–409, 2005.

22. Forsstrom E, Hakko H, Nordstrom T, Rasanen P, Mainio A. Suicide in patients with stroke: a population-based study of suicide victims during the years 1988–2007 in Northern Finland. *J Neuropsychiatry Clin Neurosci*, 22: 182–187, 2010.

23. Kummer A, Teixeira AL. Neuropsychiatry of Parkinson's disease. *Arq Neuropsiquiatr*, 67: 930–939, 2009.

24. Farabaugh AH, Yap L, McDonald WM, Alpert JE, Fava M. Pattern of depressive symptoms in Parkinson's disease. *Psychosomatics*, 50: 448–454, 2009.

25. Raskind MA. Diagnosis and treatment of depression comorbid with neurologic disorders. *Am J Med*, 121: S28–S37, 2008.

26. Slaughter JR, Slaughter KA, Nichols D, Holmes SE, Martens MP. Prevalence, clinical manifestations, etiology, and treatment of depression in Parkinson's disease. *J Neuropsychiatry Clin Neurosci*, 13: 187–196, 2001.

27. Stenager EN, Wermuth L, Stenager E, Boldsen J. Suicide in patients with Parkinson's disease. An epidemiological study. *Acta Psychiatrica Scandinavica*, 90: 70–72, 1994.

28. Nazem S, Siderowf AD, Duda JE, Brown GK, Ten Have T, Stern MB, Weintraub D. Suicidal and death ideation in Parkinson's disease. *Mov Disord*, 23: 1573–1579, 2008.

29. Kummer A, Cardoso F, Teixeira AL. Suicidal ideation in Parkinson's disease. *CNS Spectr*, 14: 431–436, 2009.

30. Kostic VS, Pekmezovic T, Tomic A, Jecmenica-Lukic M, Spica V, Svetel M, Stefanova E, Petrovic I, Dzoljic E. Suicide and suicidal ideation in Parkinson's disease. *J Neurol Sci*, 289: 40–43, 2010.

31. Merschdorf U, Berg D, Csoti I, Fornadi F, Merz B, Naumann M, Becker G, Supprian T. Psychopathological symptoms of depression in Parkinson's disease compared to major depression. *Psychopathology*, 36: 221–225, 2003.

32. Voon V, Krack P, Lang AE, Lozano AM, Dujardin K, Schupbach M, D'Ambrosia J, Thobois S, Tamma F, Herzog J, Speelman JD, Samanta J, Kubu C, Rossignol H, Poon Y, Saint-Cyr JA, Ardouin C, Moro E. A multicentre study on suicide outcomes following subthalamic stimulation for Parkinson's disease. *Brain*, 131: 2720–2728, 2008.

33. Paulsen JS, Hoth KF, Nehl C, Stierman L. Critical periods of suicide risk in Huntington's disease. *Am J Psychiatry*, 162: 725–731, 2005.

34. Paulsen JS, Ready RE, Hamilton JM, Mega MS, Cummings JL. Neuropsychiatric aspects of Huntington's disease. *J Neurol Neurosurg Psychiatry*, 71: 310–314, 2001.

35. Bird TD. Outrageous fortune: the risk of suicide in genetic testing for Huntington disease. *Am J Hum Genet*, 64: 1289–1292, 1999.

36. Maio LD, Squitieri F, Napolitano G, Campanella G, Trofatter JA, Conneally PM. Suicide risk in Huntington's disease. *J Med Genet*, 30: 293–295, 1993.

37. Lanska DJ, Lavine L, Lanska MJ, Schoenberg BS. Huntington's disease mortality in the United States. *Neurology*, 38: 769–772, 1988.

38. Schoenfeld M, Myers RH, Cupples LA, Berkman B, Sax DS, Clark E. Increased rate of suicide among patients with Huntington's disease. *J Neurol Neurosurg Psychiatry*, 47: 1283–1287, 1984.

39. Siemers E. Huntington disease. *Arch Neurol*, 58: 308–310, 2001.

40. Farrer LA. Suicide and attempted suicide in Huntington disease: implications for preclinical testing of persons at risk. *Am J Med Genet*, 24: 305–311, 1986.

41. Sorensen SA, Fenger K. Causes of death in patients with Huntington's disease and in unaffected first degree relatives. *J Med Genet*, 29: 911–914, 1992.

42. Almqvist EW, Bloch M, Brinkman R, Craufurd D, Hayden MR. A worldwide assessment of the frequency of suicide, suicide attempts, or psychiatric hospitalization after predictive testing for Huntington disease. *Am J Hum Genet*, 64: 1293–1304, 1999.

43. Bell GS, Sander JW. Suicide and epilepsy. *Curr Opin Neurol*, 22: 174–178, 2009.

44. Jones JE, Hermann BP, Barry JJ, Gilliam FG, Kanner AM, Meador KJ. Rates and risk factors for suicide, suicidal ideation, and suicide attempts in chronic epilepsy. *Epilepsy Behav*, 4: S31–S38, 2003.

45. Christensen J, Vestergaard M, Mortensen PB, Sidenius P, Agerbo E. Epilepsy and risk of suicide: a population-based case-control study. *Lancet Neurol*, 6: 693–698, 2007.

46. Nilsson L, Ahlbom A, Farahmand BY, Asberg M, Tomson T. Risk factors for suicide in epilepsy: a case control study. *Epilepsia*, 43: 644–651, 2002.

47. Kanner AM. Suicidality and epilepsy: a complex relationship that remains misunderstood and underestimated. *Epilepsy Curr*, 9: 63–66, 2009.

48. Kanner AM, Soto A, Gross-Kanner H. Prevalence and clinical characteristics of postictal psychiatric symptoms in partial epilepsy. *Neurology*, 62: 708–713, 2004.

49. Kanemoto K, Kawasaki J, Mori E. Violence and epilepsy: a close relation between violence and postictal psychosis. *Epilepsia*, 40: 107–109, 1999.

50. Fukuchi T, Kanemoto K, Kato M, Ishida S, Yuasa S, Kawasaki J, Suzuki S, Onuma T. Death in epilepsy with special attention to suicide cases. *Epilepsy Res*, 51: 233–236, 2002.

51. Pompili M, Girardi P, Tatarelli G, Angeletti G, Tatarelli R. Suicide after surgical treatment in patients with epilepsy: a meta-analytic investigation. *Psychol Rep*, 98: 323–338, 2006.

52. Hesdorffer DC, Kanner AM. The FDA alert on suicidality and antiepileptic drugs: fire or false alarm? *Epilepsia*, 50: 978–986, 2009.

53. Patorno E, Bohn RL, Wahl PM, Avorn J, Patrick AR, Liu J, Schneeweiss S. Anticonvulsant

medications and the risk of suicide, attempted suicide, or violent death. *JAMA*, 303: 1401–1409, 2010.

54. Andersohn F, Schade R, Willich SN, Garbe E. Use of antiepileptic drugs in epilepsy and the risk of self-harm or suicidal behavior. *Neurology*, 75: 335–340, 2010.

55. Arana A, Wentworth CE, Ayuso-Mateos JL, Arellano FM. Suicide-related events in patients treated with antiepileptic drugs. *N Engl J Med*, 363: 542–551, 2010.

56. Hesdorffer DC, Hauser WA, Olafsson E, Ludvigsson P, Kjartansson O. Depression and suicide attempt as risk factors for incident unprovoked seizures. *Ann Neurol*, 59: 35–41, 2006.

57. Purandare N, Voshaar RC, Rodway C, Bickley H, Burns A, Kapur N. Suicide in dementia: 9-year national clinical survey in England and Wales. *Br J Psychiatry*, 194: 175–180, 2009.

58. Schneider B, Maurer K, Frolich L. Demenz und Suizid. *Fortschr Neurol Psychiat*, 69: 164–169, 2001.

59. Draper B, Peisah C, Snowdon J, Brodaty H. Early dementia diagnosis and the risk of suicide and euthanasia. *Alzheimers Demen*, 6: 75–82, 2010.

60. Haw C, Harwood D, Hawton K. Dementia and suicidal behavior: a review of the literature. *Int Psychogeriatr*, 21: 40–453, 2009.

61. Erlangsen A, Zarit SH, Conwell Y. Hospital-diagnosed dementia and suicide: a longitudinal study using prospective, nationwide register data. *Am J Geriatr Psychiatry*, 16: 220–228, 2008.

62. Draper B, MacCuspie-Moore C, Brodaty H. Suicidal ideation and the "wish to die" in dementia patients: the role of depression. *Age Ageing*, 27: 503–507, 1998.

63. Lim WS, Rubin EH, Coats M, Morris JC. Early-stage Alzheimer disease represents increased suicidal risk in relation to later stages. *Alzheimer Dis Assoc Disord*, 19: 214–219, 2005.

64. Fang F, Valdimarsdóttir U, Fürst CJ, Hultman C, Fall K, Sparén P, Ye W. Suicide among patients with amyotrophic lateral sclerosis. *Brain*, 131: 2729–2733, 2008.

65. Albert SM, Rabkin JG, Del Bene ML, Tider T, O'Sullivan I, Rowland LP, Mitsumoto H. Wish to die in end-stage ALS. *Neurology*, 65: 68–74, 2005.

66. McCluskey L. ALS: ethical issues from diagnosis to end of life. *NeuroRehabilitation*, 22: 463–472, 2007.

67. Maessen M, Veldink JH, van den Berg LH, Schouten HJ, van der Wal G, Onwuteaka-Philipsen BD. Requests for euthanasia: origin of suffering in ALS, heart failure, and cancer patients. *J Neurol*, 257: 1192–1198, 2010.

68. Norris L, Que G, Bayat E. Psychiatric aspects of Amyotrophic Lateral Sclerosis (ALS). *Curr Psychiatry Rep*, 12: 239–245, 2010.

69. Stenager EN, Stenager E, Koch-Henriksen N, Brønnum-Hansen H, Hyllested K, Jensen K, Bille-Brahe U. Suicide and multiple sclerosis: an epidemiological investigation. *J Neurol Neurosurg Psychiatry*, 55: 542–545, 1992.

70. Brønnum-Hansen H, Stenager E, Nylev Stenager E, Koch-Henriksen N. Suicide among Danes with multiple sclerosis. *J Neurol Neurosurg Psychiatry*, 76: 1457–1459, 2005.

71. Stenager EN, Koch-Henriksen N, Stenager E. Risk factors for suicide in multiple sclerosis. *Psychother Psychosom*, 65: 86–90, 1996.

72. Carson AJ, Best S, Warlow C, Sharpe M. Suicidal ideation among outpatients at general neurology clinics: prospective study. *BMJ*, 320(7245): 1311–1312, 2000.

73. Ghaffar. O, Feinstein A. The neuropsychiatry of multiple sclerosis: a review of recent developments. *Curr Opin Psychiatry*, 20:278–285. 2007.

74. Feinstein A. Neuropsychiatric syndromes associated with multiple sclerosis. *J Neurol*, 254, Suppl. 2: II/73–II/76, 2007.

75. Cahill CM, Murphy KC. Migraine: another headache for psychiatrists? *Br J Psychiatry*, 185: 191–193, 2004.

76. Peterlin BL, Ward TN. Neuropsychiatric aspects of migraine. *Neuropsychiatr Disord*, 7: 371–375, 2005.

77. Breslau N, Davis GC, Andreski P. Migraine, psychiatric disorders, and suicide attempts: an epidemiologic study of young adults. *Psychiatry Res*, 37: 11–23, 1991.

78. Breslau N. Migraine, suicidal ideation, and suicide attempts. *Neurology*, 42: 392–395, 1992.

79. Wang SJ, Juang KD, Fuh JL, Lu SR. Migraine and suicide. *Neurology*, 68: 1468–1473, 2007.

80. Simpson G, Tate R. Suicidality in people surviving a traumatic brain injury: prevalence, risk f actors and implications for clinical management. *Brain Inj*, 21: 13335–11351, 2007.

81. Shavelle RM, Strauss D, Whyte J, Day SM, Yu YL. Long-term causes of death after traumatic brain injury. *Am J Phys Med Rehabil*, 80: 510–516, 2001.

82. Harrison-Felix C, Whiteneck G, DeVivo M, Hammond FM, Jha A. Mortality following rehabilitation in the Traumatic Brain Injury Model Systems of Care. *NeuroRehabilitation*, 19: 45–54, 2004.

83. Teasdale TW, Engberg AW. Suicide after traumatic brain injury: a population study. *J Neurol Neruosurg Psychiatry*, 71: 436–440, 2001.

84. Simpson G, Tate R. Suicidality after traumatic brain injury: demographic, injury and clinical correlates. *Psychol Med*, 32: 687–697, 2002.

85. Simpson G, Tate R. Clinical features of suicide attempts after traumatic brain injury. *J Nerv Ment Dis*, 193: 680–685, 2005.

86. Hartkopp A, Brønnum-Hansen H, Seidenschnur AM, Biering-Sørensen F. Survival and cause of death after traumatic spinal cord injury. A long-term epidemiological survey from Denmark. *Spinal Cord*, 35: 76–85, 1997.

87. Hartkopp A, Brønnum-Hansen H, Seidenschnur AM, Biering-Sørensen F. Suicide in a spinal cord injured population: its relation to functional status. *Arch Phys Med Rehabil*, 79: 1356–1361, 1998.

88. DeVivo MJ, Black KJ, Richards JS, Stover SL. Suicide following spinal cord injury. *Paraplegia*, 29: 620–627, 1991.

89. Soden RJ, Walsh J, Middleton JW, Craven ML, Rutkowski SB, Yeo JD. Causes of death after spinal cord injury. *Spinal Cord*, 38: 604–610, 2000.

90. Charlifue SW, Gerhart KA. Behavioral and demographic predictors of suicide after traumatic spinal cord injury. *Arch Phys Med Rehabil*, 72: 488–492, 1991.

91. Kennedy P, Rogers B, Speer S, Frankel H. Spinal cord injuries and attempted suicide: a retrospective review. *Spinal Cord*, 37: 847–852, 1999.

92. Jones JE, Hermann BP, Woodard JL, Barry JJ, Gilliam F, Kanner AM, Meador KJ. Screening for major depression in epilepsy with common self-report depression inventories. *Epilepsia*, 46: 731–735, 2005.

93. Spitzer RL, Kroenke K, Williams JBW, Loewe B. A brief measure for generalized anxiety disorder. *Arch Intern Med*, 166: 1092–1097, 2006.

94. Sheehan DV, Lecrubier Y, Sheehan KH, Amorim P, Janavs J, Weiller E, Hergueta T, Baker R, Dunbar GC. The Mini-International Neuropsychiatric Interview (M.I.N.I.): the development and validation of a structured diagnostic psychiatric interview for DSM-IV and ICD-10. *J Clin Psychiatry.*, 59, Suppl. 20: 22–33, 1998.

Neuropsychological Aspects of Depression: Their Relevance in Depression in Neurologic Disorders

Erica J. Kalkut[1] and Christopher L. Grote[2]
[1]Department of Neurology, Medical College of Wisconsin, Milwaukee, WI, USA
[2]Department of Behavioral Sciences, Rush University Medical Center, Chicago, IL, USA

Introduction

Depression is a psychiatric disorder that not only has a high prevalence in the general population, but that is often comorbid with other physical and psychiatric illnesses, including neurologic disorders [1]. By definition, depression has a negative impact on an individual's overall well-being through academic, occupational, interpersonal, and/or social areas of functioning. Additionally, subjective cognitive complaints are common among people with depression and can serve to further impact daily functioning. While people with depression often complain of memory problems or decreased concentration, these areas of cognitive difficulty are not always evident on objective measurement of cognitive ability. Understanding whether changes in cognition are actually occurring in the context of depression is important not only for patients, but also for the physicians and clinicians who are treating them.

A neuropsychological evaluation is useful in determining the cognitive impact of neurologic and psychiatric conditions, like depression, on an individual. First, a neuropsychological evaluation provides an assessment of a person's current neurocognitive level of functioning. This entails determining a pattern of cognitive strengths and weaknesses or areas of cognitive decline. For example, a patient may have intact intellectual ability but impaired memory. Second, neuropsychological assessments are sensitive to brain damage, lending them useful in differential diagnosis of neurobehavioral syndromes. A neuropsychologist has the skills and training to use these assessment tools in evaluating brain–behavior relationships. This ability is particularly important in evaluating the complex patient with multiple conditions such as depression and neurologic disorders.

Much information can be gleaned from a neuropsychological evaluation, which is important in understanding patients with complex psychiatric and neurologic presentations. This chapter will review the literature on cognitive performance in depression and neurologic illness and illustrate the usefulness of neuropsychological evaluations in patients with neurologic disorders, particularly those with comorbid depression. In order to achieve the first aim of this chapter, several areas of research will be reviewed: cognitive performance in depression, cognitive performance in depression and neurologic disorder, and cognitive performance following

Depression in Neurologic Disorders: Diagnosis and Management, First Edition.
Edited by Andres M. Kanner.
© 2012 Blackwell Publishing Ltd. Published 2012 by Blackwell Publishing Ltd.

treatment for depression. Broadly, this chapter aims to provide further insight into the complex nature of these patients from a neuropsychological perspective and highlight the benefit of a neuropsychological evaluation in treating such patients.

Cognitive performance in depression

The relationship between depression and cognition is one that has been investigated for a number of years, but which has not been well understood until recently. Historically, the literature on depression and cognition has been widely discrepant, with some studies reporting no effect of depression on cognition and other studies reporting significant effects. The studies that do find an effect of depression on cognition have been further complicated by inconsistencies across studies on the reported areas of cognition affected by depression (e.g., memory, language, executive functioning).

Mixed findings with regard to the relationship between depression and cognition are largely due to the failure of studies in this area to isolate cognitive impairments specific to depression. For example, examining general cognition (i.e., IQ) as opposed to individual cognitive domains, such as processing speed or attention, could mask the true impairments associated with depression. As evidence, inconsistent findings have been noted in research investigating the performance of people with depression on tests of general cognitive ability [2, 3]. Furthermore, studies that utilize heterogeneous samples of individuals with varying levels of depressive symptomatology and/or a multitude of comorbid factors could also result in variable findings with regard to cognition. Recognition of these confounds has resulted in contemporary researchers in this area to be more diligent in describing sample characteristics and using specific assessment measures.

A meta-analysis of research on the cognitive performance of depression conducted in the late 1990s revealed that impairments in patients with depression were considered global and diffuse [4], reflecting the current view at the time. However, it was further reported in this meta-analysis that while people with depression appeared to have global cognitive impairment, greater deficits were noted on tasks thought to preferentially involve the frontal lobes [4]. This led to the more modern view that although individuals with depression may show a generally suppressed overall neuropsychological profile, including a slower processing speed, performance on tasks involving frontal regions tends to be most affected.

Functional neuroimaging studies provide further information on the neurobiological aspects of depression and the involvement of the frontal lobes as they relate to brain functioning. While there is some evidence to suggest that patients with depression have a reduction in total frontal lobe brain volume, functional abnormalities appear to be more distinct [5]. Mood disorders, like depression, typically involve changes in affect, reward, motor activity, sleep, appetite, sexual interest, concentration, and memory [5]. Neuroimaging studies indicate that the anterior structures and basal ganglia-thalamocortical pathways are often most affected in depression [5]. Since the basal ganglia-thalamocortical pathways involve dorsolateral prefrontal, lateral orbitofrontal, and anterior cingulate circuits [5, 6], it is not surprising that individuals with depression also show reduced metabolic activity in the left dorsolateral prefrontal cortex, anterior–medial prefrontal cortex, the caudate nucleus, and the paralimbic cortex, including the inferior–posterior frontal cortex, anterior temporal cortex, and cingulated gyrus [4].

The frontal lobe is the primary brain region which regulates the cognitive skills known as "executive functioning" [4]. Executive functioning is a somewhat broad term to describe complex, effortful skills involved in creative thinking, planning, organization, and novel problem solving. Measurable executive functioning includes verbal fluency, set-shifting (i.e., switching from one task to another), divided attention, impulsivity/behavioral inhibition, working memory, and problem solving. The dorsolateral prefrontal cortex in particular is thought to be involved in verbal fluency tasks [5]. The anterior–medial prefrontal cortex is thought to subserve effortful processing [5]. The ventral frontal lobe, including the paralimbic cortex, appears to be involved in the expression of affect; lesions in this area can also result in disinhibition and deficits in visual discrimination [5] as well as memory functions [4].

Considering the neuroanatomical correlates in the frontal lobes in depression, it is not surprising that individuals with depression tend to demonstrate the greatest impairment on assessments sensitive to frontal lobe dysfunction, or effortful, executive functioning tasks [5–9]. Several studies have indicated that depression in young patients without brain injury interferes with performance on tasks of mental processing and attention [7, 10]. In addition to global slowing, suppressed performance is most frequently noted on executive functioning tests requiring frontal lobe involvement [4], such as mental flexibility and control, scanning and visuomotor tracking, visuospatial functions, and verbal fluency than in patients without depression.

Patients with depression have long been described as more lethargic and lower in initiation. Clinicians working with these patients also note them to be slower to respond or react. Not surprisingly, neuropsychological assessments have found similar results. Walter and colleagues demonstrated that patients with depression were significantly slower independent of the cognitive task load [9]. That is, regardless of whether patients with depression were performing tasks that were "simple" or "complex," they performed these tasks more slowly than individuals without depression. However, these researchers found that as compared with individuals without depression, patients with depression showed greater activation in the left dorsolateral prefrontal cortex while performing tasks with the highest cognitive load and greater activation in the ventromedial prefrontal cortex during the control "simple" condition, indicating that depressed patients may show a frontal compensatory mechanism.

Further research has supported the notion that patients with depression have greater difficulty on tasks involving executive functioning, including set shifting and descriptions of sorting categories [2, 11], sustained attention [2], selective attention [3], working memory [3], and verbal fluency [3].

The cognitive impairments associated with depression seem to be present regardless of patient age. Several studies with young individu-

als without brain injury have found a relationship between depression and performance on tasks of mental processing and attention [7, 10]. Similarly, older adults with depression tend to show impairments in executive and psychomotor functioning [12]. Furthermore, duration of depression does not seem to be associated with degree of cognitive impairment [13–20].

When studied as a whole, the research largely supports the finding that individuals with depression are more likely to experience cognitive impairment, particularly with regard to executive functioning. However, it is important to note that not all individuals with depression will evidence cognitive impairment. Interestingly though, these latter individuals might still report subjective cognitive impairment despite their intact cognitive functioning on objective assessment. As evidence, one study reported that while older adults with depression did not perform differently than their peers without depression on objective assessment, they did report significantly more subjective complaints of memory and language impairment than individuals without depression [21]. Similarly, another study utilizing both objective and subjective assessment found that individuals with depression reported subjective memory complaints in the context of intact performance on cognitive assessment [22]. In light of these findings, patients with depression who report cognitive impairment should undergo a neuropsychological evaluation to determine their cognitive level and the severity of their cognitive impairments, if any, to better understand their complaints and need for intervention.

Cognitive performance in depression and neurologic illness

Understanding that patients with depression are more likely to experience cognitive impairments in executive functioning and speed of processing than individuals without depression is an important starting point to evaluating and treating these patients. Yet, what about those patients with both neurologic illness and depression? As described in great detail in other chapters of this text, depression is more common in multiple neurologic disorders such as epilepsy, stroke, traumatic brain injury, multiple sclerosis, Alzheimer's dementia, and Parkinson's disease, to name a few. When a patient with any of these conditions presents to clinic and complains of cognitive problems, it is difficult to determine if their cognitive complaints are due to their neurologic disorder or their depression. The answer to this question is an important one toward understanding the course and prognosis to their complaints. For example, take a patient who has had a traumatic brain injury and complains of memory problems. If the memory problems are due to poor executive functioning secondary to depression rather than the traumatic brain injury, a better prognosis might be expected than if the executive dysfunction is the result of the traumatic brain injury.

A neuropsychological evaluation can be helpful in teasing these various factors apart. In addition to determining a pattern of cognitive strengths and weaknesses, a neuropsychological evaluation can help determine the presence of cognitive decline and aid in the differential diagnosis. Many neurologic disorders have known cognitive impairments in the absence of depression. For example, patients with multiple sclerosis tend to perform more poorly on measures of processing speed and attention. Patients with left temporal lobe epilepsy have greater impairment in language and verbal memory. Depending on the duration of the neurologic disorder, course, and severity, the level of cognitive impairment may be more or less severe.

In addition to assessing cognitive performance, a neuropsychological evaluation includes an assessment of psychological functioning. If a patient is found to have depression, as well as a neurologic disorder, it becomes necessary to understand the level of severity and course of the depression in addition to the neurologic disorder. The neuropsychologist can then attempt to distinguish the impairments that may be due to the neurologic disorder and those that are due to the depression. This determination is much easier in a patient who suffered a mild traumatic injury several years prior, an onset of depression 3 months ago, an onset of subjective memory problems 2 months ago, and a neurocognitive profile consisting of slowed processing and divided attention problems than in a patient who

has a history of depression and epilepsy for 20 years with global cognitive impairment.

Cognitive performance following treatment of depression

For those patients with depression who do experience objective cognitive impairment, an important question is what to expect with regard to their cognition following treatment for depression. Can these patients expect to experience an improvement in their cognitive symptoms following amelioration of depressive symptoms? Recent research is attempting to answer this question and this line of study hopes to provide greater insight into the prognosis for these patients.

Longitudinal follow-up of patients with depression has found that a remission in depression was associated with an increase in verbal memory performance [23]. For patients with a diagnosis of major depressive disorder who are undergoing active treatment, pharmacological treatment of depression may be effective in improving cognitive performance. A study conducted by Herrera-Guzman and colleagues compared patients with major depressive disorder and comorbid major depressive disorder and anxiety disorder on neurocognitive measures before and after pharmacological treatment for depression [24]. While there were no differences between the groups on neurocognitive measures at baseline, after 24 weeks of pharmacological treatment both groups showed improvements in depression and on tasks of attention, memory, and executive functioning. Interestingly, the patients without a comorbid anxiety disorder showed the greatest neurocognitive benefit.

Similarly, elderly patients with depression and white matter hyperintensities on brain neuroimaging performed worse than controls on neuropsychological testing during their acute depression [17]. After a 6-month remission of depressive symptoms following a treatment with antidepressants, these patients improved on all cognitive tests, with the exception of verbal memory and verbal fluency tests. Although cognitive benefit was achieved in this sample of elderly patients with depression, it was unclear why they were left with residual cognitive deficit, as this was not accounted for magnetic resonance imaging (MRI) hyperintensities or other vascular risk factors assessed. In a more recent study involving patients with depression and hyperintensities on brain MRI, baseline processing speed, executive functioning, language, and episodic memory predicted remitters from non-remitters following a 12-week treatment for depression [25].

Despite these few promising studies pointing to cognitive improvement following treatment of depression, such encouraging outcome may not be the case for all patients. For example, elderly patients with a frontal lobe syndrome or executive dysfunction [26], extrapyramidal signs, and/or specific brain lesions (i.e., in basal ganglia and the pontine reticular formation) show a poorer response to antidepressant treatment [27]. Cognitive changes in patients with depression who underwent deep brain stimulation (DBS) for treatment of depression were correlated with improvements in mood [28]. Further research is needed to determine what type of treatment for depression is likely to be effective at improving cognition for which type of patient.

The neuropsychological evaluation

A neuropsychological evaluation involves an assessment of the cognitive, social, and emotional functioning of individuals through a clinical interview and testing procedure. Typically someone is referred for a neuropsychological evaluation in response to a specific question, often related to a neurologic or psychiatric disorder. Referral questions can include diagnostic/screening, identification of treatment needs, evaluation of treatment efficacy, research, and forensic [10]. Neuropsychological evaluations can be completed in a variety of settings, such as medical centers, clinics, or private practices, and depending on the need may be completed at the bedside or in a testing room. Regardless of the specific referral question or setting, a thorough psychological assessment, which includes depression, is an important aspect of the neuropsychological evaluation.

Given the independent contribution of various neurologic disorders on cognition, providing an accurate assessment of cognitive ability in patients with these conditions and comorbid depression is challenging. Despite the challenges, determining the cause of cognitive impairment in patients with neurologic disorders has important implications for disease course, prognosis, treatment recommendations, and expectations for both the patient and the patient's family. A neuropsychological assessment is uniquely equipped to answer this question through the use of instruments sensitive to brain dysfunction and the experience of a neuropsychologist trained to evaluate brain–behavior relationships.

Patients with neurologic disorders might be referred for a neuropsychological evaluation to assess for cognitive problems or as part of a comprehensive workup with other neurodiagnostic techniques, such as neuroimaging or electrophysiological techniques. Current views of the value of neuropsychological assessments include the goal to understand the contribution of behavioral, cognitive, and psychosocial components on brain function.

The neuropsychological evaluation has several important contributions to the evaluation of patients with neurologic disorders in particular. First, as it is presented elsewhere in this text, there is a high comorbidity of depression in neurologic illness. As a result, the assessment of depression is becoming a standard of practice in neuropsychology for patients presenting with neurologic disorders. Clinicians may find it difficult to determine the relationship between depression and neurologic disorders in their patients. A neuropsychological evaluation can be useful in determining the nature of the relationship between neurologic illness and depression as they relate to a patient's level of functioning.

Second, cognitive problems are a cause for great concern among patients, their family members, and/or the physicians treating the patients. Cognitive complaints are common among individuals with neurologic disorders, but they are also common among individuals with depression. A neuropsychological evaluation can not only provide an evaluation of a patient's level of cognitive functioning, but it can also be useful in determining the contribution of depressive symptoms and neurologic problems on the cognitive level.

Finally, a neuropsychological evaluation contributes to patient care in its ability to provide information regarding the course of a diagnosed condition and inform treatment recommendations. Through a neuropsychological evaluation, a neuropsychologist can help determine a patient's level of cognitive, psychological, social, and adaptive functioning. Based on these findings, the neuropsychologist can often provide specific recommendations for psychological, psychiatric, and/or cognitive interventions.

Given the importance of assessing depression and mood problems in patients referred for neuropsychological evaluation, the clinician is confronted with the choice of how to do this. Three methods can be used.

The first consists to simply *observe*. No matter what a patient might say, or how they might respond on a test, there is no substitute for a clinician paying attention to a patient's affective presentation. While this chapter is not necessarily the place for an exhaustive review of what to look for to determine if a patient is depressed (or manic, psychotic, etc.), it is surprising that in our "modern age," behavioral observation from an attending clinician may take a back seat to the observations of junior colleagues or test results because of other demands on the time of those who seemingly would be in the best position to detect the presence of a behavioral disturbance. It is clear though that there really can be no substitute for an experienced clinician to spend the necessary amount of time with a patient to observe their level of energy, facial characteristics, motoric responses, and other mannerisms.

The second manner is to *ask*. It is not unusual for there to be a striking discrepancy between how a patient "looks" and what they say in interview or on testing regarding their mood and psychological health. It is more typical for a patient to appear to be depressed but to deny related symptoms, but it is not unusual for the converse. That is, some patients "look fine," but upon inquiry readily admit to not feeling so. Some patients might even merit a diagnosis of anosognosia, given their seeming inability to recognize and describe their mood problems. Careful and sensitive prodding of these disparities might reveal a total unawareness of how the patient appears to others and these findings might be ascribed to neurologic (sometimes localized to the right frontal lobe) dysfunction. In other cases, the patient admits to a masking or covering up of their true emotional state as it is important for them to look strong or unimpaired to family members and others that they are close to. Other patients simply don't want to admit to the existence of feelings of depression because of the possible stigma attached to such issues, or even because they fear that such disclosure would likely be followed by further inquiries or "digging around" from the clinician. This can be an overwhelming and frightening prospect for many patients.

The authors have had the experience of sharing with some patients, initially thought to be having epileptic seizures, that their presentation was more consistent with a diagnosis of psychogenic nonepileptic seizure disorder. While this often is presented to the patient as "Good news, the results indicate that you do not have brain damage!" some patients instead become angry and agitatedly hostile at such diagnostic impressions. One patient replied, "I'd rather be told that I have a brain tumor than be told these seizures have something to do with the sexual abuse I endured as a child. I don't want to deal with that and I think your results are wrong." While this may be an extreme example of the disconnect between appearance and self-report, it does serve as a reminder of the importance of the clinician conducting a verbal interview of the patient. Asking questions such as current and recent mood, sleep patterns, past/current suicidal ideation and attempts, crying, sex drive, and activity, all are vital components of the neuropsychological evaluation and should not be exclusively relegated to junior colleagues or behavioral observation. It is only in the asking of these questions, and the interplay between experienced clinician and complicated patient, that one can begin to understand the presence and significance of changes in and problems with mood.

The third arrow in the neuropsychologist's quill of mood investigation tools is that of *personality testing*. It is the availability of such a tool that might differentiate the neuropsychologist from that of other health-care providers. There is no evidence that psychologists are any better (or worse) than neurologists, psychiatrists, social workers, family members, and others in observing or asking about a patient having signs or symptoms of depression, but psychologists typically are better informed than others in both administering/interpreting psychometric instruments and in integrating these results with a patient's history and other findings. This, in part, at times may be due to the psychologist having been specifically educated about the reliability and validity of various tests, including those of cognition and depression, and in better understanding both their potential benefits and limitations.

Assessment

Psychological tests measuring depression can be delineated into at least two categories: projective and objective testing. Projective tests are those in which a patient is asked to respond to an ambiguous stimulus or stimuli. It is assumed that a patient will "project" important psychological issues in their responses, and that some of this is "unconscious" and typically not manifest otherwise. That is, the patient's response to inkblots and other ambiguous stimuli will reveal conflicts, psychological problems and issues, and personality traits not necessarily obvious or known either to the patient or the clinician. The Rorschach inkblot test, Thematic Apperception Test, and the Incomplete Sentences tests are three of the more commonly used projective instruments. While these tests have a long history in psychological assessment and can generate a rich set of hypotheses about a patient's behavior, their utility is limited by problems with their reliability and validity [29]. Despite the availability of scoring systems developed by Exner [30], it remains that the interrater reliability and construct validity of these instruments typically are not sufficiently high enough as to generate confidence. It has been further argued that projective tests may reveal more about the interpreter's (psychologist's) problems and "issues" than that of the patient. Some of this may be due to problems with the instruments themselves, but also to the fact that training in projective techniques is often given short shrift or may be an afterthought in contemporary graduate school programs. The

utility of these instruments in the hands of a well-trained and experienced psychologist logically would be much greater in comparison to that of someone who was barely taught how to administer and interpret projectives, but it seems that relatively few students in recent decades claim sufficient training in such techniques as to recommend their use in assessing depression in patients with neurologic disorders.

The second category of neuropsychological/psychological tests that might be used to assess the presence and severity of depression are termed objective. Characteristics of objective testing include clearly standardized and described instructions, manner of scoring, and guidelines on interpretation. The questions and answers often are more transparent or straightforward. A patient is asked to say "true" or "false" or "yes" or "no" to a series of questions regarding their mood, experiences, beliefs, and feelings. In contrast to a projective test such as the Rorschach inkblot test, where the patient's mood may be judged on the degree to which they responded to the color, form, or shading perceived in the stimuli, objective testing, such as on the Minnesota Multiphasic Personality Inventory-2 (MMPI-2) or the Beck Depression Inventory (BDI), simply tallies the number of times a patient endorses items such as "I feel depressed" or "I have marked difficulty in sleeping at night."

Objective personality testing has the advantage in that any test protocol administered should result in the same exact score regardless of who scored the test. The BDI simply requires that the clinician add up the value of items endorsed by the patient. The MMPI-2 typically is computer scored. The clinician enters the patient's responses to up to 567 true or false items. A computer program then calculates the resulting T-scores for a variety of clinical and validity scales. Any two people who can accurately enter the correct keystrokes will obtain the same MMPI-2 profiles. In contrast, even highly experienced clinicians who score the Rorschach are likely to obtain different scores given the inherent subjectivity of this test.

It is beyond the scope of this chapter to describe, and review the respective strengths or limitations of the MMPI-2 , BDI, Geriatric Depression Scale (GDS), and other objective measures of personality and/or mood. The interested reader can read a description and review in the fourth edition of Lezak [10]. The MMPI-2 is useful if other measures of psychopathology (including measures of anxiety, somatization, disturbed thinking, etc) are desired, but of course it may take a patient 60 minutes to complete this test. In contrast, other measures such as the BDI or GDS can be finished in 5 or 10 minutes as they focus just on depressive symptoms.

Administration of psychological tests, whether projective or objective, can be an important addition to an assessment. It quantifies the raw number of symptoms endorsed, and this raw score can often be transformed into a standardized (such as T- or percentile) score. Either the raw or transformed score offers the clinician and the patient the advantage of measuring the severity or extent of a patient's problems, and goes beyond the subjective impressions already garnered by the clinician. The availability of a standardized score allows one to objectively compare a patient's condition against other patients, or even against the patient themselves should repeat testing be done to measure the efficacy of treatment or if the patient otherwise seems to have changed across time.

Despite the possible advantages of having psychometric testing, it must always be remembered that "a test score is not a diagnosis." It can be too easy for the intellectually and clinically disengaged practitioner to let a test score substitute for a comprehensive evaluation. An MMPI-2 T-score of 73 or a BDI-II score of 24 may or may not tell a clinician what they need to know about a patient's functioning. Instead, test scores should "only" be used as a means of generating hypotheses about patients. A high BDI-II score may indeed reflect a certain number of depressive symptoms, but without proper observation and interview it may be impossible to make sense of such a score and what it implies for diagnosis and treatment.

Case studies

Case study 1: A neurologic disorder presenting as a major depressive episode

Neuropsychology was consulted to see a 51-year-old white male who was admitted as an inpatient to treat obsessional thoughts and symptoms of depression. He originally was left-handed but was forced in school to become a right-hander. This patient had been treated for the past 4 years by psychiatry because of a "nervous breakdown" that first occurred when he was 47. Up until that time, the patient reportedly had been in good physical and psychological health. He had grown up in a "normal" family with a childhood that he described as being happy and free of any type of abuse or neglect. He was a skilled draftsmen who earned a bachelor's degree who went on to a very successful career as a self-employed person specializing in services to engineering and tool and die firms as he was noted to have unusually good design skills. He denied any problems while in school, typically earning Bs and Cs in many classes, while earning straight As in those related to science, art, and drafting. At the time of evaluation he had been happily married for nearly 40 years and had two adult children.

The patient became "obsessed" for the first time in his life 4 years prior to this admission and neuropsychological evaluation. His daughter was arrested for repeated shoplifting at age 25, that had until then been unknown to the patient. The daughter was able to enter a diversionary program through the court system, and happily by all reports (from the husband and his wife) had successfully completed this. Her arrest was reportedly stricken from her record and she had been clean and sober since this incident 4 years ago, and had gone on to marry and have a baby, and was pregnant with her second child at the time of this evaluation, all while working as a highly paid commodities broker.

The patient described a second "obsession" that dated to about the time of his daughter's arrest. He had invested a large portion of his life savings in a speculative real estate venture on the advice of a friend from his church. Unfortunately, by the patient's report, this investment was nearly lost in a Ponzi-style scheme that was later publicized. While many others reportedly lost all of their investment, the patient reportedly was able to recoup over 90% of his original investment as he had been "paid out" relatively early in the process. The patient readily admitted that the money he had lost was relatively inconsequential and in no way interfered with his financial security and outlook.

The patient readily admitted that both incidents (his daughter's arrest and drug problem and his nearly failed and lost investment) turned out well in the end. His daughter went on to a happy and successful life, and the patient and his wife still enjoyed a comfortable and financially secure lifestyle. Despite this, the patient admitted to being "stuck" in his worries and reminiscences of these events. He described sitting hours on end at home, rocking back and forth or pacing, as he recounted "the horrors" of how both incidents could have turned out far worse. He would readily agree with his wife and others that things had turned out nicely and that nobody had been hurt or compromised in the long run. However, he couldn't "turn off" these negative thoughts. He gave up his consulting practice and went into an early retirement. He gave up his scratch game of golf (he had been club champion for his age range), and became very reluctant to socialize or even leave his bedroom at home without a lot of prompting from his wife.

This patient was referred to a psychiatrist 3 years prior to this admission and neuropsychological evaluation, at which time he was diagnosed with major depressive disorder. He was treated with a variety of selective serotonin reuptake inhibitor (SSRI) medications, none of which seemed to stop his perseverations about these two incidents. His day-to-day functioning fluctuated somewhat and at times he reportedly was "more like his old self" in terms of spending time with friends or golfing, but these brief remissions invariably led to him again being socially isolated and progressively more perseverative and obsessional about past incidents. He never reported suicidal thinking but his increasingly reclusive lifestyle eventually led to two other psychiatric hospitalizations, both of which included electroconvulsive treatments (ECT). The first of these treatments (about 18 months prior to the current admission and neuropsychological evaluation) reportedly led to some improvement in functioning, including a reduction in observed perseverative behavior, but these improvements evaporated in the following weeks. A second hospitalization and ECT course (about 8 months prior to this admission) did not result in any

changes in observed behavior other than the patient seemed confused for days afterward, with him returning to baseline in a week or two.

The patient and his wife were not aware of his having any cognitive problems or changes. She described him as being a life-long "worrier," but had never seen the perseverations/obsessions currently evident. He did not have any history of substance abuse and did not have any psychiatric history prior to 4 years ago. His medical history was minimal and noncontributory to his current problems.

Neuropsychology's first contact with the patient was that of viewing him in his inpatient room from outside the nearly closed room door. He could be observed sitting on the edge of his bed, saying "No, no, why, why?" He stopped this immediately upon our knocking on the door, and came over to make an appropriate greeting, and then saying he had just been thinking about his daughter's arrest and his real estate investment. The patient was slightly disheveled but otherwise appropriate in interview. He was able to recount his recent and remote history and seemed both straightforward and accurate in doing so.

The patient was estimated to have been in the high average, or better, range of cognitive function prior to his psychiatric problems 4 years ago, given his education, occupation, and predicted "premorbid" IQ of 111 (77th percentile) from the Wechsler Test of Adult Reading (WTAR). However, current cognitive testing showed him to generally be performing below this expected level. One exception was that of well-preserved Visuospatial/Constructional skills (Repeatable Battery for the Assessment of Neuropsychological Status [RBANS] index score = 116; 86th percentile). He was particularly impaired on a measure of executive functioning. On the Wisconsin Card Sorting Test, testing was discontinued after 64 cards (one deck) as he had achieved only one category at that time, and was becoming frustrated when told that most of his answers were not correct as he tried increasingly nonsensical ways of finding solutions for this task. Other assessed skills were not as impaired, but still below expectation. He did poorly in taking in or manipulating newly presented information (RBANS Immediate Memory and Attention indices were about the 15th percentile each). While he learned relatively little information on immediate recall tests, he did relatively well in holding on to this material after a delay (over 90% of initially learned material was retained after a delay). Language skills generally were intact and judged to be commensurate with premorbid abilities, although some word finding problems were noted in conversation. MMPI-2 results were valid, but 4 of the 10 clinical scales were significantly elevated (scales 2, 3, 7, and 8). This is consistent with a person endorsing many symptoms of depression and anxiety.

Given that neuropsychological test results were suggestive of executive functioning, attentional and/or "frontal system" deficits, imaging tests were ordered. MRI of the brain at the time of the neuropsychological evaluation was read as "greater than age-appropriate cerebral volume loss and chronic microvascular changes." Nuclear medicine produced a single-photon emission computed tomography (SPECT) report which read: "Compared to the temporal lobes, there is moderately decreased perfusion of both frontal lobes and slightly decreased perfusion of parietal lobes."

In conclusion, this patient was diagnosed with and treated exclusively as a person with depression for 4 years until he underwent recent neuropsychological and imaging studies. These all suggested cortical dysfunction, particularly for the bilateral frontal lobes. The patient's behavior can also be interpreted as "frontal" given the frequent and disabling perseverations noted in recent years. The degree to which this patient's "depression" is separate from, or either a cause of or effect of "brain damage" is arguable. It might be most useful to again invoke the bidirectional hypothesis in conceptualizing this patient's late-onset obsessions being a brain-related problem that causes, and in turn is worsened by, depression. The patient's diagnosis was later amended to include "frontal lobe disorder," along with depression. The take-home point for this is to encourage clinicians to remember the often inextricable link between depression and cognitive deficits, particularly those of executive functioning. Knowing which came first or which is worst, the depression or the brain damage, is often impossible, but in knowing that both are factors can lead to more effective treatments and to a better handling of the problems by both the patient's family and health-care providers.

Case study 2: Dysthymia presenting as a neurologic disorder

A 46-year-old Hispanic, right-handed woman was referred for neuropsychological evaluation as she felt that problems related to her seizure disorder and subsequent resective surgery were interfering with her ability to find new employment. The patient had undergone resection of the left temporal lobe 10 years ago and had been seizure free ever since. Postoperative testing done a year after her surgery (9 years ago) actually showed greatly improved scores in a number of areas of cognition, including learning and memory for both verbally and visually presented stimuli. The patient had a high school and trade school/electronic education, and had been employed before and after surgery as an electronics technician for a small manufacturing firm, but had been laid off a year prior to this evaluation. She recounted that, because of her seniority at that firm, she had been paid about 20% higher than those doing similar work, and that her employer for some time had been on a campaign to find a way to fire her. They came up with "nitpicky" criticisms of her job performance and finally terminated her. While she disagreed with this outcome, of course, she felt like she didn't have the energy to fight back and had resigned herself to find another job. However, she felt that her (resolved) epilepsy and related surgery had left her with cognitive deficits that would make it difficult for her to learn new skills, and so wanted this evaluation to determine the extent to which this was the case.

The patient did not have any health problems and had not undergone MRI scanning in some time given the stability of her new condition. MRI from years ago, before and after her surgery, had indicated left mesial temporal sclerosis before surgery, and the effects of a craniotomy and surgery afterwards.

Current neuropsychological test results included a prediction that "premorbid" intellectual functioning had been in the average range (WTAR predicted Full Scale IQ = 95). Most of her current scores were consistent with this expectation. Verbal abilities were an exception, however, in that she achieved a Wechsler Adult Intelligence Scale (WAIS)-III Verbal Comprehension score of 76 (fifth percentile). This was interpreted as being due both to the effects of her having had a left temporal lobe focus, and that she was raised in a bilingual household (although she now spoke English almost exclusively). Her other current cognitive test scores were within normal limits, and at expectation. Her verbal memory scores were in the low average range (between 15th and 20th percentile) and a relative weakness when compared to her scoring in the average range on measures of visual memory (about the 50th percentile), but her verbal memory was judged to be intact overall and quite similar to what was seen 9 years ago at the previous postoperative neuropsychological evaluation. In fact, all of her current cognitive test scores were similar to the most recent testing, including very good scores on measures of nonverbal ability (WAIS-III Perceptual Organization index is 114; 82nd percentile). She also did very well on measures of executive functioning (Wisconsin Card Sorting is six categories achieved; five perseverative errors was at the 68th percentile).

What had changed across time for this patient was her report of depression and psychiatric distress. While she endorsed symptoms of depression and anxiety during all three of her neuropsychological exams, the current breadth and depth of endorsement had greatly expanded. While her current MMPI-2 results were judged to be valid, she still obtained significant elevations on 6 of the 10 clinical scales (2-7-4-3-5-8), with scales 2 and 7 having a T-score of about 85. This indicates she endorsed more symptoms of depression and anxiety than did 99.9% of the females in the standardization sample. Further interview with the patient revealed the story behind this patient, who in interview did not really "look" to be depressed as she was dressed and groomed attractively and had a bright and pleasant manner. Instead, she indicated that she had largely become housebound in the months following her job termination, which also occurred about the same time that a long-term relationship with her partner had come to an end. Her current diet consisted of "whatever is laying around and doesn't need to be cooked" and her house had become "a dirty mess." She

spent most of her time laying on the couch, watching television or being on the Internet, or "whatever doesn't take any effort." She avoided physical activity, but with the encouragement of her therapist had taken a 4-hour-a-week job in an office to get out of the house. She had completely lost her libido, had not gone on a date since breaking up with her partner, and had no interest in looking for another date. She denied any active suicidal ideation but admitted to at times having wished that a tree limb would fall on her or an oncoming car would swerve into her as "what's the point of this?" She had entered into a contract with her therapist to not attempt to hurt herself, and recently had at least begun to visit her sister episodically as she had not otherwise had any contact with friends or family for some months.

Concluding remarks

This chapter has reviewed how neuropsychological deficits are common both among patients with brain damage and patients who are depressed. It is more useful in many cases to attempt to determine which portion of a patient's cognitive deficits are due to cerebral dysfunction and what portion is due to depression, and less useful to simply attempt to say that it is just one factor or the other. It is also important to remember that there is often a bidirectional relationship between depression and neurologic illness. Neuropsychological testing can be an important tool in measuring the degree to which a patient's cognition is impaired, why it is impaired, and what might be done to restore the patient to a higher level of function.

💡 **PEARLS TO TAKE HOME**

- Individuals with depression are more likely to experience cognitive impairment, particularly executive dysfunction.
- In patients with neurologic illness and depression, the degree of cognitive impairment is impacted by the duration of the neurologic disorder and its course and severity.
- Patients with neurologic illness and depression can display objective and subjective cognitive problems, but not necessarily both.

- There is the potential for cognitive improvement following treatment for depression for some patients with depression and neurologic illness.
- For these complex patients, determination of cognitive level, the severity of their cognitive impairments, and need for intervention are important.
- A neuropsychological evaluation is used to determine a patient's level of cognitive, psychological, social, and adaptive functioning, which can assist in providing specific recommendations for psychological, psychiatric, and/or cognitive interventions.
- Case studies provide a valuable source for understanding the complexities of patients presenting with neurologic illness, depression, and cognitive impairment.

References

1. Schmitz N, Wang J, Malla N, et al. Joint effect of depression and chronic conditions on disability: results from a population-based study. *Psychosomatic Medicine*, 69: 332–338, 2007.
2. Channon S. Executive dysfunction in depression. *Journal of Affective Disorders*, 39: 107–114, 1996.
3. Landro NI, Stiles TC, Sletvold H. Neuropsychological function in nonpsychotic unipolar major depression. *Neuropsychiatry, Neuropsychology, and Behavioral Neurology*, 14: 233–240, 2001.
4. Veiel HOF. A preliminary profile of neuropsychological deficits associated with major depression. *Journal of Clinical and Experimental Neuropsychology*, 19: 587–603, 1997.
5. Goodwin GM. Neuropsychological and neuroimaging evidence for the involvement of the frontal lobes in depression. *Journal of Psychopharmacology*, 11: 115–122, 1997.
6. Levin RL, Heller W, Mohanty A, et al. Cognitive deficits in depression and functional specificity of regional brain activity. *Cognitive Therapy Research*, 31: 211–233, 2007.
7. Hartlage S, Alloy LB, Vazquez C, et al. Automatic and effortful processing in depression. *Psychological Bulletin*, 113: 247–278, 1993.
8. Elliot R. The neuropsychological profile in unipolar depression. *Trends in Cognitive Sciences*, 2: 447–454, 1998.
9. Walter H, Wolf RC, Spitzer M, et al. Increased left prefrontal activation in patients with unipolar depression: an event-related, parametric, performance controlled fMRI study. *Journal of Affective Disorders*, 101: 175–185, 2007.
10. Howieson DB, Loring DW, Hannay HJ. Neurobehavioral variables and diagnostic issues. In: *Neuropsychological Assessment*, eds. MD Lezak, DB Howieson, DW Loring. New York: Oxford University Press, pp. 286–336, 2004.
11. Austin MP, Mitchell P, Wilhelm K, et al. Cognitive function in depression: a distinct pattern of frontal impairment in melancholia? *Psychological Medicine*, 29: 73–85, 1999.
12. Porter RJ, Bourke C, Gallagher P. Neuropsychological impairment in major depression: its nature, origin and clinical significance. *Australian and New Zealand Journal of Psychiatry*, 41: 115–128, 2007.
13. Burt T, Prudic J, Peyser S, et al. Learning and memory in bipolar and unipolar major depression: effects of aging. *Neuropsychiatry, Neuropsychology, and Behavioral Neurology*, 13: 246–253, 2000.
14. Grant M, Thase M, Sweeney J. Cognitive disturbance in outpatient depressed younger adults: evidence of modest impairment. *Biological Psychiatry*, 50: 35–43, 2001.
15. Lampe I, Sitskoorn M, Heeren T. Effects of recurrent major depressive disorder on behavior and cognitive function in female depressed patients. *Psychiatry Research*, 125: 73–79, 2004.
16. Neu P, Kiesslinger U, Schlattmann P, et al. Time-related cognitive deficiency in four different types of depression. *Psychiatry Research*, 103: 237–247, 2001.
17. Neu P, Bajbouj M, Schilling A, et al. Cognitive function over the treatment course of depression in middle-aged patients: correlation with brain MRI signal hyperintensities.

Journal of Psychiatric Research, 39: 129–135, 2005.

18. Reischies F, Neu P. Comorbidity of mild cognitive disorder and depression-a neuropsychological analysis. *European Archives of Psychiatry and Clinical Neuroscience*, 4: 186–193, 2000.

19. Trichard C, Martinot J, Alagille M, et al. Time course of prefrontal lobe dysfunction in severely depressed inpatients: a longitudinal neuropsychological study. *Psychological Medicine*, 25: 79–85, 1995.

20. Verdoux H, Liraud F. Neuropsychological function in subjects with psychotic and affective disorders. Relationship to diagnostic category and duration of illness. *European Psychiatry*, 15: 236–243, 2000.

21. Fischer C, Schweizer TA, Atkins JH, et al. Neurocognitive profiles in older adults with and without major depression. *International Journal of Geriatric Psychiatry*, 23: 851–856, 2008.

22. Rohling ML, Green P, Allen LM, et al. Depressive symptoms and neurocognitive test scores in patients passing symptom validity tests. *Archives of Clinical Neuropsychology*, 17: 205–222, 2002.

23. Biringer E, Mykletun A, Sundet K, et al. A longitudinal analysis of neurocognitive function in unipolar depression. *Journal of Clinical and Experimental Neuropsychology*, 29: 879–891, 2007.

24. Herrera-Guzman I, Gudayol-Ferre E, Jarne-Esparcia A, et al. Comorbidity of anxiety disorders in major depressive disorder. A clinical trial to evaluate neuropsychological deficit. *European Journal of Psychiatry*, 23: 5–18, 2009.

25. Beblo T, Baumann B, Bogerts B, et al. Neuropsychological correlates of major depression: a short-term follow-up. *Cognitive Neuropsychiatry*, 4: 333–341, 1999.

26. Kalayam B, Alexopoulos GS. Prefrontal dysfunction and treatment response in geriatric depression. *Archives of General Psychiatry*, 56: 713–718, 1999.

27. Simpson S, Baldwin RC, Jackson A, et al. Is subcortical disease associated with a poor response to antidepressants? Neurological, neuropsychological neuroradiological findings in late-life depression. *Psychological Medicine*, 28: 1015–1026, 1998.

28. McNeely HE, Mayberg HS, Lozano AM, et al. Neuropsychological impact of Cg25 deep brain stimulation for treatment-resistant depression. *The Journal of Nervous and Mental Disease*, 196: 405–410, 2008.

29. Lilienfeld SO, Wood JM, Garb HN. The scientific status of projective techniques. *Psychological Science in the Public Interest*, 1: 27–66, 2000.

30. Exner JE. *The Rorschach: Basic Foundations and Principles of Interpretation*, Vol. 1. Hoboken, NJ: John Wiley and Sons, 2002.

Depressive Disorders in Children and Adolescents with Neurologic Disorders

Rochelle Caplan
Department of Psychiatry, David Geffen School of Medicine, UCLA Semel
Institute for Neuroscience and Human Behavior, Los Angeles, CA, USA

Introduction

This chapter provides neurologists with a bird's eye view of the clinical importance, neurobiological aspects, clinical manifestations, diagnostic instruments, neuropsychological findings, and basic management principles of depression and anxiety disorders in children and adolescents with neurologic disorders. The chapter concludes with a case study that illustrates clinical management from diagnosis through treatment of a child with epilepsy referred for depression. This review is limited to the following neurologic disorders: epilepsy, traumatic brain injury (TBI), multiple sclerosis, brain tumor, and neurofibromatosis.

Clinical importance: why should neurologists care?

The Isle of Wight study [1] was the first epidemiological study to demonstrate that psychiatric diagnoses are significantly more prevalent in children with central nervous system (CNS) disorders than in those with chronic medical illness, who, in turn, have significantly higher rates than children in the general population. Since this important study, epidemiological studies over the past two decades have replicated these findings and demonstrated prevalent mood and/or emotional difficulties in pediatric chronic illness,

particularly in neurologic disorders such as epilepsy [2] and TBI [3].

These findings have important clinical and theoretical implications for neurologists treating children with these disorders. From the clinical perspective, the presence of behavioral and emotional problems rather than the severity of the neurologic illness is related to the quality of life of children with epilepsy [4] and neurofibromatosis [5] as well as to depression in the parents of children with epilepsy [6] and pediatric chronic illness [7]. In fact, extensive research on the psychosocial impact of pediatric epilepsy [8] has shown that risk factors for depression in children with this disorder include poor maternal mental health and depression, parental stress level, impaired family functioning (an indirect measure of parental psychopathology), parent perception of epilepsy-related stigma, and limited financial resources. Clinicians' awareness of the bidirectional relationship between child and parent depression and the associated poor coping [9, 10] could facilitate early psychiatric referral of children with neurologic disorders who may be at risk for depression.

In terms of patient management, children with depression and anxiety disorders may be more prone to the adverse behavioral/emotional effects of medications used to treat the primary neurologic disorders such as antiepileptic drugs

Depression in Neurologic Disorders: Diagnosis and Management, First Edition.
Edited by Andres M. Kanner.
© 2012 Blackwell Publishing Ltd. Published 2012 by Blackwell Publishing Ltd.

(AEDs), particularly levetiracetam, topiramate, phenobarbitol, or mysoline [11, 12]; benzodiazepines [13]; steroids [14]; interferon [15]; and baclofen [16]. Since these patients may also be at risk for treatment-induced increased suicidality [17], early identification and treatment of depression and anxiety disorders is essential.

Regarding the outcome of neurologic disorders, follow-up of children and adolescents with epilepsy [18–20], TBI [3, 21, 22], brain tumor [23], and multiple sclerosis [16] reveals evidence of poor educational, vocational, social, and emotional/behavioral outcomes during adulthood. The poor outcomes of these CNS disorders are associated with depression in pediatric epilepsy [18, 19], fatigue in multiple sclerosis [24], poor social skills in neurofibromatosis [25], and learning difficulties in TBI [3], rather than with the severity of neurologic symptoms. Of note, in adolescents without a neurologic disorder, untreated depression is related to adult depression in 75.2% of subjects [26], completed suicide in 2.45%, and suicide attempts in 44.5% [27], particularly in adolescents who also had conduct problems.

From the theoretical perspective, impaired stress response in depression [28], seizures [29], multiple sclerosis [30], and TBI [31] may contribute to exacerbation of symptoms in these disorders. Moreover, as described in the section "Neurobiological aspects," recent clinical, neuroimaging, and animal model results indicate that depression and anxiety disorders are comorbidities of neurologic illnesses such as epilepsy, TBI, and multiple sclerosis, rather than psychosocial responses to the disorder. As such, accurate diagnosis and treatment of all aspects of these disorders, including psychiatric aspects, is warranted.

In summary, the prevalence of mood and anxiety disorders and their role in the quality of life of children with neurologic disorders and their parents, associated risk for adverse behavioral responses to treatment of the primary neurologic disorder, and poor long-term outcomes highlight the clinical importance of early detection of psychiatric components such as depression and anxiety disorder diagnoses in pediatric neurologic disorders. The Decade of the Brain has provided evidence that these emotional problems are integral aspects of pediatric neurologic disorders.

Neurobiological aspects

Epilepsy

Although depression and anxiety disorders are found in 23% and 36%, respectively, of children and adolescents with recent onset epilepsy [32] and in 16% and 33%, respectively, of those with chronic epilepsy [33, 34], large sample studies of children have not demonstrated an association with seizure variables [35]. A history of depression prior to the first seizure in subjects with new-onset epilepsy [32] provides additional evidence that depression in these children does not reflect the effects of ongoing seizures.

Volumetric abnormalities in the limbic system and its frontal connections are found in children with CNS disorders who have depression and anxiety disorders. Thus, increased left amygdala volume in children with complex partial seizures with depression and anxiety disorder diagnoses [36], together with volumetric [37] and functional magnetic resonance abnormalities [38] in youth without epilepsy with these psychiatric diagnoses, underscore the role of the amygdala in mood regulation. Similarly, decreased hippocampal volume in children with complex partial seizures with depression and anxiety disorders [39] has also been demonstrated in children and adolescents without epilepsy who are at genetic risk for these psychiatric diagnoses [40]. Suicidal ideation is also related to decreased white matter volume of the orbital frontal gyrus in children with epilepsy [41].

These neuroimaging findings, which demonstrate amygdala, hippocampal, and orbital frontal gyrus involvement in the mood and anxiety disorders of children with epilepsy, are particularly important given the role of these brain regions in the evolution and spread of seizures as well as the response to stress [42]. Kindling of immature rats through subconvulsant electric stimulation of the ventral hippocampus increases seizure susceptibility of the hippocampus as well as animal behaviors considered equivalent to depression, such as immobility in the forced swim test and the loss of taste preference toward calorie-free saccharin [43].

Furthermore, evidence from animal models of neonatal seizures highlight alterations in developmental programs, with decreases in neurogenesis, sprouting of mossy fibers, and long-standing changes in signaling properties that also involve the hippocampus [44]. Neonatal seizures also cause abnormal development of gamma-aminobutyric acid (GABA), glutamate, and serotonin [45], which play an important role in depression [46] and anxiety disorders [47, 48]. Clearly, depression and anxiety disorders, as well as suicidal ideation, are related to structural abnormalities in the limbic system and frontal lobe rather than to seizure variables in children with epilepsy. Similarly, young animals with seizures have structural involvement of these regions, "depressed" and "anxious" behavior, and abnormal development of neurotransmitters involved in mood disorders.

Traumatic brain injury

In contrast to pediatric epilepsy, research on the comorbidities of pediatric TBI has focused primarily on attention deficit hyperactivity disorder (ADHD) [49], irritability and aggression [50], and emotional problems [51], while focusing less on depression [52], mood and anxiety disorders [31], obsessive–compulsive disorder [53], and post-traumatic stress disorder (PTSD) [54]. The majority of studies of children with TBI with mood and anxiety diagnoses were conducted on children with severe or moderate head trauma. Unlike epilepsy, the severity of head trauma is associated with post-TBI depression in children [31, 52, 54]. Little is known, however, about depression and anxiety disorders in children who experience mild head trauma.

Although children with anxiety disorders (i.e., overanxious, obsessive–compulsive, separation, and simple phobia) before head injury are more likely to have these diagnoses after TBI [55], there is also *de novo* development of depression [31], anxiety [50], and obsessive–compulsive disorder [53] following TBI. Some studies describe multiple mood and anxiety disorder diagnoses in such children [53].

Neuroimaging studies of a large number of children who sustained severe TBI have shown that PTSD is associated with temporal lobe damage. However, increased orbital frontal cortex volume and more lesions in this brain region reduced the likelihood of anxiety and PTSD [55]. Unrelated to severity of injury, temporal lobe and mesial prefrontal lesions were found in children with new post-TBI onset of obsessive–compulsive disorder [53]. Of note, structural abnormalities are found in these brain regions in children without TBI who are diagnosed with these disorders [56, 57]. In terms of white matter abnormalities, increased fractional anisotropy, decreased apparent diffusion coefficient, and radial diffusivity in adolescents shortly following mild TBI are related to postconcussion symptoms of emotional distress (depression, anxiety, irritability) thought to reflect postinjury edema [58].

In summary, severe TBI is related to depression and anxiety disorders in children with and without these diagnoses before the head injury and may reflect involvement of specific brain regions. Information is lacking on the emotional sequelae of mild head injury.

Brain tumors

Social withdrawal, depressive symptoms, anxiety, and somatic complaints are described in earlier studies of children with CNS tumors and of children treated with CNS radiation and chemotherapy for pediatric cancer [23]. However, there is no increased rate of depression in children with brain tumors treated in oncology centers compared to the general child population [59, 60]. Yet, consistent high social withdrawal and somatic complaints based on Child Behavior Checklist (CBCL) responses [61] completed by parents of children with brain tumors [59, 62, 63] are thought to underlie the higher CBCL internalizing and depression/anxiety scores found in these earlier studies [59, 62]. High scores on the Children's Depression Inventory (CDI) [64] also appear to be related to poor social skills, lower self-worth, and decreased IQ in children with brain tumors [59].

The relationship between CNS involvement and poor social skills is further highlighted by three sources of evidence. First, peer report of pediatric cancer survivors without brain tumors but treated with cranial radiation therapy and/or intrathecal chemotherapy indicates poorer peer acceptance, fewer friendships, greater social sensitivity isolation, and diminished leadership popularity compared with patients treated with systemic methotrexate [65]. Second, compared with healthy siblings, adult childhood cancer survivors demonstrate poor social functioning and physical health [66] as well as increased depression and suicidal ideation [66, 67]. Third, a Danish epidemiological follow-up study revealed higher rates of psychiatric hospitalization than in the general population for pediatric cancer survivors (mean 14.3 years follow-up after diagnosis), particularly in patients who had brain tumors [68]. The psychiatric diagnoses of these patients included psychosis and diagnoses other than affective disorders.

Thus, inconsistent findings on depression and anxiety disorders in children with brain tumors and cancer treatment involving the CNS are thought to reflect misinterpretation of poor social skills. However, adult survivors of pediatric cancer with treatment involving the CNS or primary brain tumors are more likely to be depressed and socially withdrawn.

Multiple sclerosis

Weisbrot et al. [16] reviewed the factors associated with depression and anxiety diagnoses in approximately 50% of youth with multiple sclerosis. These factors include the combined effects of severity of illness, associated cognitive deficits, adverse behavioral effects of medications used to treat the disorder (e.g., steroids, interferons, and baclofen), and fears related to the disability involved in the illness. However, the relationship of depression and anxiety comorbidities with neuroimaging structural and functional abnormalities is yet to be determined in juvenile multiple sclerosis.

Neurofibromatosis

Earlier studies reported depression (emotional difficulties) in children with neurofibromatosis [69], which is similar to the results of pediatric chronic illness research [25]. Recent methodologically refined studies that include control groups and use child self-report instruments describe social difficulties (e.g., peer rejection, social isolation) [25, 70] but not depression in children with neurofibromatosis and other chronic pediatric illnesses compared with healthy control subjects. The social difficulties of these

patients are associated with severity of their neurologic illness, learning problems, and ADHD (inattentive type). As mentioned above, earlier parent reports of internalizing emotional problems were derived from clinical CBCL T-scores for social withdrawal, which, in turn, probably reflect the social difficulties these children experience [25].

In summary, children with neurofibromatosis with social difficulties, learning problems, and inattentive ADHD may appear to be depressed.

Neurobiological aspects: conclusions

Knowledge of the similarities and differences in the neurobiological underpinnings of depression and anxiety disorders in pediatric neurologic disorders further emphasizes why neurologists should screen all children with these disorders for psychiatric comorbidities. In pediatric epilepsy, depression and anxiety disorders reflect the cellular, neurotransmitter, and microstructural volumetric, morphometric, and functional neurobiological underpinnings of epilepsy involving the limbic system and frontal connections. In contrast, as found in adults with TBI and multiple sclerosis [71, 72], the association of illness severity with depression in children with these disorders suggests effects of the extent of involved brain regions, particularly the limbic system and its frontal connections, together with the child's emotional response to the severity of symptoms and functional limitations (e.g., cognition, language, and social skills). In children with brain tumors, CNS treatment of pediatric cancer, and neurofibromatosis, studies are warranted to delineate the mechanisms underlying the apparent predilection for poor social skills during childhood and for depression during adulthood.

Clinical manifestations

This section focuses on general developmental and clinical guidelines for diagnosing depression, anxiety disorders, and suicidality in children and adolescents, the importance of differentiating symptoms of these comorbidities from the underlying neurologic disorder and its treatment, and the need to inquire about fears of death and dying.

Developmental guidelines

From the developmental perspective, pediatric depression and anxiety disorders differ from the adult and adolescent disorders in terms of clinical manifestations and children's awareness of and ability to spontaneously inform adults about their symptoms. In addition, children lack the verbal skills to describe their complaints and often do not understand the abstract language physicians use when asking about symptoms of these disorders. This is particularly relevant in CNS disorders associated with cognitive and linguistic deficits, such as epilepsy, TBI, multiple sclerosis, brain tumor, and neurofibromatosis.

In contrast to depressed adolescents and adults, depressed children do not appear sad, slowed down, without motivation, or unable to enjoy things (i.e., anhedonic). Similarly, anxious children do not seem to be worried, scared, tense, or nervous. Therefore, parents are often unaware that their children are experiencing symptoms of depression and anxiety disorders. The most common manifestations of depression and anxiety in children include irritable, oppositional, angry, aggressive, or avoidant behavior [73]. In addition, sleep problems (e.g., avoidance behavior at bedtime) may reflect the insomnia of depression, separation fears in children with separation anxiety disorder, fear of recurrent trauma-related nightmares following TBI, and fear of dying. Thus, parents often inform physicians of the "bad" rather than the "sad," "worried," or "scared" behavior of children, such as acting out or sleep refusal.

Separation fears or lack of motivation found in depression may lead to behavioral difficulties in the morning, exacerbation of symptoms of the neurologic disorder, and school refusal. Anxious and depressed children frequently report abdominal pain and headaches and avoid going to school [74]. Children may also evade homework because of difficulties concentrating due to poor quality of sleep, negative or repetitive thoughts and worries of the underlying depression or anxiety disorder, and impairments related to their neurologic disorder. In these cases, parents sometimes think their children are lazy and need a firmer hand. If teachers complain that the child is not paying attention in class, parents may tell the physician that the child has ADHD.

Confounding symptoms

Given the high rate of ADHD in children with epilepsy [75–77], TBI [49], and neurofibromatosis [78], and the familiarity of physicians with this comorbidity, it is essential to rule out the possibility of depression and anxiety disorders when parents present ADHD-like complaints about their children. Furthermore, symptoms of the underlying disorder and related treatment may mimic depression and anxiety disorder symptoms. High doses of AEDs and AED polytherapy can slow children down and make them apathetic, listless, unmotivated, and uninterested in their environment. Specific AEDs, including phenobarbital, mysoline, levetiracetam, and topiramate can trigger depression in children [79]. Benzodiazepines, felbamate, and gabapentin can increase agitation and aggression [79]. Management of multiple sclerosis with steroids and interferon can also induce depression [16].

Response to illness and/or adverse effects: death and dying

Children with the neurologic disorders described in this chapter often harbor fears of brain damage, death, deformity, and loss of skills. Often, they do not share these fears with their parents for two reasons: they do not want to burden their parents and they are scared that if they verbalize their fear of death, it might happen. Since these fears can potentiate anxiety, depression, and suicidal ideation, it is important that clinicians ask children about them without the parents present.

Although more frequent in adolescents, suicidality is found in children with depression [80] and anxiety disorders [81] who do not have neurologic disorders. Recent Food and Drug Administration (FDA) warnings about possible suicidality in patients treated with AEDs [82] and evidence for this association in patients on steroids [83] further underscore the need to screen all children with these disorders for depression and anxiety disorders. In summary, the clinical presentation of depression and anxiety disorders in children differs from that of adolescents and adults, and parents may report "bad" rather than "sad," "scared," or "worried" behavior. Symptoms related to the primary neurologic disorder or its treatment can contribute to these behaviors. It is essential to inquire about the child's concerns about death, disability, and suicidal ideation.

Diagnostic instruments

Comprehensive psychiatric evaluation of children with a primary neurologic disorder involves a detailed history obtained from the parent and the child. This should include information about the child's neurologic disorder, behavior, emotions, learning, relationships within the family and with peers, and any changes in these factors since the onset of illness and treatment. Structured psychiatric interviews, administered separately to the child or adolescent and his or her parent(s), are the gold standard for assessing *Diagnostic and Statistical Manual of Mental Disorders*, Fourth Edition (DSM-IV) diagnoses of depression and anxiety disorders in youth. Examples of these instruments are the Schedule for Affective Disorders and Schizophrenia for School-Age Children—Present and Lifetime Version (K-SADS-PL) [84] and the Diagnostic Interview Schedule for Children (DISC) [85], as well as interviews focused on depression, such as the Children's Depression Rating Scale–Revised (CDRS-R) [86], and on anxiety, such as the Anxiety Disorder Interview Schedule [87]. A parent-based questionnaire, the Child Symptom Inventory (CSI) [88], also yields DSM-IV diagnoses.

Although self-report instruments provide reliable and valid information on symptoms of depression and anxiety that are highly correlated with DSM-IV diagnoses, they are not diagnostic instruments. Frequently used self-report instruments include the CDI [64], the Multidimensional Anxiety Scale for Children (MASC) [89], and Screen for Child Anxiety Related Emotional Disorders (SCARED) [90]. Parent-based CBCL [61] and the CBCL Youth Self-Report (YSR) [91] provide a depression/anxiety *T*-score.

As previously mentioned, parents are often unaware of symptoms of depression and anxiety disorders in their children. Since depression and anxiety disorder symptoms in adolescents are more similar to those of adults, observant parents are reliable sources of this information. However, parents who have past or current diagnoses of these disorders may overrate or underrate the presence and severity of their child's symptoms.

Further, some adolescents, especially boys, under-report their symptoms [92].

For detailed clinical guidelines on how to interview young children to ascertain key diagnostic criteria of pediatric psychiatric disorders, including depression and anxiety disorders, see Kanner et al. [93]. Table 7.1 presents examples of questions clinicians can ask young children while doing the neurologic examination to screen for depression. Of note, anhedonia, weight loss, and fatigue are rare in children with depression.

Table 7.2 includes screening questions for more common anxiety disorders. Parents are sometimes a better source of information on their children's compulsions because children are embarrassed to talk about them. Treating physicians will need to modify the PTSD questions presented in Table 7.2 based on their knowledge of the TBI or traumatic medical procedures experienced by children with brain tumors or multiple sclerosis or those treated for pediatric cancer involving the CNS.

Knowledge about the neurologic and psychosocial risk factors for depression and anxiety disorders can help clinicians identify which patients with neurologic disorders should be screened for these psychiatric comorbidities. The previous section ("Neurobiological aspects") described the risk factors associated with the primary neurologic disorders. Youth without neurologic disorders are at risk for depression if they are adolescents, female, have a family history of depression, lower socioeconomic status, stressful life events, school failure, or history of depression or separation anxiety disorder during early childhood [94]. Children and adolescents with a family history of an anxiety disorder or early separation anxiety disorder are vulnerable for anxiety disorders [95].

The following are red flags for youth at risk for suicidal acts: adolescence, available guns, family history of mood disorder or suicide, past attempts, male gender, impulse control disorders, substance abuse, family problems, stressful life events, and school failure [80]. Predictors of suicidal ideation in youth are somewhat different and include childhood mood disorder, female gender, family history of mood disorder or suicide, lower socioeconomic status, family problems, romantic breakup, and school failure [96].

Table 7.1 Depression screening questions and examples for young children

Symptom	Questions
Mood	Are you happy, sad, or in between?
Sad	What makes you sad (cry)? Are you ever sad and don't know what is making you sad?
Irritable	What makes you angry? Are you ever mad and don't know at what? Do lots of things bug you?
Insomnia	Is it easy or difficult to fall asleep (stay asleep)?
Suicidality	Have you ever tried to kill yourself?
Thoughts	Do you have thoughts of wanting to die?
Plans	How would you do it?
Worthlessness	What don't you like about yourself?
Guilt	Do you feel bad if you do something wrong? If someone else gets into trouble, do you feel it might have been your fault?
Concentration	Is it easy or difficult for you to pay attention? In what subjects?
Anhedonia	What do you do for fun? Is it still fun now that you have. . . . (CNS disorder)?
Appetite/weight loss	Do you like to eat? Are your clothes getting small or too big?
Fatigue	When you want to do fun stuff, do you get tired easily?

Thus, structured psychiatric interviews are the gold standard for diagnosing depression and anxiety disorders in children. However, reliable and valid self-report questionnaires together with information on risk factors enable clinicians to screen children with neurologic disorders for these psychiatric comorbidities.

Neuropsychological findings

Although depressed adults without neurologic disorders have deficits in executive function and memory as well as psychomotor slowing [97], similar studies have not been conducted in depressed youth. However, depressed youth and children with anxiety disorders, like their adult counterparts, have cognitive biases that include dysfunctional attitudes, negative coping styles, and ruminations [98] as well as attention focused on danger [99].

As previously described, the neuropsychological deficits of children with TBI are related to ADHD [49, 52] but not to depression and anxiety disorders [31]. In children with brain tumor [59] and epilepsy [33], low IQ is associated with depression and anxiety disorders. In terms of cognitive style, negative attitude and external locus of control [34, 100] are found in youth with epilepsy with depression, particularly adolescent girls. However, similar studies have not been conducted on children with depression and anxiety disorders who have other neurologic disorders. In summary, other than low IQ in pediatric brain tumor and epilepsy and some cognitive distortions in depressed adolescent girls with epilepsy, there are limited neuropsychological data on depression and anxiety disorders associated with pediatric neurologic disorders.

Management

Psychoeducation about the possible association of the primary neurologic disorder with depression or anxiety is the first essential management step. This information helps parents and children understand that identification of the psychiatric, cognitive, and social comorbidities of the CNS disorder will optimize how they deal with the underlying neurologic disorder and its outcome.

To confirm the psychiatric diagnosis, referral to a child psychiatrist or clinical psychologist, preferably with expertise in pediatric chronic medical

Table 7.2 Anxiety disorder screening questions and examples for young children

Disorder and Symptoms	Questions
Generalized anxiety disorder	
Worry/apprehension	Do you think about things that are going to happen like tests (homework, projects, what friends think about you, what you say?
Uncontrolled	Do these thoughts keep on coming back into your head?
Irritability	Is it easy or difficult to make you angry?
Sleep disturbance	Is it easy or difficult to fall asleep (stay asleep)?
Separation anxiety disorder	When you are not with your parents:
Worry	Are you scared something bad might happen to them or to you?
Distress	Do you think about that a lot or does it make you cry?
Refusal	Are you scared to go to school because something bad might happen to you or to your parents?
Nightmares	Do you dream about not being with your parents?
Physical complaints	When you are not with your parents, do any parts of your body hurt?
Phobias	Fear + avoidance
Social	Is it easy or difficult for you to be with kids you do not know or just know a little?
Agoraphobia	When you go to places with lots of people like the mall, do you feel OK (comfortable)? So do you not go to the mall?
Specific	What things are you scared of? Do you stay away from them?
Obsessive–compulsive disorder	
Obsessions: thoughts, images, impulses	Do thoughts or pictures come in your head that you do not want to think about? That even if you don't want to think about the? What do you do to stop those thoughts?
Compulsions: Behaviors, mental acts	Do you feel you have to do things again and again that you cannot stop? For example, washing your hands, jumping over cracks, counting things, checking food for germs, and so on?
PTSD	
Traumatic event	Did something scary (car accident, someone being hit hard or in a bad fight, fire, someone touching private parts) happen to you or did you see that happen to someone else?
Recurrent recollections	Do you think about that again and again?
Recurrent nightmares	Do you have dreams about that?
Physiological reactivity	Do you scare easily, like jump when there is a big noise or shout?

and/or CNS illness, is optimal but not always feasible. Evaluation of how the child and family deal with the illness and the child's related learning and/or social deficits help the clinician decide which individual and family interventions are required. More specifically, this evaluation provides information on illness-related stress in the family, such as fears for the child's future, divisive parenting approaches, sibling rivalry, increased economic burden, or illness-related stigma. These stressors, in turn, can trigger the child's behavioral and emotional symptoms.

Neuropsychological testing is warranted for each case given the previously described role of cognitive deficits and related social difficulties in the depression and anxiety of children with neurologic disorders. Without addressing the underlying neuropsychological deficits, symptomatic psychopharmacological treatment of depression and anxiety will not improve the child's condition. In fact, sedative adverse effects of psychophotropic drugs in a child with illness-related poor concentration and fatigue may further compromise the child's already slowed and/or impaired cognitive functioning. The resulting impact on the child's self-esteem could worsen the depression and anxiety symptoms. Neuropsychological testing is also required to ensure the patient's appropriate school and class placement.

To date, other than one open uncontrolled drug study in children with epilepsy using sertraline or fluoxetine [101] and one randomized study of cognitive–behavior therapy (CBT) versus treatment as usual in youth with epilepsy and subthreshold depression [102], there have been no double–blind, randomized controlled treatment studies of children with neurologic disorders with depression and anxiety disorders. This section briefly describes treatment of pediatric depression and anxiety disorders in youth without neurologic disorders. Detailed reviews can be found on adolescent depression [103], anxiety disorders [104], obsessive–compulsive disorder [105], and PTSD [106]. Of note, all treatment studies conducted in children with these disorders have excluded children with neurologic disorders.

In terms of pharmacotherapy, selective serotonin reuptake inhibitors (SSRIs) are first-line drugs used to treat depression in childhood and adolescents and include fluoxetine (Prozac, Eli Lilly, Indianapolis, IN), sertraline (Zoloft, Pfizer, New York), paroxetine (Paxil, GlaxoSmithKline, Middlesex, UK), fluvoxamine (Luvox, Forest Laboratories, New York), citalopram (Celexa, Jazz Pharmaceuticals, Palo Alto, CA), and escitalopram (Lexapro, Forest Laboratories). Second-line drugs are mixed receptor agents or selective serotonin norepinephrine reuptake inhibitors (SSNRIs), such as venlafaxine hydrochloride (Effexor, Pfizer), mirtazapine (Remeron, Organon, Oss, The Netherlands), and duloxetine hydrochloride (Cymbalta, Eli Lilly). There is recent evidence for the efficacy of venlafaxine in adolescents with treatment-resistant depression [107]. Whereas these drugs are effective in adolescent depression, only fluoxetine has a significant treatment effect in children older than age 8 [108]. Although approved for use by the FDA, a black box warning issued in 2004 warned of a possible twofold increase in suicidal ideation and behavior in the first months of treatment [109].

The FDA provided treatment guidelines to monitor suicidality in children and adolescents treated with such drugs. These include weekly visits documenting the child's mood, sleep, activation, suicidality, adverse effects, and treatment response for the first month of treatment, followed by bimonthly visits for the next 2 months. Nevertheless, there has been a significant decrease in diagnoses of depression and prescription of these drugs in youth with depression together with a marked increase in suicidality [110–112].

In contrast to their use for depression, SSRIs are effective and suicidality does not appear to be an adverse effect for treatment of pediatric anxiety disorders [113]. The FDA approved fluoxetine for obsessive–compulsive disorder in children older than age 7, sertraline in those older than age 6, and fluvoxamine in those older than age 8 [114].

Regarding psychotherapy, CBT is effective for both depression [115] and anxiety disorders [104] in children and adolescents. Combined CBT and medication therapy appears to be superior for treatment-resistant adolescent depression [103] and pediatric anxiety disorders [113]. CBT focused on increasing competence (addresses poor self-esteem), child psychoeducation (normalizes effects of depression and anxiety), self-monitoring (increases awareness of sensitivity, cognitive distortions), relationship skills (improves social skills), communication training (helps verbalize feelings and difficulties), cognitive restructuring (corrects cognitive distortions), problem solving (counteracts passivity and avoidant behavior), and behavioral activation (helps to engage in activities that are enjoyable) is most effective in children with depression [116]. Added components in anxiety disorders include exposure to the source of anxiety [95]. Thus, management of children with neurologic disorders with depression and anxiety disorders includes psychoeducation of the child and family, comprehensive psychiatric evaluation and neuropsychological testing with school/class recommendations, choice of treatment modality for the child or adolescent (medication, CBT, or both), and family therapy.

Case study: depression in a child with epilepsy

A 10-year-old boy with difficult to control seizures presented with crying during class, refusal to go to school, and lack of interest in and motivation for things he previously enjoyed. On examination, the child appeared dull and apathetic and had great difficulty responding to questions. He would begin to answer, drift off, and lose all interest in the conversation. It was also difficult to engage him in conversation, and he initiated no conversation. When asked what he and the examiner were talking about, he began to cry. The mental exam was stopped since the child appeared zoned out. His mother reported that he would cry when told to do homework and when he had to go to school.

Based on adult criteria of depression, this child appeared to be depressed. However, the following questions needed to be answered prior to making this diagnosis:

- Why did he drift off during conversation?
- Why was he dull and lifeless?
- Why did he start to cry when the examiner tried to continue the conversation?
- Could these behaviors be adverse effects of medication, ongoing seizures, or both?

Videotelemetry demonstrated that the child was actually experiencing ongoing seizures. His "depressed" mood, lack of motivation and interest, and poor conversation skills improved following a change of his AEDs and the resulting seizure control.

Six months later, the child was seen again because of anger, irritability, failure to do his homework, refusal to go to school, and excessive tiredness when he needed to do homework. A mental status examination revealed that the child was sad and felt that he was stupid and that nothing would get better for him. He also thought it would be better if he were dead, but had no plans of trying to kill himself. He was angry with his mother and teachers for making him do homework and go to school. Although he had lost his temper with his mother and sisters, he was not aggressive at school.

He acknowledged difficulties with concentration that occurred mainly during language-based subjects (e.g., reading, writing, comprehension). At night, when he could not sleep he would think about how stupid he was and that his epilepsy had "messed up" his brain. He was also scared that he might die during a seizure. His appetite was poor and he had lost weight since the last visit. The child demonstrated no evidence of anxiety disorders or psychosis. His seizures continued to be well controlled.

The patient met criteria for depression and underwent neuropsychological testing. His test results confirmed significant learning difficulties with deficits primarily in language, and a recommendation was made for placement in a special education class. Due to his marked language difficulties, he was treated with sertraline rather than with CBT. Follow-up assessment revealed significant improvement in his depression and motivation for school.

Conclusion: take home message

Children with CNS disorders should be evaluated early in the course of their disorder to determine if they have depression and anxiety disorders. Early initiation of treatment and, when indicated, educational intervention, will improve the long-term outcome for these children.

References

1. Rutter M, Graham P, Yule W. *A Neuropsychiatric Study in Childhood*. London: S.I.M.P./William Heineman Medical Books Ltd, 1970.
2. Davies S, Heyman I, Goodman R. A population survey of mental health problems in children with epilepsy. *Dev Med Child Neurol*, 45: 292–295, 2003.
3. Hawley C, Ward AB, Magnay AR, Long J. Children's brain injury: a postal follow-up of 525 children from one health region in the UK. *Brain Inj*, 16: 969–985, 2002.
4. Sherman E, Slick DJ, Connolly MB, Eyrl KL. Neurological correlates and health-related quality of life in severe pediatric epilepsy. *Epilepsia*, 48: 1083–1091, 2007.
5. Krab LC, Oostenbrink R, de Goede-Bolder A, Aarsen FK, Elgersma Y, Moll HA. Health-related quality of life in children with neurofibromatosis type 1: contribution of demographic factors, disease-related factors, and behavior. *J Pediatr*, 154: 420–425, 2009.
6. Shore C, Austin J, Dunn D. Maternal adaptation to a child's epilepsy. *Epilepsy Behav*, 5: 557–568, 2004.
7. Wagner JL, Chaney JM, Hommel KA, Page MC, Mullins LL, White MM, Jarvis JN. The influence of parental distress on child depressive symptoms in juvenile rheumatic diseases: the moderating effect of illness intrusiveness. *J Pediatr Psychol*, 28: 453–462, 2003.
8. Austin K, Caplan R. Behavioral and psychiatric comorbidities in pediatric epilepsy: toward an integrative model. *Epilepsia*, 48: 1639–1651, 2007.
9. Austin J, Dunn DW, Johnson CS, Perkins SM. Behavioral issues involving children and adolescents with epilepsy and the impact of their families: recent research data. *Epilepsy Behav*, 5: S33–S41, 2004.
10. Hodes M, Garralda ME, Rose G, Schwartz R. Maternal expressed emotion and adjustment in children with epilepsy. *J Child Psychol Psychiatry*, 40: 1083–1093, 1999.
11. Brent D, Crumrine P, Varma R, Allan M, Allman C. Phenobarbital treatment and major depressive disorder in children with epilepsy. *Pediatrics*, 80: 909–917, 1987.
12. Mula M, Trimble MR, Sander JW. Are psychiatric adverse events of antiepileptic drugs a unique entity? A study on topiramate and levetiracetam. *Epilepsia*, 48: 2322–2326, 2007.

13. Ketter TA, Post RM, Theodore WH. Positive and negative psychiatric effects of antiepileptic drugs in patients with seizure disorders. *Neurology*, 53: S53–S67, 1999.

14. Stuart F, Segal TY, Keady S. Adverse psychological effects of corticosteroids in children and adolescents. *Arch Dis Child*, 90: 500–506, 2005.

15. Raison CL, Demetrashvili M, Capuron L, Miller AH. Neuropsychiatric adverse effects of interferon-[alpha]: recognition and management. *CNS Drugs*, 19: 105–123, 2005.

16. Weisbrot DM, Ettinger AB, Gadow KD, Belman AL, MacAllister WS, Milazzo M, Reed ML, Serrano D, Krupp LB. Psychiatric comorbidity in pediatric patients with demyelinating disorders. *J Child Neurol*, 25: 192–202, 2010.

17. Shneker B, Cios J, Elliott J. Suicidality, depression screening, and antiepileptic drugs: reaction to the FDA alert. *Neurology*, 72: 987–991, 2009.

18. Camfield C, Camfield PR. Juvenile myoclonic epilepsy 25 years after seizure onset: a population-based study. *Neurology*, 73: 1041–1045, 2009.

19. Wirrell EC, Camfield CS, Camfield PR, Dooley JM, Gordon KE, Smith B. Long-term psychosocial outcome in typical absence epilepsy. Sometimes a wolf in sheep's clothing. *Arch Pediatr Adolesc Med*, 151: 152–158, 1997.

20. Sillanpaa M, Jalava M, Kaleva O, Shinnar S. Long-term prognosis of seizures with onset in childhood. *N Engl J Med*, 338: 1715–1722, 1998.

21. Muscara F, Catroppa C, Eren S, Anderson V. The impact of injury severity on long-term social outcome following paediatric traumatic brain injury. *Neuropsychol Rehabil*, 19: 541–561, 2009.

22. Catroppa C, Anderson VA, Muscara F, Morse SA, Haritou F, Rosenfeld JV, Heinrich LM. Educational skills: long-term outcome and predictors following paediatric traumatic brain injury. *Neuropsychol Rehabil*, 19: 716–732, 2009.

23. Zeltzer LK, Recklitis C, Buchbinder D, Zebrack B, Casillas J, Tsao JCI, Lu Q, Krull K. Psychological status in childhood cancer survivors: a report from the childhood cancer survivor study. *J Clin Oncol*, 27: 2396–2404, 2009.

24. Goretti B, Ghezzi A, Portaccio E, Lori S, Zipoli V, Razzolini L, Moiola L, Falautano M, De Caro MF, Viterbo R, Patti F, Vecchio R, Pozzilli C, Bianchi V, Roscio M, Comi G, Trojano M, Amato MP. Psychosocial issue in children and adolescents with multiple sclerosis. *Neurol Sci*, 31: 467–470, 2010.

25. Noll R, Reiter-Purtill J, Moore BD, Schorry EK, Lovell AM, Vannatta K, Gerhardt CA. Social, emotional, and behavioral functioning of children with NF1. *Am J Med Genet A*, 143: 2261–2273, 2007.

26. Fombonne E, Wostear G, Cooper V, Harrington R, Rutter M. The Maudsley long-term follow-up of child and adolescent depression. 1. Psychiatric outcomes in adulthood. *Br J Psychiatry*, 179: 210–217, 2001.

27. Fombonne E, Wostear G, Cooper V, Harrington R, Rutter M. The Maudsley long-term follow-up of child and adolescent depression: 2. Suicidality, criminality and social dysfunction in adulthood. *Br J Psychiatry*, 179: 218–223, 2001.

28. Gatt JM, Nemeroff CB, Dobson-Stone C, Paul RH, Bryant RA, Schofield PR, Gordon E, Kemp AH, Williams LM. Interactions between BDNF Val66Met polymorphism and early life stress predict brain and arousal pathways to syndromal depression and anxiety. *Mol Psychiatry*, 14: 681–695, 2009.

29. Taher TR, Salzberg M, Morris MJ, Rees S, O'Brien TJ. Chronic low-dose corticosterone supplementation enhances acquired epileptogenesis in the rat amygdala kindling model of TLE. *Neuropsychopharmacology*, 30: 1610–1616, 2005.

30. Liu XJ, Ye HX, Li WP, Dai R, Chen D, Jin M. Relationship between psychosocial factors and onset of multiple sclerosis. *Eur Neurol*, 62: 130–136, 2009.

31. Luis C, Mittenberg W. Mood and anxiety disorders following pediatric traumatic brain injury: a prospective study. *J Clin Exp Neuropsychol*, 24: 270–279, 2004.

32. Jones J, Watson R, Sheth R, Caplan R, Koehn M, Seidenberg M, Hermann B. Psychiatric

comorbidity in children with new onset epilepsy. *Dev Med Child Neurol*, 49: 493–497, 2007.

33. Caplan R, Siddarth P, Gurbani S, Hanson R, Sankar R, Shields WD. Depression and anxiety disorders in pediatric epilepsy. *Epilepsia*, 46: 720–730, 2005.

34. Dunn D, Austin J, Huster G. Symptoms of depression in adolescents with epilepsy. *J Am Acad Child Adolesc Psychiatry*, 38: 1132–1138, 1999.

35. Caplan R. Pediatric epilepsy: a developmental neuropsychiatric disorder. International Review of Neurobiology. In: *Epilepsy: Scientific Foundation of Clinical Management*, eds. J Rho, R Sankar, J Cavazos. New York: Marcel Dekker, Inc, 2010.

36. Daley M, Siddarth P, Levitt J, Gurbani S, Shields WD, Sankar R, Toga A, Caplan R. Amygdala volume and psychopathology in childhood complex partial seizures. *Epilepsy Behav*, 13: 212–217, 2008.

37. Milham M, Nugent AC, Drevets WC, Dickstein DP, Leibenluft E, Ernst M, Charney D, Pine DS. Selective reduction in amygdala volume in pediatric anxiety disorders: a voxel-based morphometry investigation. *Biol Psychiatry*, 57: 961–966, 2005.

38. Brotman MA, Rich BA, Guyer AE, Lunsford JR, Horsey SE, Reising MM, Thomas LA, Fromm SJ, Towbin K, Pine DS, Leibenluft E. Amygdala activation during emotion processing of neutral faces in children with severe mood dysregulation versus ADHD or bipolar disorder. *Am J Psychiatry*, 167: 61–69, 2010.

39. Daley M, Ott D, Siddarth P, Gurbani G, Caplan R. Hippocampal volume in childhood complex partial seizures and absence epilepsy. In: Annual Meeting of the American Epilepsy Society, Washington, 2005.

40. Chen MC, Hamilton JP, Gotlib IH. Decreased hippocampal volume in healthy girls at risk of depression. *Arch Gen Psychiatry*, 67: 270–276, 2010.

41. Caplan R, Siddarth P, Levitt J, Gurbani S, Shields WD, Sankar R. Suicidality and brain volumes in pediatric epilepsy. *Epilepsy Behav*, 18: 286–290, 2010.

42. Koe AS, Jones NC, Salzberg MR. Early life stress as an influence on limbic epilepsy: an

hypothesis whose time has come? *Front Behav Neurosci*, 3: 24, 2009.

43. Mazarati A, Shin D, Auvin S, Caplan R, Sankar R. Kindling epileptogenesis in immature rats leads to persistent depressive behavior. *Epilepsy Behav*, 10: 377–383, 2007.

44. Holmes GL. The long-term effects of neonatal seizures. *Clin Perinatol*, 36: 901–914, 2009.

45. Stafstrom CE. Neurobiological mechanisms of developmental epilepsy: translating experimental findings into clinical application. *Semin Pediatr Neurol*, 14: 164–172, 2007.

46. Kalia M. Neurobiological basis of depression: an update. *Metabolism*, 54: 24–27, 2005.

47. Nikolaus S, Antke C, Beu M, Müller HW. Cortical GABA, striatal dopamine and midbrain serotonin as the key players in compulsive and anxiety disorders—results from *in vivo* imaging studies. *Rev Neurosci*, 21: 119–139, 2010.

48. Krystal J, Mathew SJ, D'Souza DC, Garakani A, Gunduz-Bruce H, Charney DS. Potential psychiatric applications of metabotropic glutamate receptor agonists and antagonists. *CNS Drugs*, 24: 669–693, 2010.

49. Levin H, Hanten G, Max J, Li X, Swank P, Ewing-Cobbs L, Dennis M, Menefee DS, Schachar R. Symptoms of attention-deficit/hyperactivity disorder following traumatic brain injury in children. *J Dev Behav Pediatr*, 28: 108–118, 2007.

50. Cole W, Gerring JP, Gray RM, Vasa RA, Salorio CF, Grados M, Christensen JR, Slomine BS. Prevalence of aggressive behaviour after severe paediatric traumatic brain injury. *Brain*, 22: 932–939, 2008.

51. Hawley C, Ward AB, Magnay AR, Long J. Outcomes following childhood head injury: a population study. *J Neurol Neurosurg Psychiatry*, 75: 737–742, 2004.

52. Bloom DR, Levin HS, Ewing-Cobbs L, Saunders AE, Song J, Fletcher JM, Kowatch RA. Lifetime and novel psychiatric disorders after pediatric traumatic brain injury. *J Am Acad Child Adolesc Psychiatry*, 40: 572–579, 2001.

53. Grados M, Vasa RA, Riddle MA, Slomine BJ, Salorio C, Christensen J, Gerring J. New

onset obsessive-compulsive symptoms in children and adolescents with severe traumatic brain injury. *Depress Anxiety*, 25: 398–407, 2008.

54. Levi R, Drotar D, Yeates KO, Taylor HG. Posttraumatic stress symptoms in children following orthopedic or traumatic brain injury. *J Clin Child Psychol*, 28: 232–243, 1999.

55. Vasa R, Gerring JP, Grados M, Slomine B, Christensen JR, Rising W, Denckla MB, Riddle MA. Anxiety after severe pediatric closed head injury. *J Am Acad Child Adolesc Psychiatry*, 41: 148–156, 2002.

56. MacMaster F, Vora A, Easter P, Rix C, Rosenberg D. Orbital frontal cortex in treatment-naive pediatric obsessive-compulsive disorder. *Psychiatry Res*, 181: 97–100, 2010.

57. Carrion VG, Weems CF, Watson C, Eliez S, Menon V, Reiss AL. Converging evidence for abnormalities of the prefrontal cortex and evaluation of midsagittal structures in pediatric posttraumatic stress disorder: an MRI study. *Psychiatry Res*, 172: 226–234, 2009.

58. Wilde EA, McCauley SR, Hunter JV, Bigler ED, Chu Z, Wang ZJ, Hanten GR, Troyanskaya M, Yallampalli R, Li X, Chia J, Levin HS. Diffusion tensor imaging of acute mild traumatic brain injury in adolescents. *Neurology*, 70(12): 948–955, 2008.

59. Barrera M, Schulte F, Spiegler B. Factors influencing depressive symptoms of children treated for a brain tumor. *J Psychosoc Oncol*, 26: 1–16, 2008.

60. Noll RB, Kupst MJ. Commentary: the psychological impact of pediatric cancer hardiness, the exception or the rule? *J Pediatr Psychol*, 32: 1089–1098, 2007.

61. Achenbach T. *Manual for the Child Behavior Checklist and Revised Child Behavior Profile.* Burlington, VT: Department of Psychiatry, University of Vermont, 1991.

62. Papazoglou A, King TZ, Morris RD, Krawiecki N. Parent report of attention problems predicts later adaptive functioning in children with brain tumors. *Child Neuropsychol*, 15: 40–52, 2009.

63. Schultz KAP, Ness KK, Whitton J, Recklitis C, Zebrack B, Robison LL, Zeltzer L, Mertens AC. Behavioral and social outcomes in adolescent survivors of childhood cancer: a report from the childhood cancer survivor study. *J Clin Oncol*, 25: 3649–3656, 2007.

64. Kovacs M. The Children's Depression Inventory (CDI). *Psychopharmacol Bull*, 21: 995–998, 1985.

65. Vannatta K, Gerhardt CA, Wells RJ, Noll RB. Intensity of CNS treatment for pediatric cancer: prediction of social outcomes in survivors. *Pediatr Blood Cancer*, 49: 716–722, 2007.

66. Zebrack BJ, Gurney JG, Oeffinger K, Whitton J, Packer RJ, Mertens A, Turk N, Castleberry R, Dreyer Z, Robison LL, Zeltzer LK. Psychological outcomes in long-term survivors of childhood brain cancer: a report from the childhood cancer survivor study. *J Clin Oncol*, 22: 999–1006, 2004.

67. Recklitis CJ, Diller LR, Li X, Najita J, Robison LL, Zeltzer L. Suicide ideation in adult survivors of childhood cancer: a report from the childhood cancer survivor study. *J Clin Oncol*, 28: 655–661, 2010.

68. Ross L, Johansen C, Dalton SO, Mellemkjaer L, Thomassen LH, Mortensen PB, Olsen JH. Psychiatric hospitalizations among survivors of cancer in childhood or adolescence. *N Engl J Med*, 349: 650–657, 2003.

69. Johnson H, Wiggs L, Stores G, Huson SM. Psychological disturbance and sleep disorders in children with neurofibromatosis type 1. *Dev Med Child Neurol*, 47: 237–242, 2005.

70. Barton B, North K. Social skills of children with neurofibromatosis type 1. *Dev Med Child Neurol*, 46: 553–563, 2004.

71. Jorge R, Robinson RG, Moser D, Tateno A, Crespo-Facorro B, Arndt S. Major depression following traumatic brain injury. *Arch Gen Psychiatry*, 61: 42–50, 2004.

72. Sicotte N, Kern KC, Giesser BS, Arshanapalli A, Schultz A, Montag M, Wang H, Bookheimer SY. Regional hippocampal atrophy in multiple sclerosis. *Brain*, 131: 1134–1141, 2008.

73. Garland EJ, Garland OM. Correlation between anxiety and oppositionality in a children's mood and anxiety disorder clinic. *Can J Psychiatry*, 46: 953–958, 2001.

74. Feldman J, Ortega AN, Koinis-Mitchell D, Kuo AA, Canino G. Child and family psychi-

atric and psychological factors associated with child physical health problems: results from the Boricua youth study. *J Nerv Ment Dis*, 198: 272–279, 2010.

75. Caplan R, Siddarth P, Gurbani S, Ott D, Sankar R, Shields WD. Psychopathology In pediatric complex partial seizure: seizure-related, cognitive, and linguistic variables. *Epilepsia*, 45: 1273–1281, 2004.

76. Caplan R, Siddarth P, Stahl L, Lanphier E, Vona P, Gurbani S, Koh S, Sankar R, Shields WD. Childhood absence epilepsy: behavioral, cognitive, and linguistic comorbidities. *Epilepsia*, 49: 1838–1846, 2008.

77. Dunn D, Austin J, Harezlak J, Ambrosius W. ADHD and epilepsy in childhood. *Dev Med Child Neurol*, 45: 50–54, 2003.

78. Hyman S, Arthur E, North KN. Learning disabilities in children with neurofibromatosis type 1: subtypes, cognitive profile, and attention-deficit- hyperactivity disorder. *Devl Med Child Neurol*, 48: 973–977, 2006.

79. Austin J, Caplan R. Behavioral and psychiatric comorbidities in pediatric epilepsy: toward an integrative model. *Epilepsia*, 48: 1639–1651, 2007.

80. Asarnow J, Baraf LJ, Berk M, Grob C, Devich-Navarro M, Suddath R, Piacentini J, Tang L. Pediatric emergency department suicidal patients: two-site evaluation of suicide ideators, single attempters, and repeat attempters. *J Am Acad Child Adolesc Psychiatry*, 47: 958–966, 2008.

81. Strauss J, Birmaher B, Bridge J, Axelson D, Chiappetta L, Brent D, Ryan N. Anxiety disorders in suicidal youth. *Can J Psychiatry*, 45: 739–745, 2000.

82. FDA public health advisory: suicidal thoughts and behavior antiepileptic drugs. http://www.fda.gov/Drugs/DrugSafety/PostmarketDrugSafetyInformationfor PatientsandProviders/DrugSafety InformationforHeathcareProfessionals/PublicHealthAdvisories/ucm054709.htm, 2008.

83. Fietta P, Fietta P, Delsante G. Central nervous system effects of natural and synthetic glucocorticoids. *Psychiatry Clin Neurosci*, 63: 613–622, 2009.

84. Kaufman J, Birmaher B, Brent D, Rao U, Flynn C, Moreci P, Williamson D, Ryan N. Schedule for Affective Disorders and Schizophrenia for School-Age Children-Present and Lifetime version (K-SADS-PL): initial reliability and validity data. *J Am Acad Child Adolesc Psychiatry*, 36: 980–988, 1997.

85. Shaffer D, Fisher P, Lucas CP, Dulcan MK, Schwab-Stone ME. NIMH Diagnostic Interview Schedule for Children Version IV (NIMH DISC-IV): description, differences from previous versions, and reliability of some common diagnoses. *J Am Acad Child Adolesc Psychiatry*, 39: 28–38, 2000.

86. Poznanski EO, Mokros HB. *Children's Depression Rating Scale–Revised (CDRS-R)*. Los Angeles, CA: Western Psychological Services, 1996.

87. Silverman W, Albano AM. The Anxiety Disorders Interview Schedule for Children (DSM-IV). San Antonio, TX: Psychological Corporation, 1997.

88. Sprafkin J, Gadow KD, Salisbury H, Schneider J, Loney J. Further evidence of reliability and validity of the Child Symptom Inventory-4: parent checklist in clinically referred boys. *J Clin Child Adolesc Psychol*, 31: 513–524, 2002.

89. March J, Parker D, Sullivan K, Stallings P, Conners C. The Multidimensional Anxiety Scale for Children (MASC): factor structure, reliability, and validity. *J Am Acad Child Adolesc Psychiatry*, 36: 554–565, 1997.

90. Birmaher B, Khetarpal S, Brent D, Cully M, Balach L, Kaufman J, Neer SM. The Screen for Child Anxiety Related Emotional Disorders (SCARED): scale construction and psychometric characteristics. *J Am Acad Child Adolesc Psychiatry*, 36: 545–553, 1997.

91. Achenbach T. *Manual for the Youth Self-Report and 1991 Profile*. Burlington, VT: Department of Psychiatry, University of Vermont, 1991.

92. Grills A, Ollendick T. Issues in parent-child agreement: the case of structured diagnostic interviews. *Clin Child Fam Psychol Rev*, 5: 57–83, 2002.

93. Kanner A, Caplan R, Dunn D. Epilepsy and psychiatric comorbidities counseling points. Psychiatric Comorbidities in Children with

Epilepsy Postgraduate Institute for Medicine, Delaware Media Group, Delaware, 2009.

94. Mazza J, Fleming C, Abbott R, Haggerty K, Catalano R. Identifying trajectories of adolescents' depressive phenomena: an examination of early risk factors. *J Youth Adolesc*, 39: 579–593, 2010.

95. Keeton CP, Kolos AC, Walkup JT. Pediatric generalized anxiety disorder. *Pediatr Drugs*, 11: 171–183, 2009.

96. Peter T, Roberts LW, Buzdugan R. Suicidal ideation among Canadian youth: a multivariate analysis. *Arch Suicide Res*, 12: 263–275, 2008.

97. Basso MR, Lowery N, Ghormley C, Combs D, Purdie R, Neel J, Davis M, Bornstein R. Comorbid anxiety corresponds with neuropsychological dysfunction in unipolar depression. *Cognit Neuropsychiatry*, 12: 437–456, 2007.

98. Hankin B, Oppenheimer C, Jenness J, Barrocas A, Shapero BG, Goldband J. Developmental origins of cognitive vulnerabilities to depression: review of processes contributing to stability and change across time. *J Clin Psychol*, 65: 1327–1338, 2009.

99. Cisler J, Koster EHW. Mechanisms of attentional biases towards threat in anxiety disorders: an integrative review. *Clin Psychol Rev*, 30: 203–216, 2010.

100. Austin J, Huberty T. Development of the Child Attitude Toward Illness Scale. *J Pediatr Psychol*, 18: 467–480, 1993.

101. Thomé-Souza M, Kuczynski E, Valente KD. Sertraline and fluoxetine: safe treatments for children and adolescents with epilepsy and depression. *Epilepsy Behav*, 10: 417–426, 2007.

102. Martinovic Z, Simonovic P, Djokic R. Preventing depression in adolescents with epilepsy. *Epilepsy Behav*, 9: 619–624, 2006.

103. March JS, Vitiello B. Clinical messages from the Treatment for Adolescents With Depression Study (TADS). *Am J Psychiatry*, 166: 1118–1123, 2009.

104. Sakolsky D, Birmaher B. Pediatric anxiety disorders: management in primary care. *Curr Opin Pediatr*, 20: 538–543, 2008.

105. Bloch MH, McGuire J, Landeros-Weisenberger A, Leckman JF, Pittenger C. Meta-analysis of the dose-response relationship of SSRI in obsessive-compulsive disorder. *Mol Psychiatry*, 15: 850–855, 2009.

106. Donnelly CL, Amaya-Jackson L. Post-traumatic stress disorder in children and adolescents: epidemiology, diagnosis and treatment options. *Pediatr Drugs*, 4: 159–170, 2002.

107. Brent D, Emslie G, Clarke G, Wagner KD, Asarnow JR, Keller M, Vitiello B, Ritz L, Iyengar S, Abebe K, Birmaher B, Ryan N, Kennard B, Hughes C, DeBar L, McCracken J, Strober M, Suddath R, Spirito A, Leonard H, Melhem N, Porta G, Onorato M, Zelazny J. Switching to another SSRI or to venlafaxine with or without cognitive behavioral therapy for adolescents with SSRI-resistant depression: the TORDIA randomized controlled trial. *JAMA*, 299: 901–913, 2008.

108. Bridge JA, Iyengar S, Salary CB, Barbe RP, Birmaher B, Pincus HA, Ren L, Brent DA. Clinical response and risk for reported suicidal ideation and suicide attempts in pediatric antidepressant treatment: a meta-analysis of randomized controlled trials. *JAMA*, 297: 1683–1696, 2007.

109. Hammad TA, Laughren T, Racoosin J. Suicidality in pediatric patients treated with antidepressant drugs. *Arch Gen Psychiatry*, 63: 332–339, 2006.

110. Libby AM, Brent DA, Morrato EH, Orton HD, Allen R, Valuck RJ. Decline in treatment of pediatric depression after FDA advisory on risk of suicidality with SSRIs. *Am J Psychiatry*, 164: 884–891, 2007.

111. Gibbons RD, Brown CH, Hur K, Marcus SM, Bhaumik DK, Erkens JA, Herings RMC, Mann JJ. Early evidence on the effects of regulators' suicidality warnings on SSRI prescriptions and suicide in children and adolescents. *Am J Psychiatry*, 164: 1356–1363, 2007.

112. Morrato EH, Libby AM, Orton HD, Degruy FV, III, Brent DA, Allen R, Valuck RJ. Frequency of provider contact after FDA advisory on risk of pediatric suicidality With SSRIs. *Am J Psychiatry*, 165: 42–50, 2008.

113. Walkup JT, Albano AM, Piacentini J, Birmaher B, Compton SN, Sherrill JT, Ginsburg GS, Rynn MA, McCracken J, Waslick B, Iyengar S,

March JS, Kendall PC. Cognitive behavioral therapy, sertraline, or a combination in childhood anxiety. *N Engl J Med*, 359: 2753–2766, NEJMoa0804633. 2008.

114. Wagner K, Ambrosini PJ. Childhood depression: pharmacological therapy/treatment. *J Clin Child Psychol*, 30: 88–97, 2001.

115. David-Ferdon C, Kaslow NJ. Evidence-based psychosocial treatments for child and adolescent depression. *J Clin Child Adolesc Psychol*, 37: 62–104, 2008.

116. McCarty C, Weisz JR. Effects of psychotherapy for depression in children and adolescents: what we can (and can't) learn from meta-analysis and component profiling. *J Am Acad Child Adolesc Psychiatry*, 46: 879–886, 2007.

Basic Principles in the Management of Depression in Neurologic Disorders

Marco Mula
Department of Clinical and Experimental Medicine, Amedeo Avogadro University; Division of Neurology, University Hospital Maggiore della Carità, Novara, Italy

Introduction

Depression commonly complicates neurologic diseases, impairing quality of life, speed of recovery, independence, and survival [1]. Generally, depression is the result of a number of components (i.e., biological, psychological, and genetic factors) that interface with the acquired brain disorder. Although depression is highly treatable, it still remains undetected and undertreated because of two main problems: first, clinicians and patients often falsely accept depression as a "normal response" to the disease; second, the majority of neurologists are not familiar with the use of psychotropic medications (e.g., antidepressant drugs, antipsychotic drugs, mood stabilizers) in terms of prescription and indications. In fact, pharmacological therapy of depression is warranted for patients with both reactive and "endogenous" depression, and the ultimate goal should be full remission of symptoms.

Depression can be unipolar or bipolar. Unipolar depression can be subcategorized into major depression (severe depression lasting at least 2 weeks) or dysthymia (lower grade unremitting chronic depression lasting at least 2 years) [2]. Atypical depression identifies a subgroup of patients with severe depression characterized by mood reactivity and a tendency to overeat, gain weight, and oversleep.

There are a few differences in response to therapy between the different types of depression. Patients with bipolar depression may switch into manic excitement with antidepressant drugs, especially when mood-stabilizing agents are not included. Paradoxically, dysthymia can be more difficult to treat than severe depression, while atypical depression seems to respond to a specific group of antidepressant drugs such as monoamine oxidase inhibitors (MAOIs) [3].

Classification of antidepressant drugs

Antidepressants can be classified as first- or second-generation drugs (Table 8.1). This classification is based on two main factors: (1) the progressive importance of drug design in developing chemical compounds and (2) the evolution of the hypotheses on the neurobiology of depression, from the monoaminergic hypothesis to the monoaminergic receptor hypothesis, to the signaling adaptation hypothesis and neuromodulation [4] (Table 8.2).

First-generation antidepressants

MAOIs became available for therapy in the 1960s. They inhibit the main metabolic enzymes of the monoamine neurotransmitters norepinephrine (NE), serotonin (5-HT), and dopamine (DA), resulting in a generalized increase of monoamine

Depression in Neurologic Disorders: Diagnosis and Management, First Edition.
Edited by Andres M. Kanner.
© 2012 Blackwell Publishing Ltd. Published 2012 by Blackwell Publishing Ltd.

Table 8.1 Classification of antidepressant drugs

Irreversible Inhibitors of Monoamine Oxidase A (IMAOIs)
Tranylcypromine
Reversible Inhibitors of Monoamine Oxidase A (RIMAs)
Moclobemide
Tricyclic Antidepressant Drugs (TCAs)
Amitriptyline
Clomipramine
Desipramine
Imipramine
Maprotiline
Nortriptyline
Protriptyline
Trimipramine
Selective Serotonin Reuptake Inhibitors (SSRIs)
Citalopram
Escitalopram
Fluoxetine
Fluvoxamine
Paroxetine
Sertraline
Selective Noradrenergic Reuptake inhibitors (NRIs)
Reboxetine
Norepinephrine and Dopamine Reuptake Blockers (NDRIs)
Bupropion
Dual Serotonin and Norepinephrine Reuptake Inhibitors (SNRIs)
Duloxetine
Venlafaxine
Noradrenergic and Specific Serotoninergic Antidepressants (NaSSAs)
Mianserin[a]
Mirtazapine
Dual Serotonin 2 Antagonists/Serotonin Reuptake Inhibitors (SARIs)
Nefazodone
Trazodone

[a]Not marketed in the United States.

levels throughout the central nervous system (CNS). Among MAOIs, it is possible to identify irreversible inhibitors (irreversible monoamine oxidase inhibitors, IMAOIs) such as hyproniazide or tranylcypromine, and reversible inhibitors (reversible inhibitors of monoamine oxidase A, RIMAs) such as moclobemide. There are two sub-types of MAOIs: A and B. The A form metabolizes mostly 5-HT and NA, while the B form is thought to be linked to DA. This is one of the reasons why

Table 8.2 Hypotheses on the pathophysiology of depression and drug strategies

Period	Hypotheses	Role of Antidepressants
1960s–1970s	*Monoaminergic hypothesis*: Decreased availability of monoamines	Increase monoamine levels
1980s	*Monoaminergic receptor hypothesis*: Abnormalities in monoamine receptors	Modify sensitization state of receptors
1990s	*Signaling adaptation hypothesis*: Abnormalities in gene expression and intracellular signaling	Induce adaptive changes in postreceptor signaling cascades
2000s	*Neuroplasticity hypothesis*: Functional and structural changes in targeted areas	Induce changes in cellular resilience and synaptic plasticity

MAO-B inhibitors, such as selegiline, are used to treat Parkinson's disease. Both forms are inhibited by the IMAOIs, which are nonselective, while RIMAs are considered selective for the A form.

As a group, MAOIs are powerful drugs in terms of therapeutic efficacy, but their use has been limited by the pronounced and potentially lethal adverse effects, including hypertension during intake of food containing tyramine. Such effects are commonly reported with IMAOIs, while they are less pronounced with RIMAs. Nowadays, IMAOIs are rarely prescribed, though they are still in use in some countries because they are less expensive than new agents. RIMAs are still used for the treatment of specific conditions such as atypical depression [5, 6].

Tricyclic antidepressants (TCAs) are familiar to the majority of clinicians, having represented the mainstay of pharmacological treatment of depression for decades. Introduced shortly after MAOIs, they primarily block the reuptake of both 5-HT and NA and, to a lesser extent, that of DA. Some molecules have more marked inhibition properties for the 5-HT reuptake (e.g., clomipramine), while others are more selective for the NA reuptake (e.g., desipramine, nortriptyline, protriptyline, maprotiline). However, the majority of TCAs block both 5-HT and NA reuptake. In addition, all of these compounds have at least three other actions: the blockade of muscarinic cholinergic receptors (M1), the blockade of histamine receptors (H1), and the blockade of alpha1 adrenergic receptors. These actions account for the majority of side effects of TCAs; however, they also account for the efficacy of TCAs on different psychiatric symptoms [5, 6].

Viloxazine is a bicyclic antidepressant that shares some mechanisms of actions with TCAs, imipramine in particular, with special attention to the effect on the NA and 5-HT systems. However, unlike any other TCA, viloxazine showed no activity on M1 receptors and seems to upregulate gamma-aminobutyric acid-B (GABA-B) receptors in the frontal cortex [5, 6].

Second-generation antidepressants

Selective serotonin reuptake inhibitors (SSRIs) are represented by fluoxetine, fluvoxamine, sertraline, paroxetine, citalopram, and escitalopram. Although each of these molecules belongs to a chemically distinct family, all of them share the same major pharmacological feature, that is, the selective and potent inhibition of 5-HT reuptake, which is more powerful than their actions on NA reuptake or on alpha-1, H1, or M1 receptors, and with virtually no ability to block sodium channels, even in overdose. As such, SSRIs are considered much safer than TCAs, not only with regard to the spectrum of side effects, but also in overdose [5, 6].

Reboxetine is the logical pharmacological complement to SSRIs. In fact, it is a selective norepinephrine reuptake inhibitor (NRI) with low affinity for H1, M1, DA, and alpha-1 receptors. Interestingly, reboxetine was developed from viloxazine, but the mechanism of action is different. It appears to be equally effective as TCAs in treating depression, but without several undesirable side effects [5, 6].

The mechanism of action of bupropion remained unclear for many years. Bupropion has weak reuptake properties for DA and even weaker for NA [5, 6]; however, it has always appeared to be more powerful than these weak properties could explain in potentiating NA and DA neurotransmission and is considered the prototype of a specific class of antidepressants, that is, NE and dopamine reuptake blockers (NDRIs) (see Table 8.1) [5, 6].

Dual serotonin and norepinephrine reuptake inhibitors (SNRIs) is a class of antidepressants that combines the actions of both SSRIs and NRIs [5, 6]. What is unique about these drugs compared to TCAs, which actually act on both neurotransmission systems, is the lack of alpha-1, M1, or H1 blocking properties. Thus, SNRIs are not only dual-action agents, but are also selective for this dual action [5, 6].

Mirtazapine is currently classified among noradrenergic and specific serotoninergic antidepressants (NaSSAs). Its primary therapeutic action is the alpha-2 antagonism that disinhibits NA and 5-HT neurons [5, 6]. However, because mirtazapine also blocks 5-HT2 and 5-HT3 receptors, the increased serotonin turnover only stimulates 5-HT1 receptors. It is free of side effects related to M1, alpha-1, and 5HT2 and 5HT3, but its effects on H1 receptors can cause sedation and weight gain [5, 6].

Nefazodone is the prototypical member of the dual-serotonin 2 antagonists/serotonin reuptake inhibitors (SARIs). It is a powerful 5-HT2a antagonist with secondary actions as an SNRI [5, 6]. This activity of blockade at the 5-HT2a postsynaptic receptor site leads to a dual mechanism of action on the 5-HT system involving both 5-HT1 and 5-HT3 subsites, representing the major distinctive property of this class of antidepressant drugs. NA reuptake inhibition is minimal, and there is no interaction with H1 or M1 receptors [5, 6].

Basic issues in the pharmacological treatment of depression

Remission and recovery are the main goals of the acute treatment of depression, while avoiding its recurrence is the primary objective of long-term treatment [7]. The term *response* means that a patient experienced at least 50% reduction in symptoms of depression as assessed on a standardized psychiatric rating scale, while *remission* is used when all symptoms disappear. The term *recovery* is used when a remission lasts for 6–12 months, while *relapse* is used in case of worsening symptoms before remission or before a remission has turned into a recovery. *Recurrence* refers to worsening symptoms a few months after a complete recovery is achieved [7].

In general terms, it is estimated that the percentage of response to one treatment or a combination of therapeutic interventions is up to 90% of patients with depression. Among these subjects, approximately 50% may recover within 6 months and up to 75% within 2 years [8]. The probability of recurrence depends on a number of factors, such as the presence of multiple prior episodes, long-lasting episodes, incomplete recovery from prior episodes, and bipolar or psychotic features [8].

Moreover, it is important to point out that treatment of depression should not focus only on depressed mood, but also on associated symptoms such as insomnia, circadian desynchronization, sexual dysfunction, cognitive impairment, and pain. In fact, up to 50% of patients who respond to treatment nevertheless fail to attain remission, with maintenance of illness involving a milder form or modification into a new clinical phenotype. Depressed mood can be controlled, but the patient may complain of continuing anhedonia, lack of motivation, decreased libido, cognitive slowing, decreased concentration, generalized anxiety, insomnia, or somatic symptoms. Several reasons may account for such a partial remission, including inadequate early treatment, underlying dysthymia, or personality disorders. However, it is important to identify these patients because partial remission is associated with increased relapse risk, continuing functional impairment, and increased suicidal rate.

The use of MAOIs

Acute administration of RIMAs causes significant increases in NA and 5-HT in synaptic terminals but a reduction in NA synthesis, with acute euphoria and decreased rapid eye movement (REM) sleep. On the other hand, chronic administration is associated with reduction in NA-stimulated cyclic adenosine monophosphate (cAMP) and downregulation of beta-adrenergic and 5-HT2 receptors [5, 6].

RIMAs should be used cautiously due to a number of possible negative drug interactions with compounds that directly or indirectly act on the adrenergic system, including SSRIs, TCAs, opioid analgesics, nasal decongestants, sympathomimetics, and amphetamines. Hypotension, hepatotoxicity, and sedation may be clinically relevant side effects [5, 6].

The use of TCAs

All TCAs have a wide therapeutic window, with a therapeutic dose ranging between 50 and 150 mg daily. It is possible to identify two main drug groups of TCAs based on their chemical structure: tertiary and secondary amines (Figure 8.1). Those in the former group have been shown to be more serotoninergic than those in the latter group, which have been shown to be more noradrenergic. All tertiary amines are metaboli-

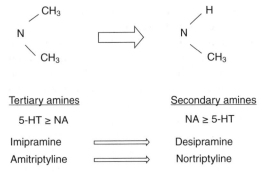

Tertiary amines   Secondary amines

5-HT ≥ NA   NA ≥ 5-HT

Imipramine   ⟹   Desipramine

Amitriptyline   ⟹   Nortriptyline

Figure 8.1 Tricyclic antidepressant drugs: tertiary and secondary amines and their relative effects on the noradrenergic (NA) and serotoninergic (5-HT) systems.

cally transformed into secondary amines, thus creating a complex equilibrium between the action on the 5HT and the NA systems [5, 6]. It goes without saying that the coadministration of inducers such as carbamazepine or barbiturates may alter this equilibrium, leading to prominent NA effects instead of the 5HT effects initially presumed. Such a balance is of relevance not only for the specific antidepressant effect, but also and especially for the spectrum of side effects and associated properties. In fact, a low NA profile associated with a high 5-HT and M1 profile is usually sedative and anxiolytic associated with cognitive slowing and sedation [5, 6].

The relative activity on different receptor groups is of importance regarding side effects. In fact, dry mouth, paradoxical excessive perspiration, constipation, blurred vision, mydriasis, metallic taste, and urinary retention are related to M1 blockade; orthostatic hypotension to the alpha-1 and possibly alpha-2 blockade; drowsiness, sedation, and weight gain to the H1 blockade; palpitation, tachycardia, and dizziness to heart-specific NA receptors; and sexual dysfunction, loss of libido, impaired erection or ejaculation, and anorgasmia to 5-HT2 stimulation [5, 6]. Therefore, it is possible to suppose the relative spectrum of side effects of different TCAs based on their relative activity on different receptor groups (Table 8.3).

The use of SSRIs

SSRIs have been claimed to be selective, but it seems well established that the majority of these compounds have a peculiar spectrum of activity on different receptors apart from their major

Table 8.3 Sedative properties of TCAs in relationship with their relative activity on different neurotransmitter systems

	NA	5-HT	Acetylcholine	Sedation
Amitriptyline	Low	High	High	High
Clomipramine	Low	High	High	High
Desipramine	High	Low	Low	Low
Imipramine	Low	Low	Mod	Mod
Nortriptyline	Mod	Low	Mod	Mod
Proptriptyline	High	Low	Mod	Low
Trimipramine	Low	Low	High	High

mechanism of action on 5-HT reuptake. Fluoxetine partially inhibits NA reuptake and has a specific activity on the 5-HT2c receptors; paroxetine blocks M1 receptors and partially inhibits NA reuptake; sertraline has peculiar DA properties, with some activity on sigma-receptors of the opioid system, which is also shared by fluvoxamine [5, 6].

Moreover, SSRIs have significant differences in terms of half-life. Paroxetine and fluvoxamine have a half-life of less than 24 hours, thus explaining the possibility of uncomfortable symptoms when some doses are missed. On the contrary, fluoxetine has a long half-life, limiting the possible impact of missed doses [5, 6]. All of this evidence clearly suggests that the prescription of one SSRI cannot be considered equivalent to another; instead, the specific compound should be chosen according to the specific needs of the patient.

Adverse effects of SSRIs include hyponatremia, sexual dysfunction, bleeding, and extrapyramidal symptoms [5, 6]. In case of malaise or confusion, electrolytes should be tested. Particular attention is required when SSRIs are prescribed in combination with oxcarbazepine or carbamazepine, which are both associated with hyponatremia. Sexual dysfunction is caused by 5-HT2 stimulation and has been reported in up to 70% of male patients taking SSRIs [9]. In young males, the use of SSRIs should be carefully considered, and other compounds such as bupropion or duloxetine may be taken due to the relatively low prevalence of adverse events on sexuality (less than 30%) [9]. Bleeding may be a concern especially in elderly patients. Platelets release 5-HT to initiate aggregation, and the inhibition of 5-HT reuptake may result in increased risk of bleeding. Relative risk has been estimated at 1 out of 8000 prescription of SSRIs [10], but such risks can be significantly increased when SSRIs are administered in association with salicylates or nonsteroidal inflammatory drugs. Finally, extrapyramidal symptoms such as dystonic reactions, akathisia, or even a Parkinsonism must be considered. The estimated rate is 1 case per 1000 treated patients [11]. The mechanism is unclear, but it has been suggested that overactive 5-HT neurons inhibit DA synapses in the basal ganglia. This seems to occur quite early in treatment (usually the first month), especially when rapid titration schedules are adopted [12].

The use of selective antidepressants

Novel, selective antidepressants, comprising SSRIs, are not more effective than TCAs in treating depression; however, the "clean" mechanism of action and relatively simple pharmacokinetics make SSRIs easier to use and more tolerable than old compounds [5, 6]. Among the new class of antidepressants, some have advantages over others. For example, NARIs such as reboxetine and NDRIs such as bupropion seem to be almost completely free of sexual dysfunction as a side effect. SARIs have been shown to be effective in treating anxiety disorders (e.g., generalized anxiety disorders or panic disorders), but without the 5-HT2a activating side effects associated with SSRIs, which can cause worsening of anxiety symptoms at the very beginning of the antidepressant drug treatment. Thus, it is clear that selective compounds present a number of favorable aspects, which must be balanced with the more limited existing literature and experience compared to those of classic antidepressant drugs [5, 6].

Antidepressant drugs in neurologic disorders

For patients with neurologic disorders, the use of antidepressants could, on occasion, have a negative impact on the underlying neurologic condition or cause adverse effects from their pharmacodynamic and pharmacokinetic interactions with concomitant medications. Specific treatment strategies will be discussed in each chapter regarding individual diseases. Therefore, this section will review the basic pharmacological issues of antidepressant drugs that are relevant to some of the major neurologic disorders.

Migraine and other headaches

Migraine has a high comorbidity with unipolar and bipolar mood disorders [13]. Accordingly, antidepressant drugs should be used with great caution in patients with migraine and bipolar depression (see also Chapter 3).

The use of antidepressant drugs in patients with headaches has implications on two different treatment strategies, namely prophylaxis and acute treatment. For example, triptans are used for acute treatment of migraines. Clinicians must consider the theoretical risk of serotoninergic syndrome when triptans and SSRIs or SNRIs are used together; however, no definite data are available regarding this issue [14]. Likewise, the use of sumatriptan and rizatriptan in combination with SSRIs or RIMAs remains controversial [15]. In general terms, almotriptan is considered to yield a low risk when coprescribed with antidepressants but is contraindicated in patients taking lithium [15].

Regarding prophylactic treatment strategies, calcium antagonists, beta-blockers, and topiramate should be avoided or carefully considered in depressed patients. In contrast, SSRIs, SNRIs, TCAs, or valproate may be successfully used for depressed patients, although some of these drugs are still off label in some countries [16].

Finally, migraine resulting from excessive use of analgesic medications is an emerging issue with theoretical therapeutic implications. Although no controlled studies are available, DA antidepressants may be considered as a potential option because they showed favorable effects in patients with substance abuse problems [17].

Multiple sclerosis

In patients with multiple sclerosis (MS), depressive episodes may include a number of symptoms also associated with either the underlying immune system disease (e.g., fatigue), CNS damage (cognitive slowing, sexual dysfunction), or iatrogenic causes. For example, some of the drugs used to prevent relapse of MS, such as the family of interferon drugs, may be associated with treatment-emergent depressive symptoms. Interferon beta is generally less depressogenic than alpha interferon, which should be considered when treating depressed patients [18].

Given some of the frequent neurologic symptoms of MS, TCAs with prominent anticholinergic properties (i.e., desipramine) or SSRIs associated with sexual problems (i.e., paroxetine and sertraline) should be avoided [19]. NARIs may be promising, but controlled studies are lacking.

Parkinson's disease and other neurodegenerative disorders

The issue of 5-HT/DA balance in patients with Parkinson's disease (PD) is still controversial.

Although some authors have suggested that SSRIs may aggravate motor symptoms [20], data are still limited. Theoretically, NARIs, NDRIs, or TCAs with prominent NA properties (i.e., nortriptyline) are indicated in this population of patients [21], but controlled studies are lacking. Pharmacological combinations that should be avoided include SSRIs and selegiline, L-DOPA and RIMAs, and TCAs and anticholinergic drugs [22].

In patients with other neurodegenerative disorders such as Alzheimer's disease and other dementias, it is important to consider the issues shared with the general elderly population, including differences in pharmacokinetic and pharmacodynamic properties that could lead to potential detrimental adverse effects (e.g., on electrocardiography [EKG] and blood pressure). For example, trazodone has an immediate impact (minutes to hours) on the QT interval of the EKG, while TCAs have short-term effects (<12 weeks of treatment). In general terms, QT prolongation is more pronounced with tertiary TCAs than with secondary ones. Therefore, the use of such drugs may be limited in this population of patients [23]. Bupropion, sertraline, and most antidepressants with a selective mechanism of action (e.g., citalopram or escitalopram) have no effect on the QT interval [23] and can be reasonably considered first options.

"Start low, go slow" is definitely appropriate here, but it is important to keep in mind that low starting doses do not necessarily mean low target doses.

Epilepsy

Two main issues are relevant when using antidepressants in patients with epilepsy: pharmacological interactions (both pharmacodynamic and pharmacokinetic) and the potential impact on seizure threshold [24]. In general terms, the new families of antidepressants have a favorable pharmacokinetic profile with a low risk of interactions. The issue of worsening seizures has been a source of major concern for many clinicians. However, available data derived from research studies in animal models of epilepsy and/or depression, studies using *in vitro* techniques, and trials in humans with psychiatric disorders [25] have shown that for the majority of antidepressants prescribed at dosages within the therapeutic range, the incidence of seizures is comparable with that of the general population or lower (less than 0.5%) when other risk factors are excluded.

Conclusions

Major depression represents an important complication of several neurologic disorders that may significantly affect morbidity, mortality, and quality of life. Neurologists are rightly concerned about the underlying brain disorder, but full symptom remission and complete recovery should always represent the main goal of the pharmacological treatment of depression, without considering such comorbidity as a secondary outcome. A variety of compounds are currently available and should be used according to good clinical practice guidelines, with a focus on the balance among efficacy, side effects, and impact on the neurologic condition (see "Pearls to Take Home" section). Novel, more selective antidepressants are easier to use and better tolerated compared with older drugs. Clinical guidelines in patients with comorbid neurologic and psychiatric conditions are urgently needed to develop a rational and standardized approach to the problem.

💡 PEARLS TO TAKE HOME

- Full remission and complete recovery should be the first goal in the treatment of comorbid depression
- New antidepressant drugs are not more effective than older compounds but are easier to use and better tolerated
- Antidepressant drugs should be slowly introduced and slowly titrated according to clinical response
- Low starting doses do *not* necessarily mean low target doses.
- The choice of antidepressant drugs should take into account the balance among clinical efficacy, side effects, and potential detrimental effects on the underlying neurologic disorders

---

References

1. Evans DL, Charney DS, Lewis L et al. Mood disorders in the medically ill: scientific review and recommendations. *Biol Psychiatry*, 58: 175–189, 2005.
2. American Psychiatric Association. *Diagnostic and Statistical Manual of Mental Disorders*, 4th ed. Text Revision. Washington, DC: American Psychiatric Association, 2000.
3. Nutt DJ, Davidson JR, Gelenberg AJ et al. International consensus statement on major depressive disorder. *J Clin Psychiatry*, 71, Suppl. E1: e08, 2010.
4. Racagni G, Popoli M. Cellular and molecular mechanisms in the long-term action of antidepressants. *Dialogues Clin Neurosci*, 10: 385–400, 2008.
5. Schatzberg AF, Cole JO, Debattista C. *Manual of Clinical Psychopharmacology*, 6th ed. Arlington, TX: American Psychiatric Publishing Inc., 2007.
6. Stahl SM. *Stahl's Essential Psychopharmacology*, 3rd ed. Cambridge, UK: Cambridge University Press, 2008.
7. Thase ME. Diagnosis and treatment of a major depressive episode. *J Clin Psychiatry.*, 70: e37, 2009.
8. Thase ME. Long-term nature of depression. *J Clin Psychiatry*, 60, Suppl. 14: 3–9, 1999.
9. Gregorian RS, Golden KA, Bahce A et al. Antidepressant-induced sexual dysfunction. *Ann Pharmacother*, 36: 1577–1589, 2002.
10. de Abajo FJ, Rodríguez LA, Montero D. Association between selective serotonin reuptake inhibitors and upper gastrointestinal bleeding: population based case-control study. *BMJ*, 319: 1106–1109, 1999.
11. Extrapyramidal effects of SSRI antidepressants. *Prescrire Int*, 10(54): 118–119, 2001.
12. Caley CF. Extrapyramidal reactions and the selective serotonin-reuptake inhibitors. *Ann Pharmacother*, 31: 1481–1489, 1997.
13. Breslau N, Merikangas K, Bowden CL. Comorbidity of migraine and major affective disorders. *Neurology*, 44(10 Suppl. 7): S17–S22, 1994.
14. Wenzel RG, Tepper S, Korab WE. Serotonin syndrome risks when combining SSRI/SNRI drugs and triptans: is the FDA's alert

warranted? *Ann Pharmacother*, 42: 1692–1696, 2008.

15. Millson DS, Tepper SJ, Rapoport AM. Migraine pharmacotherapy with oral triptans: a rational approach to clinical management. *Expert Opin Pharmacother*, 1: 391–404, 2000.

16. Moja PL, Cusi C, Sterzi RR et al. Selective serotonin re-uptake inhibitors (SSRIs) for preventing migraine and tension-type headaches. *Cochrane Database Syst Rev*, (3): CD002919, 2005.

17. Wilkes S. Bupropion. *Drugs Today (Barc)*, 42: 671–681, 2006.

18. Patten SB. Psychiatric side effects of interferon treatment. *Curr Drug Saf*, 1: 143–150, 2006.

19. Schiffer RB, Wineman NM. Antidepressant pharmacotherapy of depression associated with multiple sclerosis. *Am J Psychiatry*, 147: 1493–1497, 1990.

20. Veazey C, Aki SO, Cook KF et al. Prevalence and treatment of depression in Parkinson's disease. *J Neuropsychiatry Clin Neurosci*, 17: 310–323, 2005.

21. Chung TH, Deane KH, Ghazi-Noori S et al. Systematic review of antidepressant therapies in Parkinson's disease. *Parkinsonism Relat Disord*, 10: 59–65, 2003.

22. Schneider F, Althaus A, Backes V et al. Psychiatric symptoms in Parkinson's disease. *Eur Arch Psychiatry Clin Neurosci*, 258, Suppl. 5: 55–59, 2008.

23. Sala M, Coppa F, Cappucciati C et al. Antidepressants: their effects on cardiac channels, QT prolongation and Torsade de Pointes. *Curr Opin Investig Drugs*, 7: 256–263, 2006.

24. Mula M, Schmitz B, Sander JW. The pharmacological treatment of depression in adults with epilepsy. *Expert Opin Pharmacother*, 9: 3159–3168, 2008.

25. Alper K, Schwartz KA, Kolts RL et al. Seizure incidence in psychopharmacological clinical trials: an analysis of Food and Drug Administration (FDA) summary basis of approval reports. *Biol Psychiatry*, 62: 345–354, 2007.

Part Two

Depression and Neurologic Disorders

Depression and Migraine

Joan Roig Llesuy

Neuropsychiatry and Addiction Institute, Hospital del Mar, Barcelona, Spain

Case study

A 31-year-old female has suffered from migraine with aura since the age of 18. She has a family history of migraine and major depression. A structured psychiatric interview, however, failed to identify any Axis I diagnosis according to the *Diagnostic and Statistical Manual of Mental Disorders*, Fourth Edition (DSM-IV). She typically experienced an aura at the onset of her migraines consisting of a blind spot in her right visual field of approximately 5-minute duration, followed by a moderately severe throbbing pain behind the right eye with an average frequency of two per month and lasting up to 48 hours, with partial response to nonsteroidal anti-inflammatory medication or triptans. At the age of 23 she experienced one depressive episode consisting of symptoms of anhedonia, fatigue, constant crying, early night insomnia and middle-of-the-night awakening of several hours duration, loss of appetite with 10 pounds of weight loss and loss of sexual drive, and symptoms of constant worrying and restlessness. She was diagnosed with a major depressive episode (MDE) and treated with fluoxetine for 6 months by her primary care physician. Complete symptom remission was achieved 6 weeks after the start of therapy. At the age of 24 she started to experience daily tension-like headaches, with an increase in the frequency of her typical migraines to four per month. Associated with these headaches, she reported early night insomnia and symptoms of anxiety, described as constant worrying without any

apparent reason. She was treated with gabapentin up to a maximal daily dose of 1200 mg/day, which decreased the frequency and severity of tension headaches and migraines.

At the age of 29 she developed another MDE associated with anxiety symptoms and, consisting of depressive mood, anhedonia, early night insomnia, excessive guilt, constant worrying with agoraphobic symptoms, inability to concentrate, and suicidal thoughts. Fluoxetine was restarted and increased to daily doses of 60 mg/day without achieving complete symptom remission, for which she was switched to venlafaxine, up to a daily dose of 225 mg/day. The symptoms of depression and anxiety progressively remitted, and the patient was kept on venlafaxine and gabapentin up to the present.

Relation between migraines and mood disorders: an epidemiologic perspective

Depressive disorders and migraine are two common conditions. The lifetime prevalence of depressive disorders has been estimated to be 26% in women and 12% in men [1], while the prevalence of migraine has been estimated to range between 10% and 12% in population-based studies conducted in Europe and North America [2]. The World Health Organization classified migraine as the 19th leading cause of years lived with a disability worldwide [2]. Several epidemiologic studies have found that migraine is associated with mood and anxiety disorders. In a

Depression in Neurologic Disorders: Diagnosis and Management, First Edition.

Edited by Andres M. Kanner.

© 2012 Blackwell Publishing Ltd. Published 2012 by Blackwell Publishing Ltd.

Canadian population study of 36,984 subjects, migraine was diagnosed in 15.2% of females and 6.1% of males; the prevalence of major depressive disorder (MDD), bipolar disorder, panic disorder, and social phobia was more than two times higher in patients with migraine than in those without [3].

While depressive disorders and migraine are common, their comorbidity has been found to be higher than by chance occurrence. In fact, patients with major depression have higher prevalence of comorbid migraine and vice versa. Furthermore, current evidence shows that there is a significant bidirectional relationship between major depression and migraine. That is, not only are patients with migraine at higher risk of developing an MDE, but patients with MDE have an increased risk of developing migraines. A 2-year follow-up study by Breslau and colleagues [4] found that patients with migraine had significantly higher rates of first-onset depression than healthy controls, and patients with major depression also had significantly higher rates of first-onset migraine than healthy controls at follow-up. This bidirectional relationship was not observed for other chronic headaches and depression. This relation does not imply causality, but rather suggests that migraine and major depression could share some pathogenic mechanisms.

Other types of headache have been linked to depressive disorders, but migraine seems to be the one with the closest relationship. To identify the type of headache more commonly associated with depression, Saaman and colleagues [5] conducted a case-control study of 1259 patients with recurrent MDE and compared their headache type with 859 healthy controls. Compared to healthy controls, patients with recurrent MDE had more than a fivefold higher prevalence of migraine with aura, more than a threefold higher prevalence of migraine without aura, and a twofold higher prevalence of other non-migraine chronic headaches; all of these differences were statistically significant. The authors concluded that while all types of headache were linked to MDEs, the one with the highest association was migraine with aura.

Anxiety disorders and MDDs are often comorbid entities. A close relationship between anxiety disorders and migraine has also been identified. Anxiety disorders are more prevalent in patients with migraine than in healthy controls, but, according to several studies, the association with migraine is not specific. One study found that the lifetime prevalence of panic disorder was higher in patients with chronic migraine, while the lifetime prevalence of migraine was higher in patients with panic disorder. Further, significantly higher rates of new onset panic disorder were found in patients with migraine, and significantly higher rates of new onset migraine were found in patients with panic disorder. However, the same statistically significant relationships were found between other types of headache and panic disorder [6].

Depressive episodes can be an expression of an underlying MDD, but can also be caused by a bipolar disorder, which is a common but under-recognized diagnosis. Epidemiologic studies have demonstrated that the prevalence of migraine is more than two times higher in patients with bipolar disorder than in healthy controls, and the prevalence of bipolar disorder is also significantly higher in patients with migraine than in healthy controls [3]. In fact, a study found no significant differences in the prevalence of migraine in patients with MDD compared with patients with bipolar disorder [7]. Unfortunately, there is a lack of prospective studies that could clarify if there is a bidirectional relationship between bipolar disorder and migraine. However, in patients with bipolar disorder, research data suggest that the prevalence of migraine is significantly higher in patients diagnosed with a non-bipolar type I disorder when compared with patients diagnosed with bipolar type I disorder. Non-bipolar type I disorder includes patients with bipolar type II disorder, bipolar not otherwise specified, or cyclothimia [7].

Several research studies have shown that suicide attempts seem to be more frequent in young patients suffering from migraine with aura. Breslau and colleagues [8] conducted a study of 1007 young adults and found that persons with migraine had higher rates of suicide attempts than persons without migraine, with patients with migraine with aura being at significantly higher risk of suicide (odds ratio [OR] for suicide attempts in migraine with aura: 3.0 [95%

confidence interval, 1.4–6.6], after adjusting for coexisting major depression and other psychiatric disorders). Migraine without aura was not associated with an increase in suicide risk. The striking relationship between migraine with aura and increased risk of suicide was also found in a recent study by Wang and colleagues of 121 adolescents with chronic daily headache, in which patients with migraine were found to have significantly higher suicidal risk [9]. In this study, migraine with aura was the only subtype of headache that was found to be statistically significantly an independent predictor of a high suicidal risk after controlling for gender, depression, and anxiety disorders. Suicide risk was not significantly associated with other types of headache, headache frequency, or medication overuse headache. Clearly, these epidemiologic data point to a high comorbidity between migraine and mood and anxiety disorders.

Clinical manifestations

Prospective studies have found that depressive disorders can either precede or follow the onset of migraine [4]. There seem to be some differences when comparing the subtypes of depressive symptoms in patients with MDD with or without comorbid migraine. Hung and colleagues [10] investigated the impact of migraine in patients with MDD and found that 50% of patients with a current depressive episode and comorbid migraine had worsening of headaches during the depressive episodes, and that migraine in patients with MDD was associated with more frequent somatic and anxiety symptoms compared to the nonmigraine group.

The International Headache Society (IHS) published a revised classification system for headache disorders in 2004 [11]. Table 9.1 summarizes the diagnostic criteria for migraines with and without aura. Patients with migraine are likely to experience anxiety symptoms or changes in mood as a prodromal or accompanying feature of migraine attacks. Other psychiatric symptoms include hyperactivity, hypoactivity, craving for particular foods, and depressive mood, occurring from hours to days [11].

Patients with migraine can also experience symptoms of anxiety or depressive disorders that may or may not meet DSM-IV diagnostic criteria of these conditions [12]. In patients whose psychiatric symptomatology fails to meet DSM-IV criteria, anxiety or depressive symptoms tend to fluctuate in severity over time, which has also been found in patients with other neurologic disorders. Kraepelin, and then Bleuler and Gastaut described a constellation of mood and anxiety symptoms that were found to be highly prevalent in patients with epilepsy. Blumer and colleagues named it interictal dysphoric disorder of epilepsy (IDD), which includes at least three of the following symptoms occurring intermittently but with a significant negative impact: irritability, depressed mood, anergia, insomnia, atypical pain, anxiety, phobic fears, and euphoric mood [13]. The prevalence of IDD has been estimated to be approximately 30% in people with epilepsy [14]. It was thought that IDD was a specific disorder affecting only patients with epilepsy, but it seems that IDD is also very prevalent in patients with migraine. Indeed, a study of 229 patients found no significant differences in the prevalence of IDD in patients with migraine compared with patients with epilepsy [15].

Other authors have linked the irritability and affective instability that is seen in patients with migraine to bipolar illness traits. For example, Oedegaard and Fasmer [16] conducted a study to characterize the symptoms of depression in patients with MDD with and without comorbid migraine. Compared with the group of patients with MDE without comorbid migraine, the group of patients with MDE and migraine had a higher frequency of depressive episodes, a significantly higher prevalence of "affective" temperament, irritability, seasonal mood variation, agoraphobia, and migraine in family. The authors concluded that clinical features of patients with MDD with comorbid migraine are very similar to the clinical characteristics of patients with bipolar type II disorder. Thus, the presence of comorbid psychiatric disorders should be investigated in the presence of migraine, particularly with aura.

Table 9.2 lists some the self-administered screening instruments that can be helpful in the identification of mood and anxiety disorders and migraine as well as in the assessment of suicidal risk.

Table 9.1 IHS diagnostic criteria for migraine with aura and migraine without aura [11]

Migraine with aura: diagnostic criteria (subform typical aura with migraine headache)
A. At least two attacks fulfilling criteria B–D:
B. Aura consisting on one of the following, but no motor weakness: 1. Fully reversible visual symptoms including positive features (e.g., flickering lights, spots, or lines) and/or negative features (e.g., loss of vision) 2. Fully reversible sensory symptoms including positive features (e.g., pins and needles) and/or negative features (i.e., numbness) 3. Fully reversible dysphasic speech disturbance
C. At least two of the following: 1. Homonymous visual symptoms and/or unilateral sensory symptoms 2. At least one aura symptom develops gradually over ≥5 minutes and/or different aura symptoms occur in succession over ≥5 minutes. 3. Each symptom lasts more than 5 and less than 60 minutes.
D. Headache fulfilling criteria B–D for migraine without aura begins during the aura or follows aura within 60 minutes.
E. Not attributed to another disorder.
There are five other subforms of migraine with aura. Please consult IHS for a full criteria description [11].

Migraine without aura diagnostic criteria
A. At least five attacks fulfilling criteria B–D.
B. Headache attacks lasting 4–72 hours (untreated or unsuccessfully treated)
C. Headache has at least two of the following characteristics: 1. Unilateral location 2. Pulsating quality 3. Moderate or severe pain intensity 4. Aggravation by or causing avoidance of routine physical activity (e.g., walking or climbing stairs)
D. During the headache at least one of the following: 1. Nausea and/or vomiting 2. Photophobia and phonophobia
E. Not attributed to another disorder.

Modified from the International Headache Society (http://ihs-classification.org/en).

The negative impact of depression on the quality of life of patients with migraine

Migraine is a leading cause of disability. In approximately half of patients, the severity of the migrainous attack is likely to interfere with their daily activities. The presence of a comorbid MDD has been shown to worsen the quality of life in patients with migraine. In a population-based case-control study of 389 subjects with migraine and 379 controls, Lipton and colleagues [17] found significantly worse quality of life in patients with migraine, both in mental and physical health-related parameters. The presence of comorbid MDE significantly increased the differences of quality of life measurements between patients and healthy controls. In fact, migraine and depression independently

Table 9.2 Self-administered questionnaires useful for migraine or psychiatric disorder screening

Questionnaire	Suspected Diagnosis	Time Required	Score Suggestive of Illness
ID migraine [33]	Migraine	2 minutes	2 or more affirmative responses
Hospital Anxiety Depression Scale–Depression (HADS-D) [34]	Major depression and generalized anxiety disorder	5 minutes	>8 points
Beck Depression Inventory-II (BDI-II) [35]	Major depression	10 minutes	>13 points
Mood Disorder Questionnaire (MDQ) [36]	Bipolar disorder	10 minutes	>6 affirmative responses and relevant functional impairment
Mini International Neuropsychiatric Interview (MINI) Suicidal Module [37]	Suicide risk evaluation	2 minutes	>3 moderate risk

exerted a significant negative influence on health-related quality of life parameters in this study. Significant differences were maintained after controlling for age, gender, and education.

The negative impact of depression in the course of migraine

In general, juvenile onset migraine has a benign course. However, there is growing evidence that patients with migraine and psychiatric comorbidities have a worse outcome and tend to respond less to medications. An 8-year follow-up study by Guidetti and Galli [18] of 100 young adults with migraine or tension-type headache found that psychiatric comorbidities worsen the course of the headache illness. In that study, psychiatric comorbidities were more prevalent in the group of patients with migraine, and the higher the number of psychiatric disorders at initial evaluation, the worse the migraine status at follow-up. Similar results were found in the epidemiologic study by Jette and colleagues of 36,984 persons in Canada, in which health-related outcomes were significantly worse in patients with both migraine and a psychiatric disorder compared to those with either condition alone [3].

On the one hand, the severity of migraine attacks seems to have some relationship with the presence of depression and psychiatric comorbidities. On the other hand, the recurrence of migraine attacks does not seem to be related to depressive or anxiety symptoms. According to the study by Breslau and colleagues, patients with migraine and lifetime history of MDD reported a significantly higher severity of migraine attacks compared with patients without any past depressive episode. In that study, the recurrence of migraine attacks was not related to the presence of depression [4].

As stated above, there is a big concern regarding the increased risk of suicide that has been found in patients with migraine with aura. Two epidemiologic studies of people aged 12–28 years found that patients diagnosed with migraine with aura had a higher suicidal risk, independent of the psychiatric comorbidities [8, 9]. Accordingly, screening for suicidality should be conducted in young patients with migraine with aura. Further studies are needed to assess the risk of suicide in different age groups.

In addition to the increased risk of suicide, one study identified an increased risk for the development of epilepsy in patients diagnosed with migraine with aura and MDE. Indeed, Hesdorffer and colleagues [19] found that the co-occurrence of MDE and migraine with aura significantly increased the risk for developing unprovoked seizures more than did either MDE or migraine with aura alone. They also found a significant association between suicide attempts, migraine with aura, and unprovoked seizures. In contrast, migraine without aura was not associated with an increased risk of unprovoked seizures. This study suggests that migraine with aura, major depression disorder, suicide attempts, and epilepsy share common pathogenic mechanisms. Clearly, these data suggest that migraine, in association with psychiatric disorders, results in poorer health-related outcomes compared with migraine or a psychiatric condition alone.

Common pathogenic mechanisms operant in depression and migraine

As discussed above, a bidirectional relationship between migraine and MDD has been suggested in several studies, which is probably the expression of shared pathogenic mechanisms. Here are some of the data that support this hypothesis:

1. Serotonin disturbances have been identified in the central nervous system of patients with MDD and migraines. Some cerebral structures linked with pain regulation are rich in serotonin receptors, and in migraine attacks, circulating levels of serotonin and its metabolites have been described [20]. Similarly, it has been proposed that serotonin disturbances could play a role in the relationship between suicidality and migraine, as low levels of serotonin were found in cerebrospinal fluid samples of patients with suicide attempts [21].

2. A genetic study found that the dopamine D2 receptor gene is linked to migraine with aura, MDD, and other psychiatric disorders [22]. In this study, generalized anxiety disorder, MDD, migraine with aura, obsessive–compulsive disorder, panic disorder, and phobias were associated with the NcoI C allele frequency, which was significantly higher in individuals with these disorders than in healthy controls. A recent study by Stam and colleagues [23] also found that the shared genetic mechanisms between migraine and depression could partially explain their bidirectional relationship. In this study, comparison of the heritability scores for depression between patients with migraine and controls showed a significant genetic correlation between depression scores and migraine with aura.

Twin studies are helpful in highlighting the role of environmental or shared genetic factors in the pathogenesis of an illness. A recent twin study has found evidence that migraine and MDD share some significant genetic susceptibility that could explain their comorbidity [24]. In this study, an estimated 20% of the variability in depression and migraine was due to shared genetic factors, whereas 4% was due to shared unique environmental factors.

3. New data from different studies suggest that mitochondrial dysfunction and inflammatory processes could also play an important role in the pathogenesis of both illnesses [25]. While the efficacy of antidepressant treatment in both depression and migraine suggested a dysfunction of monoaminergic systems (serotonin, norepinephrine, and dopamine) in both disorders [26], antidepressant treatment has also been shown to exert effects on mitochondria and inflammation response [25].

Treatment strategies

In patients with migraine and mood disorders, the choice of treatment should be based on the type of comorbid psychiatric conditions, requiring the involvement of a multidisciplinary team constituted by a neurologist and a psychiatrist. Unfortunately, despite the high comorbidity between migraine and psychiatric disorders, it is estimated that less than 2% of patients with migraine are referred to a psychiatrist [27]. The majority of patients with migraine are treated by the primary care physician, and less than 25% are referred to a neurologist [27]. Our case study exemplifies the difficulties in the assessment and management of comorbid MDD and migraines. General strategies and recommendations that can be given to patients with migraine and depression include regular and sufficient sleep, avoidance of alcohol and other drugs, moderate physical exercise, and maintenance of a headache diary.

The pharmacological treatment of migraine can be separated into symptomatic (aimed at aborting the migraine attack) or prophylactic (designed to prevent it). The latter is recommended for patients with four or more migrainous attacks per month and requires daily administration for several months. A study of 102 patients with migraine found that quality of life and ability to function improved significantly after 3 months of prophylactic pharmacological treatment of migraine [28]. There are different medications useful for the prophylactic treatment of comorbid depressive disorders and migraine [29], but a combination of agents with specific therapeutic efficacy in the migrainous and the depressive disorders is frequently required. Therefore, knowing the pharmacokinetic and pharmacodynamic interactions of the different type of agents is mandatory. Table 9.3 lists the main prophylactic drugs used for migraine that also have a therapeutic effect in comorbid psychiatric disorders.

Several studies support the efficacy of amitriptyline, a tryciclic antidepressant (TCA), to treat depression and prevent migraine attacks

Table 9.3 Comparative profile of migraine prophylaxis medications useful for psychiatric symptoms management

Drug (Daily Dose)	Efficacy in Neuropsychiatric Disorders	Efficacy in Migraine Prophylaxis	Side Effects Severity	Main Side Effects
Beta blockers: Propranolol (80–240 mg) Timolol (20–30 mg)	Anxiety symptoms	++++[a]	++	Nausea, fatigue, sexual dysfunction, bronchial spasm, bradycardia
Valproic acid (500–1500 mg)	Bipolar disorder[a], epilepsy[a]	+++	+++	Tremor, hair weakness, weight gain, hepatotoxicity, teratogenic
Topiramate (100 mg)	Epilepsy[a], binge eating	+++[a]	++	Weight decrease, cognitive side effects, kidney stones
Gabapentin (900–2400 mg)	Epilepsy[a], generalized anxiety disorder	++	++	Dizziness, drowsiness, peripheral edema
Amitriptyline (30–150 mg)	Major depression[a]	++++	+++	Anticholinergic effects: constipation, drowsiness, dry mouth, body weight gain, heart blockade
SSRIs: fluoxetine (20–40 mg)	Major depression,[a] anxiety disorders[a]	+/−	+	Nausea, dyspepsia
SNRIs: venlafaxine (150 mg)	Major depression,[a] anxiety disorders[a]	+	+	Nausea, high blood pressure, few interactions

[a]With the indication by the Food and Drug Administration.
SSRIs, serotonin selective reuptake inhibitors; SNRIs, serotonin norepinephrine reuptake inhibitors.

[26, 27, 29]. However, amitriptyline is no longer widely prescribed because of its poor profile with respect to side effects and narrow therapeutic window [27]. In our case study, the patient could probably have benefited earlier from antidepressant drug therapy. Unfortunately, amitryptiline, which could have been the best therapeutic option for this patient since she had a recurrent MDE and migraines, was not well tolerated. When this (or other psychotropic agents) is used, treatment should start with low doses and increase slowly to avoid side effects. Yet, it is also important to remember that therapeutic doses have to be reached. Venlafaxine, a serotonin norepinephrine reuptake inhibitor (SNRI), has been found to be an effective prophylactic treatment for migraine in a controlled trial [29], while also showing good efficacy in the treatment of depressive and anxiety disorders. Other antidepressants, such as serotonin selective reuptake inhibitors (SSRI), seem to be a good adjunctive treatment to migraine prophylactic treatment in patients with an MDE, and can also improve migraine outcomes in some patients [29]. No studies on the treatment of IDD in patients with migraine have been carried out, but epileptic patients with IDD seem to benefit from receiving an SSRI [13].

In the assessment of the patient with migraine who presents with a depressive episode, the differential diagnosis between MDD and bipolar disorder has important clinical repercussions. A self-administered screening instrument forbipolar disorder (the Mood Disorder Questionnaire) can be useful.

The serotonergic syndrome is a life-threatening but very rare adverse reaction of the combination of serotonergic antidepressant drugs, with triptans, lithium, ergotaminics, or other antidepressants (see also Chapter 8).

Some antiepileptic drugs, such as valproic acid, gabapentin, and topiramate, have an excellent profile as prophylactic treatment for migraine [29]. However, these agents also have a psychotropic effect. Valproic acid is the most widely studied antiepileptic drug for migraine prophylaxis and has been found to be an excellent mood-stabilizing agent in bipolar disorder. However, the use of this drug in women at child-bearing age is limited to exceptional circumstances and must be carefully monitored because of its risk of severe teratogenic effects and an increased risk of polycystic ovarian syndrome when taken between menarche and the age of 26 [30]. While it was not a first-line option in our patient, it could be the first-line treatment for male patients with migraine and bipolar disorder because of its mood-stabilizing properties. Topiramate is indicated for the prophylactic treatment of migraine and also for epilepsy treatment. On the other hand, it is associated with cognitive side effects and an increased risk of depressive disorders [31]. Furthermore, its efficacy for bipolar disorder was not supported in controlled trials [29]. Gabapentin has efficacy in migraine treatment and is indicated as a first-line treatment for several anxiety disorders. Lamotrigine seems to have efficacy in the treatment of the aura related to migraine and can be used to prevent depressive recurrences in patients with bipolar disorder [29].

Patients with migraine and comorbid anxiety disorders or high blood pressure should benefit from propranolol treatment. Moreover, the extended opinion that propranolol and other beta blockers could induce depression has been questioned by several studies. A quantitative review of different double-blind controlled trials [32] of the risk of depression in more than 35,000 persons with heart failure, hypertension, or myocardial infarction found no significant differences in the prevalence of major depression between the group treated with placebo and the group treated with beta blockers. Thus, no evidence links propranolol and beta blockers with depression, and from the author's point of view, these drugs can be used as an adjunctive treatment to antidepressants in patients with migraine and comorbid depression, along with serving as an excellent first-line treatment in patients with migraine and comorbid anxiety disorders.

Psychotherapy is a nonpharmacological therapeutic option, which has demonstrated efficacy for both migraine and depression treatment. Cognitive–behavioral therapy and biobehavioral training (i.e., biofeedback, relaxation techniques, and stress management) have demonstrated efficacy in the preventive treatment of migraine and depression and may be used as adjunctive treatment to medications in patients with these comorbid disorders. Therefore, a multidisciplinary therapeutic approach can be necessary, including a neurologist, a psychiatrist, and a psychologist in the therapeutic team [1, 29].

Acknowledgments

The author does not report any financial disclosure or conflict of interests.

Permissions

None requested.

PEARLS TO TAKE HOME

- There is high comorbidity of depressive, bipolar, and anxiety disorders in patients with migraine.
- Migraine with aura is independently linked with an increased risk of suicide in young patients, whether or not there is comorbid depression.
- Psychiatric comorbidities worsen the course of migraine illness and the quality of life of these patients.
- Several self-administered screening tools are available to identify the presence of migraine, depressive and anxiety disorders, and suicidal risk.
- Common pathogenic mechanisms operant in depressive disorders and migraine include abnormalities of serotonin and other neurotransmitter systems, mitochondrial dysfunction, and inflammatory neuromodulator disturbances, which are probably associated with a bidirectional relationship between major depression and migraine.
- Treatment of depressive disorders in patients with migraine must aim for the total remission of psychiatric symptoms.

References

1. Akiskal H. Mood disorders. In: *Comprehensive Textbook of Psychiatry*, eds. B Sadock and V Sadock. New York: Lippincott Williams & Williams, pp. 1559–1575, 2005.
2. World Health Organization. *The World Health Report 2001*. Geneva, Switzerland: World Health Organization, 2001.
3. Jette N, Patten S, Williams J, et al. Comorbidity of migraine and psychiatric disorders—a national population-based study. *Headache*, 48(4): 501–516, 2008.
4. Breslau N, Lipton RB, Stewart WF, et al. Comorbidity of migraine and depression: investigating potential etiology and prognosis. *Neurology*, 60(8): 1308–1312, 2003.
5. Saaman Z, Farmer A, Craddock N, et al. Migraine in recurrent depression: case-control study. *Br J Psychiatry*, 194(4): 350–354, 2009.
6. Breslau N, Schultz LR, Stewart WF, et al. Headache types and panic disorder: directionality and specificity. *Neurology*, 56(3): 350–354, 2001.
7. Fasmer OB. The prevalence of migraine in patients with bipolar and unipolar affective disorders. *Cephalalgia*, 21(9): 894–895, 2001.
8. Breslau N, Davis GC, Andreski P. Migraine, psychiatric disorders, and suicide attempts: an epidemiologic study of young adults. *J Psychiatry Res*, 37(1): 11–23, 1991.
9. Wang S, Juang KD, Fuh J, et al. Psychiatric comorbidity and suicide risk in adolescents with chronic daily headache. *Neurology*, 68: 1468–1473, 2007.
10. Hung CI, Liu CY, Juang YY, et al. The impact of migraine on patients with major depressive disorder. *Headache*, 46(3): 469–477, 2006.
11. Headache Classification Subcommittee of the International Headache Society. The International Classification of Headache Disorders. 2nd ed. *Cephalalgia*, 24, Suppl. 1: 9–160, 2004.
12. American Psychiatric Association. *Diagnostic and Statistical Manual of Mental Disorders*, 4th ed. Text Revised. Washington,

DC: American Psychiatric Association, 2000.

13. Blumer D, Montouris G, Davies K. The interictal dysphoric disorder: recognition, pathogenesis, and treatment of the major psychiatric disorder of epilepsy. *Epilepsy Behav*, 5(6): 826–840, 2004.

14. Sandstrom SA, Bowman ES, Johnson CS, et al. Interictal mood disorder and quality of life in active epilepsy. *Epilepsy Behav*, 17(2): 199–204, 2010.

15. Mula M, Jauch R, Cavanna A, et al. Clinical and psychopathological definition of the interictal dysphoric disorder of epilepsy. *Epilepsia*, 49(4): 650–656, 2008.

16. Oedegaard KJ, Fasmer OB. Is migraine in unipolar depressed patients a bipolar spectrum trait? *J Affect Disord*, 84(2–3): 233–242, 2005.

17. Lipton RB, Hamelsky SW, Kolodner KB, et al. Migraine, quality of life, and depression: a population-based case-control study. *Neurology*, 55: 629–635, 2000.

18. Guidetti V, Galli F. Psychiatric comorbidity in chronic daily headache: pathophysiology, etiology, and diagnosis. *Curr Pain Headache Rep*, 6(6): 492–497, 2002.

19. Hesdorffer DC, Lúdvígsson P, Hauser WA, et al. Co-occurrence of major depression or suicide attempt with migraine with aura and risk for unprovoked seizure. *Epilepsy Res*, 75(2–3): 220–223, 2007.

20. D'Andrea G, Welch K, Riddle J, et al. Platelet serotonin metabolism and ultrastructure in migraine. *Arch Neurol*, 46: 1187–1189, 1989.

21. Lidberg L, Belfrage H, Bertilsson L, et al. Suicide attempts and impulse control disorder are related to low cerebrospinal fluid 5-HIAA in mentally disordered violent offenders. *Acta Psychiatr Scand*, 101: 395–402, 2000.

22. Peroutka SJ, Price SC, Wilhoit TL, et al. Comorbid migraine with aura, anxiety, and depression is associated with dopamine D2 receptor (DRD2) NcoI alleles. *Mol Med*, 4: 14–21, 1998.

23. Stam AH, de Vries B, Janssens AC, et al. Shared genetic factors in migraine and depression: evidence from a genetic isolate. *Neurology*, 74: 288–294, 2010.

24. Schur EA, Noonan C, Buchwald D, et al. A twin study of depression and migraine: evidence for a shared genetic vulnerability. *Headache*, 49: 1493–1502, 2009.

25. Gardner A, Boles RG. Beyond the serotonin hypothesis: mitochondria, inflammation and neurodegeneration in major depression and affective spectrum disorders. *Prog Neuropsychopharmacol Biol Psychiatry*, 35(3): 730–743, 2010 [Epub ahead of print].

26. Bendsten L, Jensen R, Olesen J. A non-selective (amytriptiline), but not a selective (citalopram), serotonin reuptake inhibitor is effective in the prophylactic treatment of chronic tension-type headache. *J Neurol Neurosurg Psychiatry*, 61: 285–290, 1996.

27. Cascade E, Kalali AH, Smitherman TA. Treatment of migraine and the role of psychiatric medications. *Psychiatry (Edgmont)*, 5(10): 20–22, 2008.

28. D'Amico D, Solari A, Usai S, et al. Improvement in quality of life and activity limitations in migraine patients after prophylaxis. A prospective longitudinal multicentre study. *Cephalalgia*, 26: 691–696, 2006.

29. D'Amico D, Tepper SJ. Prophylaxis of migraine: general principles and patient acceptance. *Neuropsychiatr Dis Treat*, 4: 1155–1167, 2008.

30. Morrell MJ, Hayes FJ, Sluss PM, et al. *Ann Neurol*, 64(2): 200–211, 2008.

31. Mula M, Sander JW. Negative effects of antiepileptic drugs on mood in patients with epilepsy. *Drug Saf*, 30(7): 555–567, 2007.

32. Ko DT, Hebert PR, Coffey CS, et al. Beta blocker therapy and symptoms of depression, fatigue, and sexual dysfunction. *JAMA*, 288: 351–357, 2002.

33. Lipton RB, Dodick D, Sadofsky R, et al. A self-administered screener for migraine in primary care: the ID migraine validation study. *Neurology*, 61(3): 375–382, 2003.

34. Bjelland I, Dahl AA, Haug TT, et al. The validity of the Hospital Anxiety and Depression Scale. An updated literature review. *J Psychosom Res*, 52(2): 69–77, 2002.

35. Arnau RC, Meagher MW, Norris MP, et al. Psychometric evaluation of the Beck Depression Inventory-II with primary care

medical patients. *Health Psychol*, 20(2): 112–119, 2001.

36. Twiss J, Jones S, Anderson I. Validation of the Mood Disorder Questionnaire for screening for bipolar disorder in a UK sample. *J Affect Disord*, 110(1–2): 180–184, 2008.

37. Sheehan DV, Lecrubier Y, Sheehan KH, et al. The Mini International Neuropsychiatric Interview (M.I.N.I.): the development and validation of a structured diagnostic psychiatric interview for DSM-IV and ICD-10. *J Clin Psych*, 59, Suppl. 20: 22–33, quiz 34–57, 1998.

Poststroke Depression

Andres M. Kanner
Departments of Neurological Sciences and Psychiatry, Rush Medical College at Rush University; Laboratory of Electroencephalography and Video-EEG-Telemetry; Section of Epilepsy and Rush Epilepsy Center, Rush University Medical Center, Chicago, IL, USA

Introduction

Poststroke depression (PSD) is the most frequent psychiatric complication of stroke [1]. It is associated with a worse recovery of motor and cognitive deficits and a higher mortality risk [1]. Yet, the relation between depression and stroke is not unidirectional, but bidirectional, as not only patients who suffer a stroke have a high prevalence of depression, but patients with depression have a higher risk of suffering from a stroke, even after controlling for the usual risk factors (see below). This chapter provides a very practical review of the epidemiologic aspects of PSD, its most frequent clinical presentations, and the potential pathogenic mechanisms that may explain the bidirectional relation between the two entities. It highlights the negative impact of PSD on the quality of life of these patients, its association with an increased mortality risk and with a lesser likelihood for recovery with respect to cognitive and motor functions, and reviews therapeutic strategies of PSD.

Epidemiologic aspects

The prevalence rates of PSD have ranged between 30% and 50% of patients in several cross-sectional studies [1–4], depending on the patient population studied. One study estimated a pooled prevalence rate of all types of depression at 31.8%

(range: 30–44%) in population-based studies [1, 4–7], with prevalence rates of major depression ranging from 11% to 15%, and minor depression from 8% to 12% [4–7]. In hospital-based studies, the overall prevalence rates ranged from 25% to 47% [3, 8–10], with those of major depressive episodes ranging from 10% to 27% and minor depression between 11% and 20% [3, 8–10]. In studies done in rehabilitation institutions, overall rates ranged from 35% to 72% [11–15], with rates of major depressive episodes ranging from 10% to 40% and of minor depression from 21% to 44% [11–15]. The occurrence of PSD peaks between 3 and 6 months after a stroke [16].

A bidirectional relation between depression and stroke

The term of PSD implies that the depressive episode follows the occurrence of a stroke and/or is one its "complications." Yet, an analysis of the literature included two meta-analyses, both of which suggested that patients with a history of depressive episodes and/or symptoms of depression may be at higher risk of suffering from a stroke [17, 18]. The most recent meta-analysis included the studies used for the first one and reviewed data from 28 prospective cohort studies that encompassed 317,540 subjects among whom 8478 stroke cases were identified during a

Depression in Neurologic Disorders: Diagnosis and Management, First Edition.
Edited by Andres M. Kanner.
© 2012 Blackwell Publishing Ltd. Published 2012 by Blackwell Publishing Ltd.

follow-up period ranging from 2 to 29 years. The investigators found depression is prospectively associated with a significantly increased risk of developing a stroke. For example, pooled adjusted hazard ratios were: 1.45 for total stroke (95% confidence interval [CI], 1.29–1.63), 1.55 for fatal stroke (95% CI, 1.25–1.93), and 1.25 for ischemic stroke (95% CI, 1.11–1.40) [18].

This bidirectional relation does not necessarily establish causality, but is suggestive of the existence of common pathogenic mechanisms that are operant in the two conditions and that when present in one may facilitate the development of the other. The next section summarizes these data.

Depressive episodes may increase the risk of stroke through intrinsic and extrinsic pathogenic mechanisms. The intrinsic mechanisms have the potential to facilitate and/or worsen (1) cardiovascular disease and hypertension, (2) cardiac arrhythmias, (3) diabetes, and (4) immunological disturbances. The extrinsic mechanisms include poor compliance with diet and medication.

Intrinsic mechanisms

Impact of depression on hypertension and cardiovascular disease

A Canadian population-based study followed 12,270 subjects who did not report high blood pressure or the use of antihypertensive medications for a 10-year period. People with a history of major depression had a significantly higher risk of developing high blood pressure, even after adjusting for age (hazard ratio: 1.6 [95% CI 1.2–2.1], $p = 0.001$), indicating a 60% increase in risk [19]. Two other studies found that a history of depression was associated with an increased risk of developing hypertension at follow-up [20, 21], but a prospective study failed to support these data [22]. In addition, five studies found that depression predicted a worse prognosis of coronary artery disease and/or cardiac mortality [23–27].

The potential pathogenic mechanisms operant in depression that can contribute to the development and/or worsening of vascular disease include: (1) a hyperactive hypothalamic–pituitary–adrenal (HHPA) axis, which can facilitate the development of cardiac arrhythmias and

a hypercoagulable state; and (2) immunological disturbances leading to a microvascular inflammation.

An HHPA axis has been demonstrated in 50% of patients with major depressive disorders (see also Chapter 2). It causes elevation of the serum cortisol, which in turn has been associated with an increased risk of atherosclerosis and sympathoadrenal hyperactivity. The latter mechanism yields an increased secretion of catecholamines that leads to vasoconstriction, platelet activation, and an elevated heart rate [28].

Increased sympathetic or decreased parasympathetic activities have been associated with a decreased heart rate variability (HRV) and have been blamed for the development of cardiac arrhythmias and sudden death. For example, in a study of 700 patients with postmyocardial infarction, those with depression had significantly decreased HRV than controls [29]. Other studies have found an association between depressive symptoms and a 30% decrease of baroreflex sensitivity [30], a higher QT variability [31, 32], and a higher risk of ventricular tachycardia [21].

A *hypercoagulable state* has also been associated with an HHPA axis and sympathoadrenal hyperactivity, as hypercortisolism can cause elevation of factor VIII and von Willebrand factor, while catecholamines can lead to an increase in fibrinolysis [33]. In addition, abnormal platelet function has been identified in untreated depressed patients in whom a platelet reactivity of up to 40% greater than controls has been reported [34]. Abnormal platelet function has been associated with abnormalities in platelets' serotonin receptors [35], while treatment with a selective serotonin reuptake inhibitor (SSRI) has been shown to normalize platelet activation [36–38].

Diabetes mellitus is a well-recognized stroke risk factor. Depression has been found to be an independent risk factor for the development of type 2 diabetes after controlling for confounding factors such as race, age, gender, socioeconomic status, level of education, and body weight [39]. The mechanisms responsible for this risk include an increased release of counterregulatory hormones (glucocorticoids, growth hormone, and glucagon) and catecholamines, which counteract the hypoglycemic action of insulin by raising levels of glucagon. These hormonal changes may be responsible, in turn, for the development of insulin resistance. Furthermore, once patients develop diabetes, the presence of depression may be associated with worse glycemic controls, related to an increased difficulty to adhere to a proper diet and worse compliance with hypoglycemic agents.

Inflammatory process

The pathogenic role of inflammatory processes has been identified in the development of primary depressive disorders as well as of stroke. This pathogenic mechanism may therefore play a key role in the development of PSD and of stroke in patients with depression. Thus, stroke has been associated with an increased synthesis of proinflammatory cytokines such as interleukin-1β (IL-1β), tumor necrosis factor-alpha (TNF-α), or IL-18. For example, 108 patients with stroke admitted to the hospital within the first 24 hours after stroke onset were followed for up to 6 months; 37 patients were found to meet criteria for a major depression at 2 weeks. Serum IL-18 on day 7 was significantly higher in patients with PSD than those without, while serum IL-18 >377.84 pg/mL on day 7 was independently associated with PSD at the acute stage of stroke (odds ratio [OR]: 12.280, 95% CI: 3.848–39.190, $p < 0.001$ after adjustment) [40]. At 6 months, 31 patients (33.0%) were diagnosed with major depression. Serum IL-18 >376.67 pg/mL on day 7 was also independently associated with PSD at 6 months (OR: 7.431, 95% CI: 1.741–31.712, $p = 0.007$ after adjustment).

Spalletta et al. have postulated that the development of PSD can be related to an amplification of the inflammatory process by the above cited cytokines, particularly in limbic areas, and widespread activation of indoleamine 2,3-dioxygenase (IDO) and subsequently to depletion of serotonin in paralimbic regions such as the ventral lateral frontal cortex, polar temporal cortex, and basal ganglia [41]. Likewise, the pathogenic role of cytokines has been documented as increased plasma concentrations of IL-1β and TNF-α have been found in patients with dysthymia or major depressive disorder, while IL-6 and IL-18 have been found to be overexpressed in patients with depression in general.

Extrinsic factors

Depression has been associated with poor compliance with pharmacotherapy and other treatments. For example, in a meta-analysis that included 20 studies of adult and pediatric patients with a variety of diseases , patients with depression were three times more likely than patients without depression to be nonadherent to medical treatment recommendations including medications, diet, and behavior changes [42]. In another study, the existence of symptoms of depression was investigated in 2180 older adults with hypertension with the Center for Epidemiologic Studies Depression Scale (CES-D), the Medical Outcomes Study Social Support Index, and the hypertension-specific Morisky Medication Adherence Scale at baseline and 1 year later [43]. After multivariable adjustment, the OR that participants with depressive symptoms would have low medication adherence were 1.96 (95% CI 1.43, 2.70) at baseline and 1.87 (95% CI 1.32, 2.66) at 1-year follow-up.

Stroke-related pathogenic factors operant in PSD

The various factors associated with PSD have included location and size of the stroke, timing of PSD relative to the stroke, and size of the lateral ventricles. The relationship between location of stroke and PSD has been the most extensively investigated, yielding contradictory findings. For example, Robinson et al. reported a relationship between PSD and a left hemispheric stroke, in particular involving left frontal dorsal–lateral cortical regions [44] and left (but not right) basal ganglia. Robinson and Szetela had also observed an inverse relationship between the severity of PSD and the proximity of the stroke to the frontal pole [45]. Yet, in a review of data from 12 studies, Singh et al. found that only four studies supported these data, six studies failed to support any relationship between location of stroke and PSD, while two studies suggested a higher likelihood of PSD in right-sided stroke [8]. Another study found that small subcortical lesions of the left hemisphere were associated with a higher frequency of depression than right-sided lesions [46].

Based on a review of the PSD literature, Cummings and Mega concluded that the relationship between location of stroke and PSD was tied to timing of the onset of depressive symptoms after the stroke [47]. Thus, in the first 10 days following a stroke, there is a higher frequency of PSD associated with left than right hemisphere lesions, while this relationship disappears if the onset of symptoms of depression takes place 3 months after the stroke. Furthermore, these authors reported that when symptoms of depression appear more than 1 year after the stroke, right-sided lesions are more frequent.

The presence of cortical atrophy and enlarged ventricles has been suggested as a potential risk factor for PSD. Starkstein et al. compared the magnitude of subcortical atrophy in brain computed tomography (CT) studies obtained immediately after the stroke [48]. Patients with PSD had a significantly greater degree of atrophy than those without depression.

Two studies have demonstrated a significant correlation between severity of disability and depression [49, 50], but this association has been inconsistent in studies in which the poststroke follow-up evaluation time was longer [51]. These data suggest that disability may cause a reactive depressive process in the early stages after stroke, but probably does not mediate the development of PSD in the long term. In a review of the literature, Robinson and Szetela concluded that the severity of impairment in activities of daily living (ADL) has a limited impact on PSD [45]. For example, Robinson and Benson reported a significantly higher prevalence of PSD among patients with nonfluent aphasia but not among patients with fluent aphasia [52].

Clinical manifestations

Major depression and minor depression are the most frequently recognized expressions of PSD, although the existence of a depressive disorder specific to stroke, also referred to as vascular depression (VD), has been described.

In general, the clinical semiology of PSD is similar to that of primary late-onset depression, with the caveat that psychomotor retardation may be more frequently identified among patients with PSD. In fact, the presence of slowness or psychomotor retardation in patients with

PSD was the only symptom distinguishing PSD from idiopathic depressed patients who, in turn, reported more anhedonia and more difficulty with concentration [53]. Catastrophic depressive reactions, hyperemotionalism, and diurnal mood variation were also found to be more common in PSD than idiopathic depression in one study [54]. The severity of PSD has been found to correlate with the degree of impairment of ADL during both its acute and chronic phases. In addition, the presence of PSD can enhance the severity of vegetative symptoms. In fact, in a study by Fedoroff and colleagues, vegetative symptoms consisting of disturbances of sleep, libido, and level of energy were significantly more frequent among patients with depression than patients without depression at initial evaluation, and at 3, 6, 12, and 24 months [3].

PSD is likely to occur in the first months after a stroke. In a study of 100 patients with stroke followed for 18 months, symptoms of PSD were identified in 46% of patients during the first 2 months, while only 12% of patients experienced their first symptoms 12 months after their stroke [55]. Among the patients with early-onset PSD, symptoms of depression persisted 12 and 18 months later. In addition, the course of PSD can be rather lengthy. For example, symptoms of major depression identified in 27% of patients with a stroke persisted for approximately 1 year, while symptoms of minor depression in 20% of patients with stroke lasted for more than 2 years [13].

Duration of PSD symptoms appears to depend on the vascular territory of the stroke, with longer durations being identified in patients with a stroke in the territory of the middle cerebral artery than in the posterior circulation. In one study, 82% of patients with middle cerebral artery stroke continued to be symptomatic at 6-month follow-up visits versus 20% of those with posterior circulation strokes, while at 12 and 24 months none of the latter exhibited symptoms, but 62% of the former did [56].

VD was described by Alexopoulos et al. [57] as consisting of symptoms of depression beginning after the age of 65 that include mood abnormalities, neuropsychological disturbances with impairment of executive functions, a greater tendency to psychomotor retardation, poor insight, and impaired ADL. A family history of depression has been found to be less frequent in VD.

This form of depression has been identified in patients with clinical and/or neuroradiologic evidence of diffuse bilateral white matter small vessel disease who present chronic cerebrovascular risk factors such as hypertension, diabetes, carotid stenosis, atrial fibrillation, and hypelipidemia [58]. Yet, these patients may or may not have experienced an overt stroke, or may have reported only a transient ischemic attack.

Impact of PSD on the course of the stroke

The presence of PSD affects the course of stroke at various levels, including a worse recovery of cognitive impairments and impairment in ADL and an increased mortality risk. For example, one study found that patients with major PSD had significantly more cognitive deficits than patients without depression with similar location and size strokes in the left hemisphere but not in right hemisphere strokes [48]. In a follow-up study of 140 patients, Robinson et al. also found that the presence of major PSD was associated with greater cognitive impairment 2 years after a stroke [9]. Likewise, in-hospital PSD was the most important predictor of poor recovery of ADL in a study that followed patients over a 2-year period [59]. In fact, the score of in-hospital ADL was not associated with the 2-year recovery.

Early poststroke symptoms of depression have been associated with a worse course of the neurologic disturbances. In a population-based study (Northern Manhattan Stroke Study) conducted in a multiethnic urban population, the existence of depressed mood within 7–10 days after stroke was investigated in 340 of 655 patients with ischemic stroke enrolled, and 139 reported that they felt depressed. Participants were followed every 6 months the first 2 years and yearly thereafter for 5 years for death and disability measured by the Barthel Index. Depressed mood was associated with a greater odds of severe disability compared with no disability at 1 (OR 2.91, 95% CI 1.07–7.91) and 2 years (OR 3.72, 95% CI 1.29–10.71) after stroke [60].

The presence of PSD has been associated with a higher mortality risk. For example, a higher 3-year mortality risk was found in patients with PSD despite the fact that these patients were younger and had fewer chronic conditions than the comparison group [61]. In a population-based study of 10,025 subjects, the existence of symptoms of depression was identified with the CES-D. Four groups were created based on history of stroke and depression status at baseline: (1) no stroke, no depression (reference group); (2) no stroke, depression present; (3) history of stroke, no depression; and (4) stroke present, depression present. A total of 1925 deaths were documented over an 8-year period, with the highest mortality rate found in the group with both a history of stroke and depression at baseline. The following are the hazard rates relative to the reference group: no stroke, depression present, 1.23 (95% CI 1.08–1.40); stroke present, no depression 1.74 (1.06–2.85); and stroke present, depression present, 1.88 (1.27–2.79) [40]. Another study found that patients with PSD were 3.4 times more likely to die during a 10-year follow-up period than patients without depression, after adjusting for other common stroke risk factors [62].

The use of antidepressant drugs has been found to be associated with a decrease in the mortality rate of patients with stroke. In one study, 104 patients with stroke were randomly assigned to receive a 12-week double-blind course of nortriptyline, fluoxetine, or placebo early in the recovery period [63]. Mortality data were obtained for all patients 9 years after initiation of the study. Fifty (48.1%) had died during the follow-up period. Thirty-six of the 53 patients randomized to antidepressants (67.9%) were alive at follow-up, compared with only 10 (35.7%) of 28 placebo-treated patients. The protective effect of antidepressants was not limited to patients with depression. Likewise, Robinson et al. found that patients treated with fluoxetine or nortriptyline had an increased survival probability at 6 years (61%) compared with that of patients given placebo (34%) [64].

Treatment of PSD

Despite the high prevalence of PSD, the number of controlled trials of antidepressant drugs remains small. For example, a recent meta-analysis identified 10 studies, of which six compared their efficacy to that of placebo [65]. The investigators concluded that antidepressants were superior to placebo (OR: 2.58, 95% CI: 1.56–4.26, $p = 0.0002$). For example, in a double-blind placebo-controlled study of fluoxetine (at doses of 20 mg/day), patients on active drug and placebo experienced comparable improvement during the first 4 weeks; by 12 weeks, however, patients on fluoxetine continued to improve while those on placebo had experienced recurrence of their depressive symptoms [66]. Robinson et al. compared fluoxetine at 40 mg/day, nortriptyline at 100 mg/day, and placebo in 56 patients with PSD [64]. Patients on placebo and fluoxetine did not differ in their response to therapy, while those on nortriptyline showed a significant improvement. Wiart et al. found a superior response to fluoxetine at 10 mg/day than to placebo in 31 patients with PSD [67], while Lipsey et al. demonstrated efficacy of nortriptyline in a double-blind, placebo-controlled study carried out in 34 patients, 14 of whom were on active drug and 20 of whom were on placebo [68]. Patients on nortriptyline showed a significantly greater improvement in their depression after 6 weeks of therapy.

As with the treatment of primary depressive disorder, the treatment of PSD is aimed at achieving complete symptom remission. In PSD, a successful treatment can be associated with a better recovery of neurologic deficits. For example, Kimura et al. showed that responders to treatment with antidepressant medication had higher scores in the Mini-Mental State Exam compared with nonresponders [69]. Chemerinski et al. found that successful treatment of PSD with nortriptyline was significantly associated with recovery of ADL [70, 71]. Likewise, in a study of 49 patients with PSD, 25 were treated with antidepressant medication and 24 were not. Treated patients were significantly more likely to achieve symptom remission and recovery of motor deficits and disability than those untreated. Furthermore, patients who were not treated had a worse recovery than those without depression [40, 72]. However, a positive impact of antidepressant treatment on neurologic deficits has not been shown in all studies; double-blind controlled studies of citalopram and nortriptyline failed to show improvement in cognitive deficits even in the presence of improvement of depression [64, 68].

Prevention of PSD with antidepressant medication has been shown in two controlled studies. In one study, 137 patients were randomized to sertraline (at doses of 50–150 mg/day) and placebo within the first month after their stroke, and were treated for 1 year [47, 73]. Among the treated patients, 8.3% of patients developed a PSD compared to 22.8% of patients on placebo ($p = 0.037$). In a separate study, 48 patients without depression were randomized to receive fluoxetine, nortriptyline, and placebo for a 3-month period [48, 74]. Patients on placebo were more likely to develop a PSD than those treated with the antidepressant drugs ($p = 0.036$).

Concluding remarks

The data reviewed in this chapter show that PSD is relatively frequent and associated with a worse course of the neurologic disorder. Its treatment seems to yield a remission of psychiatric symptoms and an improvement in the neurologic deficits, though these findings were not supported by all studies and need to be replicated in larger cohorts.

Depressive disorders and stroke have a bidirectional relationship which results from the existence of common pathogenic mechanisms operant in both disorders, which may also account for the worse course of the stroke in patients with PSD. Sadly, depression remains underrecognized and undertreated both by clinicians and investigators of stroke treatments. Furthermore, despite the unquestionable data of the impact of depression on the risk of stroke, the presence of a PSD is yet to be included among the variables associated with outcome in most of the randomized studies of stroke therapies. It is time that neurologists recognize depression as an expression of brain disease and not as a mere reactive process to an adverse situation.

Illustrative case

A 66-year-old gentleman with a prior history of type 2 diabetes and hypertension woke up with a right hemiplegia (affecting the arm more than the leg) and an expressive aphasia and was taken to the emergency room. He was somnolent, but easily arousable on admission and was able to follow commands. A brain magnetic resonance imaging (MRI) revealed an ischemic stroke in the left frontal region, in addition to bilateral lacunar infarcts in periventricular regions. After 3 days in the intensive care unit he was transferred to the neurology floor where speech, occupational, and physical therapies were started. Two weeks later he was moved to a rehabilitation facility, where he was noted to be making steady progress in the recovery of motor and language functions. He was discharged 6 weeks later to an outpatient rehabilitation program. Five months after his stroke, he was noted by his wife to become more withdrawn and to be more tired than usual after his physical therapy. Two weeks later he started to cry constantly without any reason; he refused to eat and to leave his room. His wife reported that he started to wake up around 3:00 A.M. and stay awake for the rest of the night.

When he was evaluated by his physiatrist, he was found to have lost most of the gains he had made in motor functions of the right hand. He had lost 15 pounds of weight, relative to his weight at the time of discharge from the inpatient rehabilitation facility. A diagnosis of PSD was made and he was started on fluoxetine at a dose of 20 mg/day, with subsequent increments 4 weeks later to 40 mg/day and then to 60 mg/day 3 weeks later because of no clinical improvement. He was then switched to duloxetine, starting with a dose of 30 mg/day, which was then increased to 60 mg/day. On this antidepressant, the patient appeared less withdrawn, displayed a better appetite and gained 5 pounds over 2 weeks and started to participate more in his physical, occupational, and speech therapy. Unfortunately, he developed an acute severe pain in the right eye which was found to be caused by narrow angle glaucoma and for which the duloxetine had to be discontinued. One week later, his symptoms of depression recurred and he started to refuse to participate in any activity, eat, and had to be hospitalized in an inpatient psychiatric unit where he underwent nine courses of electroshock therapy over a 3-week period, which resulted in the remission of the depressive disorder.

PEARLS TO TAKE HOME

- PSD is a common psychiatric comorbidity, with prevalence rates ranging between 30% and 50%, which peaks 3–6 months after a stroke.
- Depression and stroke have a bidirectional relationship, as not only patients with stroke are at greater risk of developing depression, but patients with depression have a twofold greater risk of developing a stroke even after controlling for other risk factors of stroke.
- Common pathogenic mechanisms operant in both conditions explain the bidirectional relation between stroke and depression and include immunological, cardiovascular, and coagulation disturbances.
- The clinical manifestations of PSD are similar to those of primary late-onset depression, with major and minor depressive episodes being the most frequent presentations of PSD.
- VD is a particular form of late-onset PSD (after the age of 65) identified in patients that may have had overt or silent stroke(s) or subcortical bilateral white matter ischemic disease, presenting with mood and cognitive disturbances with impairment of executive functions, psychomotor retardation, poor insight, and impaired ADL.
- PSD impacts a negative impact on the quality of life of patients with stroke and is associated with a worse recovery of cognitive deficits, impaired ADL, and with an increased mortality risk.
- Pharmacological treatment with antidepressant drugs can facilitate the remission of depressive episodes and decrease the mortality risk of these patients.

References

1. Robinson RG. Poststroke depression: prevalence, diagnosis, treatment and disease progression. *Biol Psychiatry*, 54: 376–387, 2003.

2. Eastwood MR, Rifat SL, Nobbs H, et al. Mood disorder following cerebrovascular accident. *Br J Psychiatry*, 154: 195–200, 1989.

3. Fedoroff JP, Starkstein SE, Parikh RM, et al. Are depressive symptoms non-specific in patients with acute stroke? *Am J Psychiatry*, 148: 1172–1176, 1991.

4. Burvill PW, Johnson GA, Jamrozik KD, et al. Prevalence of depression after stroke: the Perth Community Stroke Study. *Br J Psychiatry*, 166: 320–327, 1995.

5. House A, Dennis M, Mogridge L, et al. Mood disorders in the year after first stroke. *Br J Psychiatry*, 158: 83–92, 1991.

6. Kotila M, Numminen H, Waltimo O, et al. Depression after stroke. Results of the FINNSTROKE study. *Stroke*, 29: 368–372, 1998.

7. Wade DT, Legh-Smith J, Hewer RA. Depressed mood after stroke, a community study of its frequency. *Br J Psychiatry*, 151: 200–205, 1987.

8. Singh A, Black SE, Herrmann N, et al. Functional and neuroanatomic correlations in poststroke depression. The Sunnybrook Stroke Study. *Stroke*, 31: 637–644, 2000.

9. Robinson RG, Starr LB, Kubos KL, et al. A two year longitudinal study of post-stroke mood disorders: findings during the initial evaluation. *Stroke*, 14: 736–744, 1983.

10. Ebrahim S, Barer D, Nouri F. Affective illness after stroke. *Br J Psychiatry*, 151: 52–56, 1987.

11. Eastwood MR, Rifat SL, Nobbs H, et al. Mood disorder following cerebrovascular accident. *Br J Psychiatry*, 154: 195–200, 1989.

12. Folstein MF, Maiberger R, McHugh PR. Mood disorder as a specific complication of stroke. *J Neurol Neurosurg Psychiatry*, 40: 1018–1020, 1977.

13. Morris PLP, Robinson RG, Raphael B. Prevalence and course of depressive disorders in hospitalized stroke patients. *Intl J Psychiatr Med*, 20: 349–364, 1990.

14. Schubert DSP, Taylor C, Lee S, et al. Physical consequences of depression in the stroke patient. *Gen Hosp Psychiatry*, 14: 69–76, 1992.

15. Schwartz JA, Speed NM, Brunberg JA, et al. Depression in stroke rehabilitation. *Biol Psychiatry*, 33: 694–699, 1993.

16. Huff W, Steckel R, Sistzer M. Poststroke depression: risk factors and effects on the course of the stroke. *Nervenarzt*, 74: 104–114, 2003.

17. Van Der Kooy K, van Hout H, Marwijk H, et al. Depression and the risk for cardiovascular diseases: systematic review and meta analysis. *Int J Geriatr Psychiatry*, 22(7): 613–626, 2007.

18. Pan A, Sun Q, Okereke OI, et al. Depression and risk of stroke morbidity and mortality: a meta-analysis and systematic review. *JAMA*, 306(11): 1241–1249, 2011.

19. Patten SB, Jwilliams JVA, Lavorato DH, et al. Major depression as a risk factor for high blood pressure: epidemiologic evidence from a national longitudinal study. *Psychosom Med*, 71(3): 273–279, 2009.

20. Davidson K, Jonas BS, Dixon KE, et al. Do depression symptoms predict early hypertension incidence in young adults in the CARDIA study? Coronary Artery Risk Development in Young Adults. *Arch Intern Med*, 160: 1495–1500, 2000.

21. Carney RM, Freedland KE, Rich MW, et al. Ventricular tachycardia and psychiatric depression in patients with coronary artery disease. *Am J Med*, 95: 23–28, 1993.

22. Jonas BS, Lando JF. Negative affect as a prospective risk factor for hypertension. *Psychosom Med*, 62: 188–196, 2000.

23. Lesperance F, Frasure-Smith N, Juneau M, et al. Depression and 1-year prognosis in unstable angina. *Arch Intern Med*, 160: 1354–1360, 2000.

24. Lesperance F, Frasure-Smith N, Talajic M. Major Depression before and after myocardial infarction: its nature and consequences. *Psychosom Med*, 58: 99–110, 1996.

25. Carney RM, Rich MW, Freedland KE, et al. Major depressive disorder predicts cardiac events in patients with coronary artery disease. *Psychosom Med*, 50: 627–633, 1988.

26. Carney RM, Rich MW, Tevelde A, et al. Major depressive disorder in coronary artery disease. *Am J Cardiol*, 60: 1273–1275, 1987.

27. Frasure-Smith N, Lesperance F, Talajic M. Depression following myocardial infarction. Impact on 6 month survival. *JAMA*, 270: 1819–1825, 1993.

28. Troxler RG, Sprague EA, Albanese RA, et al. The association of elevated plasma cortisol

and early atherosclerosis as demonstrated by coronary angiography. *Atherosclerosis*, 26: 151–162, 1977.

29. Carney RM, Blumenthal JA, Stein PK, et al. Depression, heart rate variability, and acute myocardial infarction. *Circulation*, 104: 2024–2028, 2001.

30. Watkins LL, Grossman P. Association of depressive symptoms with reduced baroreflex cardiac control in coronary artery disease. *Am Heart J*, 137: 453–457, 1999.

31. Yeragani VK, Pohl R, Jampala VC, et al. Increased QT variability in patients with panic disorder and depression. *Psychiatry Res*, 93: 225–235, 2000.

32. Nahshoni E, Aizenberg D, Strasberg B, et al. QT dispersion in the surface electrocardiogram in elderly patients with major depression. *J Affect Disord*, 60: 197–200, 2000.

33. Musselman DL, Tomer A, Manatunga AK, et al. Exaggerated platelet reactivity in major depression. *Am J Psychiatry*, 153: 1313–1317, 1996.

34. Kuijpers PM, Hamulyak K, Strik JJ, et al. Beta-thromboglobulin and platelet factor 4 levels in post-myocardial infarction patients with major depression. *Psychiatry Res*, 109: 207–210, 2002.

35. Mendelson SD. The current status of the platelet 5-HT(2A) receptor in depression. *J Affect Disord*, 57: 13–24, 2002.

36. Serebruany VL, O'Connor CM, Gurbel PA. Effect of selective serotonin reuptake inhibitors on platelets in patients with coronary artery disease. *Am J Cardiol*, 87: 1398–1400, 2001.

37. Serebruany VL, Gurbel PA, O'Connor CM. Platelet inhibition by sertraline and N-demethylsertraline: a possible missing link between depression, coronary events, and mortality benefits of selective serotonin reuptake inhibitors. *Pharmacol Res*, 43: 453–462, 2001.

38. Musselman DL, Marzec UM, Manatunga A, et al. Platelet reactivity in depressed patients treated with paroxetine: preliminary findings. *Arch Gen Psychiatry*, 57: 875–882, 2000.

39. Eaton WW, Armenian H, Gallo J, et al. Depression and risk for onset of type II diabetes: a prospective population-based study. *Diabetes Care*, 22: 1097–1102, 1996.

40. Ellis C, Zhao Y, Egede LE. Depression and increased risk of death in adults with stroke. *J Psychosom Res*, 68(6): 545–551, 2010.

41. Spalletta G, Bossu P, Ciaramella A, et al. The etiology of poststroke depression: a review of the literature and a new hypothesis involving inflammatory cytokines. *Molecular Psychiatry*, 11: 984–991, 2006.

42. DiMatteo MR, Giordani PJ, Lepper HS, et al. Patient adherence and medical treatment outcomes: a meta-analysis. *Med Care*, 40: 794–811, 2002.

43. Krousel-Wood M, Islam T, Muntner P, et al. Association of depression with antihypertensive medication adherence in older adults: cross-sectional and longitudinal findings from CoSMO. *Ann Behav Med*, 40(3): 248–257, 2010.

44. Robinson RG, Kubos KL, Starr LB, et al. Mood changes in stroke patients: relation to lesion location. *Brain*, 107: 81–93, 1984.

45. Robinson RG, Szetela B. Mood changes following left hemisphere brain injury. *Ann Neurol*, 91: 447–453, 1981.

46. Starkstein SE, Robinson RG, Berther ML, et al. Depressive disorders following posterior circulation as compared with middle cerebral artery infarcts. *Brain*, 11: 375–387, 1988.

47. Cummings JL, Mega JL. Disturbances of mood and affect: cerebrovascular Disease. In: *Neuropsychiatry and Behavioral Neuroscience*. New York: Oxford University Press, pp. 206–207, 2003.

48. Starkstein SE, Robinson RG, Price TR. Comparison of patients with and without post-stroke major depression matched for age and location of lesion. *Arch Gen Psychiatry*, 45: 247–252, 1988.

49. Starkstein SE, Moran TH, Bowersox JA, et al. Behavioral abnormalities induced by frontal cortical and nucleus accumbens lesions. *Brain Res*, 473: 74–80, 1988.

50. Bolla-Wilson K, Robinson RG, Starkstein SE, et al. Lateralization of dementia of depression in stroke patients. *Am J Psychiatry*, 146: 627–634, 1989.

51. Downhill J, Robinson RG. Longitudinal assessment of depression and cognitive

impairment following stroke. *J Nerv Ment Dis*, 182: 425–431, 1994.

52. Robinson RG, Benson DF. Depression in aphasic patients: frequency, severity and clinical pathological correlations. *Brain Lang*, 14: 282–291, 1981.

53. Lipsey JR, Robinson RG, Pearlson GD, et al. Nortriptyline treatment of post-stroke depression. A double-blind study. *Lancet*, 1(8372): 297–300, 1984.

54. Gainotti G, Azzoni A, Marra C. Frequency, phenomenology and anatomical-clinical correlates of major post-stroke depression. *Br J Psychiatry*, 175: 163–167, 1999.

55. Berg A, Palomaki H, Letitihalmes M, et al. Post stroke depression: an 18-month follow-up. *Stroke*, 34: 138–143, 2003.

56. Robinson RG, Price TR. Post-stroke depressive disorders: a follow-up study of 103 outpatients. *Stroke*, 13: 635–641, 1982.

57. Alexopoulos GS, Meyers BS, Young RC, et al. Vascular depression hypothesis. *Arch Gen Psychiatry*, 54: 915–922, 1997.

58. Mast BT, MacNeill SE, Lichtenberg PA. Poststroke and clinically-defined vascular depression in geriatric rehabilitation patients. *Am J Geriatr Psychiatry*, 12: 84–92, 2004.

59. Parikh RM, Robinson RG, Lipsey JR, et al. The impact of post-stroke depression on recovery in activities of daily living over two year follow-up. *Arch Neurol*, 47: 785–789, 1990.

60. Willey JZ, Disla N, Moon YP, et al. Early depressed mood after stroke predicts long-term disability: the Northern Manhattan Stroke Study (NOMASS). *Stroke*, 41(9): 1896–1900, 2010.

61. Williams LS, Ghose SS, Swindle RW. Depression and other mental health diagnoses increase mortality risk after ischemic stroke. *Am J Psychiatry*, 161: 1090–1095, 2004.

62. Morris PL, Robinson RG, Andrzejewski P, et al. Association of depression with 10-year poststroke mortality. *Am J Psychiatry*, 150: 124–129, 1993.

63. Jorge RE, Robinson RG, Arndt S, et al. Mortality and poststroke depression: a placebo-controlled trial of antidepressants. *Am J Psychiatry*, 160(10): 1823–1829, 2003.

64. Robinson RG, Schultz SK, Castillo C, et al. Nortriptyline versus fluoxetine in the treatment of depression and in short term recovery after stroke: a placebo controlled, double-blind study. *Am J Psychiatry*, 157: 351–359, 2000.

65. Price A, Rayner L, Okon-Rocha E, et al. Antidepressants for the treatment of depression in neurological disorders: a systematic review and meta-analysis of randomised controlled trials. *J Neurol Neurosurg Psychiatry*, 82: 914–923, 2011.

66. Fruehwald S, Gatterbauer E, Rehak P, et al. Early fluoxetine treatment of poststroke depression: a three month double-blind-placebo-controlled study with an open-label long-term follow-up. *J Neurol*, 250: 347–351, 2003.

67. Wiast L, Petit H, Joseph PA, et al. Fluoxetine in early post-stroke depression: a double-blind-placebo-controlled study. *Stroke*, 31: 1829–1832, 2000.

68. Lipsey JR, Robinson RG, Pearlson GD, et al. Nortriptyline treatment of post-stroke depression: a double-blind study. *Lancet*, 1: 297–300, 1984.

69. Kimura M, Robinson RG, Kosier T. Treatment of cognitive impairment after poststroke depression. *Stroke*, 31: 1482–1486, 2000.

70. Chemerinski E, Robinson RG, Arndt S, et al. The effect of remission of poststroke depression on activities of daily living in a double-blind randomized treatment study. *J Nerv Ment Dis*, 189: 421–425, 2001.

71. Chemerinski E, Robinson RG, Kosier JT. Improved recovery in activities of daily living associated with remission of post-stroke depression. *Stroke*, 32: 113–117, 2001.

72. Gainotti G, Antonucci G, Marra C, et al. Relation between depression after stroke, antidepressant therapy and functional recovery. *J Neurol Neurosurg Psychiatry*, 71: 258–261, 2001.

73. Rasmussen A, Lunde M, Poulsen DL, et al. A double-blind-placebo-controlled study of sertraline in the prevention of depression in stroke patients. *Psychosomatics*, 44: 216–222, 2003.

74. Narushima K, Kosier JT, Robinson RG. Preventing of Poststroke depression. A 12-week double-blind randomized treatment trial with 21 month follow-up. *J Nerv Ment Dis*, 190: 296–303, 2002.

Depressive Disorders in Epilepsy

Andres M. Kanner
Departments of Neurological Sciences and Psychiatry, Rush Medical College at
Rush University; Laboratory of Electroencephalography and Video-EEG-
Telemetry; Section of Epilepsy and Rush Epilepsy Center, Rush University Medical
Center, Chicago, IL, USA

Introduction

Depressive disorders (DDs) are the most common comorbid psychiatric disorder in patients with epilepsy (PWE) [1]. While their clinical manifestations may be identical to those of primary DD, they often have an atypical presentation with pleomorphic symptomatology, including prominent symptoms of anxiety and irritability, and fail to meet any diagnostic classification listed in the *Diagnostic Statistical Manual of Mental Disorders*, Fourth Edition, Text Revision (DSM-IV-TR) [2]. DDs in epilepsy are the expression of interplay between neurobiological (including genetic), iatrogenic, and psychosocial pathogenic mechanisms. In the last two decades, several studies have suggested the existence of a bidirectional relationship between DD and epilepsy [3–5], which probably results from the presence of common pathogenic mechanisms [6].

DDs can have significant negative impact in the life of PWE, including a worse quality of life, increased suicidal risk, and worse tolerance to antiepileptic drugs (AEDs), and have been associated with an increased risk of treatment-resistant epilepsy and a lower probability of becoming completely seizure free after epilepsy surgery. This chapter reviews the most relevant epidemiologic and clinical aspects of DDs in epilepsy, the pathogenic mechanisms that explain their high comorbidity and worse course of the seizure disorder, and the therapeutic strategies of which neurologists should be aware.

Epidemiologic aspects

Population-based studies have shown that one in three to one in four PWE have experienced a DD in the course of their life [1]. In a Canadian study, the lifetime prevalence of mood disorders was 24% in PWE compared with 13% in controls, while 17% had a lifetime history of a major depressive disorder compared with 10% of controls [1]. Including dysthymia, the lifetime prevalence rate of DD increased to 34.2% (25.0–43.3%). Of note, depressive and anxiety disorders frequently occur together. In the Canadian study, the prevalence rate of lifetime comorbid anxiety and DDs was 34.2% (25.0–43.3%) in PWE versus 19.6% (19.0-20.2%) in people without epilepsy.

Studies conducted in epilepsy centers, which provide treatment to patients with more severe seizure disorders, also reveal a high comorbid occurrence of DD, often with anxiety disorders. In a study of 188 consecutive outpatients with epilepsy from five tertiary epilepsy centers, 57 (30%) were found to be suffering from a current depressive episode [7]. Of those, 31 (16%) met diagnostic criteria for a major depressive episode, 21 of whom were also experiencing one or more

Depression in Neurologic Disorders: Diagnosis and Management, First Edition.
Edited by Andres M. Kanner.
© 2012 Blackwell Publishing Ltd. Published 2012 by Blackwell Publishing Ltd.

anxiety disorders, while 26 (14%) presented with a subsyndromic form of a depressive episode, 12 of whom were also experiencing a comorbid anxiety disorder.

Despite their relatively high prevalence, DDs remain underrecognized and undertreated in PWE. Wiegartz et al. reported that 38% of 76 PWE with lifetime histories of major depressive episodes had never been referred for treatment [8]. In a study of 97 children and adults with epilepsy and a DD severe enough to warrant pharmacotherapy, Kanner et al. determined that 63% of patients with spontaneous depression and 54% of patients with an iatrogenic depression were symptomatic for more than 1 year before treatment was initiated [9]. Ettinger et al. identified symptoms of depression in 26% of 44 children with epilepsy—all were undiagnosed and untreated [10].

Negative impact of DDs in the life of PWE

Impact on treatment response of the seizure disorder

Two studies have shown that a history of depression and/or the presence of symptoms of depression at the time of diagnosis of epilepsy can be associated with a higher risk of pharmacoresistance to AEDs [11, 12]. In a study of 780 patients with new onset epilepsy, Hitiris et al. found that individuals with a history of psychiatric disorders, particularly depression, were twofold less likely to be seizure free with AEDs after a median follow-up of 79 months compared to patients without a psychiatric history [11]. Likewise, in a study of 138 patients with new onset epilepsy, Petrovski et al. found that patients with symptoms of depression and anxiety at the time of diagnosis of epilepsy were significantly less likely to be seizure free at the 1-year follow-up evaluation [12]. Furthermore, a lifetime history of depression has been found to be associated with a worse postsurgical seizure outcome following an anterotemporal lobectomy. In a study of 100 consecutive patients with treatment-resistant temporal lobe epilepsy (TLE) who had an anterotemporal lobectomy, Kanner et al. found a lifetime history of depression in only 12% of patients who became free of auras and disabling seizures

in contrast to 79% of patients with persistent disabling seizures [13]. Likewise, in a study of 121 patients who underwent a temporal lobectomy, Anhoury et al. found a significant association between presurgical psychiatric history and worse postsurgical seizure outcome [14].

Increased suicidality risk

Suicide is one of the most serious complications of DDs in PWE. In a population-based study conducted in Denmark, Christensen et al. found that PWE without any psychosocial problems had a twofold higher risk of committing suicide; this risk increased by 32-fold in the presence of a mood disorder [15]. In a review of 11 studies, Harris and Barraclough [16] found the overall suicide rate in PWE to be five times higher than in the general population and 25 times greater for patients with TLE. In a review of 21 published studies that investigated the frequency of death by suicide, Jones et al. [17] found that a mean of 11.5% of all deaths among PWE were attributed to suicide (compared with 1.1–1.2% in the general population).

The relationship between suicidality and epilepsy is complex and multifactorial. First, a bidirectional relationship exists between epilepsy and suicidality, as shown in one population-based study in which patients with suicidal behavior had a 3.5fold higher risk of developing epileptic seizures compared with controls [5]. Second, suicidal ideation is not rare as a postictal phenomenon; indeed, in a study of 100 consecutive patients with treatment-resistant epilepsy, Kanner et al. identified a 13% prevalence of habitual postictal suicidal ideation [18]. Completed suicide in the postictal period has been reported in patients who suffer from postictal psychosis [19]. Third, suicidality as an iatrogenic complication of pharmacological and surgical therapies has been reported in several studies. In fact, completed suicide has been identified in several case series of patients who developed severe depression following epilepsy surgery, in particular temporal lobectomy [20].

In January of 2008, the Food and Drug Administration (FDA) issued an alert regarding the association between increased suicidal risk and exposure to AEDs based on the results of a meta-analysis that included data from 199 randomized clinical trials of 11 AEDs [21]. The meta-analysis encompassed a total of 43,892 patients treated for epilepsy, psychiatric disorders, and other disorders, predominantly pain. The FDA concluded that there was a statistically significant 1.80-fold increased risk of suicidality (defined as suicidal ideation, suicidal behavior, and completed suicide), as suicidality occurred in 4.3 per 1000 patients treated with AEDs in the active arm, compared with 2.2 per 1000 patients in the comparison arm. Of all the suicidality reported, suicidal ideation accounted for 67.6%, preparatory acts for 2.8%, attempts for 26.8%, and completed suicide for 2.8%. AEDs were associated with a greater risk for suicidality with epilepsy (odds ratio [OR], 3.53; 95% confidence interval [CI]: 1.28–12.10) than with psychiatric disorders (OR, 1.51; 95% CI: 0.95–2.45) or other disorders (OR, 1.87; 95% CI: 0.81–4.76). Yet, the validity of the results of this meta-analysis has been questioned because of several methodological problems, including the fact that the assessment of suicidality was based on "spontaneous" reports of patients and not gathered in a systematic prospective manner [22]. Furthermore, the FDA associated the increased risk of suicide with *all* AEDs, despite the fact that statistical significance was found in only one (i.e., topiramate) of the 11 AEDs studied after a reevaluation by two independent neurobiostatistitians [21]. Two other AEDs, valproic acid and carbamazepine, actually yielded a "small protective effect." The FDA's decision to present the risk as involving all AEDs stemmed from a concern that singling out specific AEDs may only change prescribing practices, rather than emphasize the suicide risk. In addition, most epilepsy trials (92%) included patients on adjunctive therapy (compared with 14% of psychiatric trials and 15% of other medical trials). It is unclear whether the higher suicidality rates in the epilepsy trials were due to drug interactions, given the high proportion of epilepsy trials designed with polytherapy, or whether they were due to the low suicidality risk associated with carbamazepine and valproate, since both drugs are protective for suicidality and are the most common comparison drugs in these trials. Finally, suicidal behavior was greater in certain geographic regions (e.g., the OR of suicidality was 1.38 [95% CI: 0.9–2.13] in North American studies

and 4.53 [95% CI: 1.86–3.18] in studies done elsewhere). Such differences strongly suggest serious methodological errors in data gathering.

Since then, five large studies have tried to reproduce the FDA findings [22–26]. However, a careful review of these studies yielded contradictory findings [27]. Clearly, the results of the FDA's meta-analysis must be considered with great caution at this time. In fact, only a study in which suicidality data are collected in a systematic and prospective manner can help determine whether a specific AED increases or decreases the risk. Yet, these data cannot be disregarded because the FDA has decided to insert suicide warnings in the packages of all AEDs; thus, physicians will need to identify patients with increased risks of suicide.

A review of the clinical literature has yielded a paucity of data regarding the increased suicidal risk associated with AED exposure. Still, several drugs are known to cause psychiatric adverse events that could facilitate the development of suicidal ideation and behavior. These include gamma-aminobutyric acid (GABA)ergic drugs (e.g., barbiturates, benzodiazepines, vigabatrin, and tiagabine) and AEDs such as topiramate, zonisamide, and levetiracetam [28–31]. Symptoms of depression have been attributed to an inhibition of serotonergic secretion by increased GABAergic synaptic concentrations [32]. Studies done with phenobarbital, topiramate, and levetiracetam have found an increased risk of psychiatric adverse events in patients with a prior psychiatric history or a family psychiatric history. Thus, such information is essential when planning to use any of these AEDs.

Impact on quality of life

Five studies involving patients with treatment-resistant epilepsy demonstrated that DD is the most powerful predictor of poor quality of life, even after controlling for seizure frequency, severity, and other psychosocial variables [32–36]. Cramer et al. determined that depression was significantly associated with poor quality of life scores on the Quality of Life in Epilepsy Inventory-89, independent of seizure type; however, the investigators found that seizure freedom for the last 3 months improved the quality of life ratings [36].

Of note, the comorbid occurrence of depressive and anxiety disorders has a worse impact on the quality of life of PWE than the presence of a depressive or anxiety disorder alone [7]. This phenomenon is observed particularly when a major depressive episode is comorbid with more than one anxiety disorder.

In addition, DDs in PWE significantly increase the health-care costs associated with the management of the seizure disorder, as shown by Cramer et al., who found that patients with untreated depression used significantly more health resources of all types, independent of seizure type or latency [37]. Furthermore, mild to moderate depression was associated with a twofold increase in medical visits compared with nondepressed controls, while severe depression was associated with a fourfold increase. The presence and severity of depression was a predictor of worse disability scores, irrespective of the duration of the seizure disorder. Also, DDs have been found to worsen the tolerance of AEDs.

A bidirectional relationship between DDs and epilepsy: Does it account for the high comorbidity?

The recognition of a bidirectional relationship between DDs and epilepsy dates back to Hippocrates, when 26 centuries ago he wrote, "Melancholics ordinarily become epileptics, and epileptics melancholics: what determines the preference is the direction the malady takes; if it bears upon the body, epilepsy, if upon the intelligence, melancholy." And yet, this bidirectional relationship was forgotten until the last two decades, when population-based studies demonstrated that not only are PWE at higher risk of developing a DD, but that people with a history of depression have a three- to sevenfold higher risk of developing epilepsy [3–5]. This bidirectional relationship does not imply causality, but rather suggests the existence of common pathogenic mechanisms operant in both conditions. These include: (1) abnormal transmission of several neurotransmitters, such as decreased transmission of serotonin (5-hydroxytryptamine, 5-HT), norepinephrine (NE), dopamine (DA), GABA, and increased transmission of glutamate; (2) hyperactive hypothalamic–pituitary–adrenal

axis, resulting in high cortisol serum concentrations, which are neurotoxic and can impact several neurotransmitters (e.g., 5-HT, GABA and glutamate) as well as result in neuropathological and structural abnormalities of temporal and frontal lobe and subcortical structures presenting as atrophy of temporal and frontal lobe structures (identified by high-resolution magnetic resonance imaging [MRI] and volumetric measurements) in the amygdala, hippocampus, entorhinal cortex, and temporal lateral neocortex, as well as in the prefrontal, orbitofrontal, and mesialfrontal cortex and, to a lesser degree, in the thalamic nuclei and basal ganglia. AS shown below, the bidirectional relationship between DD and epilepsy can be demonstrated in animal models of epilepsy and depression [38].

Epilepsy causes psychiatric disturbances

Mazarati et al [39] used an animal model of lithium and pilocarpine-induced status epilepticus (SE) (a common animal model of TLE) with male Wistar rats. Post-SE animals exhibited phenomena equivalent to symptoms of depression, including increased immobility time in the forced swim test and decreased consumption of saccharin in the saccharin consumption test. Furthermore, in the rats with spontaneous clinical or electrographic seizures, a decrease of 5-HT concentration and turnover in the hippocampus and of 5-HT release from the hippocampus was demonstrated in response to raphe nuclei stimulation.

Psychiatric disturbances facilitate the development of epileptic activity

Three studies have suggested that early postnatal life stress consisting of maternal separation (MS) can accelerate the kindling process in rats [40–42]. In two studies, male and female nonepileptic rats were exposed to MS or early handling (EH) and brief separation. At 7 weeks of age, rats of both genders exposed to MS displayed significantly increased anxiety, as evidenced by reduced time spent in the open arms of the elevated plus maze compared with EH rats. In females but not in males, less stimulation were required following MS than EH to reach the fully kindled state (39.6 ± 6.4 vs. 67.1 ± 9.4; $p < 0.0001$) [40, 41]. In the third study, investigators used cross-fostering as a model for early life stress in seizure-prone and seizure-resistant rats, which underwent amygdala kindling until six class V seizures were recorded. An increased kindling rate was observed among all cross-fostered rats compared with nonfostered rats [42]. The common pathogenic mechanisms have been reviewed in great detail in previous reviews by this author [6, 38, 43–46]. Additional data can be found in Chapter 2 of this book and will be briefly summarized below.

Neurotransmitter disturbances

Serotonin and NE

The pathogenic role of these two neurotransmitters in DD has been recognized for a long time, as increasing 5-HT and NE synaptic activity has been the target of most psychopharmacological treatments [47]. Deceased 5-HT and NE activity has been demonstrated in animal models of epilepsy, in particular the two strains of genetic epilepsy-prone rats (GEPRs), GEPR-3 and GEPR-9, which are characterized by predisposition to sound-induced generalized tonic–clonic seizures [47, 48] and, particularly in GEPR-9s, a marked acceleration of kindling. Noradrenergic deficiencies in GEPRs appear to result from deficient arborization of neurons arising from the locus coeruleus, coupled with excessive presynaptic suppression of NE release in the terminal fields and lack of postsynaptic compensatory upregulation. GEPR-9 rats have a more pronounced NE transmission deficit and, in turn, exhibit more severe seizures than do GEPR-3 rats [48]. There is also evidence of deficits in serotonergic arborization in the GEPR's brain and deficient postsynaptic serotonin$_{1A}$ receptor density in the hippocampus [47]. Increments of either NE or 5-HT transmission can prevent seizure occurrence, while reduction will have the opposite effect [47]. The 5-HT precursor 5-hydroxy-L-tryptophan (5-HTP) has anticonvulsant effects in GEPRs when combined with the selective serotonin reuptake inhibitor (SSRI) fluoxetine [47]. SSRIs and monoamino oxidase inhibitors (MAOIs) can exert anticonvulsant effects in experimental animals, such as mice and baboons, that are genetically prone to epilepsy as well as in nongenetically prone cats, rabbits, and rhesus monkeys [49–52].

Serotonin's anticonvulsant effect may be also mediated through direct and indirect mechanisms, the latter including inhibition of voltage-gated ion channels and an effect on inhibitory neurotransmitter receptors (GABA), excitatory receptors (e.g., glutamate), and neurosteroid synthesis [53, 54]. Of note, the serotonergic anticonvulsant effect appears to have an "inverted U-shaped" concentration–response effect, as suggested by a study of pilocarpine-induced seizures in which hippocampal perfusion of 5-HT up to extracellular concentrations ranging from 80% to 350% of baseline levels protected these rats from seizures, while concentrations >900% of baseline worsened seizures [55]. Of note, the high extracellular 5-HT concentrations were associated with significant increases in extracellular glutamate.

In humans, a common pathogenic role of 5-HT has been suggested by data from several functional neuroimaging studies with positron emission tomography (PET) targeting the 5-HT$_{1A}$ receptor, which demonstrated a decreased binding of 5-HT$_{1A}$ in common mesial temporal structures, cingulate gyrus, and raphe nuclei in both disorders [56–59]. Furthermore, a significant reduction of seizure frequency reported in three open trials with SSRIs (two with fluoxetine and one with citalopram) in patients with treatment-resistant epilepsy may support the pathogenic role of 5-HT in epilepsy [60–62]. These data, however, must be confirmed in double-blind, randomized studies. Furthermore, one study compared the seizure incidence between patients with primary DD randomized to an antidepressant drug versus placebo in psychopharmacological clinical trials from the FDA Phase II and III clinical trials. The trials included several SSRIs, the serotonin norepinephrine reuptake inhibitor (SNRI) venlafaxine, and the alpha-2 antagonist mirtazapine [63]. The incidence of seizures was significantly lower among patients randomized to antidepressants than in those randomized to placebo (standardized incidence ratio = 0.48; 95% CI, 0.36–0.61). Of note, in patients randomized to placebo, the seizure incidence was 19-fold higher than the published incidence of unprovoked seizures in community nonpatient samples.

Glutamate

In epilepsy, glutamate is the excitatory neurotransmitter "par excellence." In DDs, the potential pathogenic role of glutamate has been suggested by data from experimental animal models of depression as well as functional neuroimaging studies and therapeutic studies using glutamate antagonists. Of note, glutamatergic and monoaminergic systems are closely interconnected, as evidenced by the projection of glutamatergic neurons from the cortex to the locus coeruleus, raphe nucleus, and substantia nigra. Likewise, serotonergic and noradrenergic agents can interfere with the neurotransmission of glutamate. For example, chronic treatment with the SSRI fluoxetine, the SNRI reboxetine, and the NE reuptake inhibitor desipramine caused a reduction of depolarization-evoked release of glutamate [64].

Three sources of evidence support a pathogenic role of glutamate and GABA in DD: (1) dysfunction of glutamate transporter proteins; (2) increased concentrations of cortical glutamate; and (3) antidepressant effects of glutamate receptor antagonists [65].

Dysfunction of glutamate transporter proteins vGluT1 and excitatory amino acid transporters EAAT-1, EEAT-2 (found primarily in glial cells), EEAT-3 (localized principally in neurons), and EEAT-4 (localized in the cerebellum) have been identified in animal models of depression [65, 66]. These proteins play pivotal roles in the maintenance of glutamate's low extracellular concentrations through a reuptake process into glial and neuronal cells, a mechanism through which they protect neurons from excitotoxic damage and limit the amplitude and duration of excitatory postsynaptic currents in glutamatergic synapses [67]. In humans, reduced expression of EAAT-1, EAAT-2, and glutamine synthetase has been found in the frontal cortex in postmortem brain tissue from individuals with major depressive disorders, along with decreases in EAAT-3 and EAAT-4 mRNA expression in the striatum of individuals with mood disorders that resulted in elevated synaptic glutamate concentrations [68]. Likewise, in a study of 12 patients with treatment-resistant TLE, decreased expression of EAAT-1 and EAAT-2 was found to be associated with decreased extracellular clearance of glutamate in CA1 of the hippocampus by approximately 40% and 25%, respectively [69].

Abnormal concentrations of cortical glutamate and GABA were identified with magnetic resonance spectroscopy studies (H1-MRS) in humans with major depressive and bipolar disorders, which used the combined measure of intracellular and extracellular pools of glutamate, glutamine, and GABA due to their overlapping concentration peaks, but which in fact reflect an overwhelming expression of intracellular pools in neurons and glia [70, 71]. One study revealed elevated glutamate concentrations in the occipital cortex [65].

Antidepressant effects of glutamate receptor antagonists and metabotropic antagonists (including MK-801, ketamine, mGluR5 antagonist 2-methyl-6-(phenylethynyl)-pyridine [MPEP], and the mGluR2/3 antagonists LY341495 and MGS0039) have been shown in animal models of depression including the forced swim test and the tail suspension-induced immobility test as well as in learned helplessness models of depression [65, 72]. In humans, the NMDA antagonist ketamine has shown antidepressant effects in two double-blind placebo-controlled studies carried out in patients with pharmaco-resistant depression [73, 74]. One of these studies included 18 patients with treatment-resistant major depressive disorder and assessed the response to treatment for a 2-week period of the NMDA antagonist ketamine in a double-blind placebo crossover study. An antidepressant effect was found within 2 hours of a single administration of an intravenous subanesthetic dose, as 50% of patients met response criteria within 2 hours and 71% by 24 hours. The antidepressant effect persisted for 1–2 weeks [74]. In 30% of patients, all symptoms remitted during the observation period.

Riluzole (2-amino-6-(trifluoromethoxy) benzothiazole) is a drug that inhibits glutamate transmission and also affects AMPA receptor trafficking and glutamate reuptake. The antidepressant effects of this drug were suggested in open trials, particularly a 7-week open-label monotherapy trial carried out in 19 patients with treatment-resistant major depressive disorder [75]. Another trial of 10 patients with treatment-resistant major depressive disorder with riluzole as add-on therapy to antidepressant drugs therapy resulted in a significant improvement in depressive symptoms after 6–12 weeks of treatment [76]. These findings must be replicated in double-blind placebo-controlled studies.

GABA

In contrast to glutamate, GABA is the neurotransmitter with inhibitory properties of neuronal hyperexcitability "par excellence," and for this reason, it has been the target of several AEDs (e.g., barbiturates, benzodiazepines, vigabatrin, and tiagabine). On the other hand, the pathogenic role of GABA in DDs is still poorly understood. Studies in unmedicated adults with major depressive disorders have revealed decreased GABA levels in dorsomedial, dorsal anterolateral prefrontal, and ventromedial prefrontal regions and occipital regions [71]. Likewise, a study of the GABA-synthesizing enzyme glutamic acid decarboxylase (GAD) and its two isoforms, GAD_{65} and GAD_{67}, found a decrease of the density of GAD_{65} and GAD_{67} mRNA-positive neurons by 45% and 43%, respectively, in the hippocampus, as well as a decrease in the density of GAD_{65} in the cingulate and prefrontal cortices of patients with bipolar disorder [77]. Furthermore, Mason et al. [78] found decreased GABA synthesis in depressed subjects using carbon13C-MRS, while Sanacora et al. showed a normalization of GABA concentrations with the SSRI citalopram [79]. Nonetheless, GABAergic agents have not been found to have an antidepressant effect. On the contrary, GABAergic AEDs such as barbiturates, vigabatrin, and tiagabine have been associated with significant psychiatric adverse events, including depressive episodes, which have been associated with GABA's inhibition of 5-HT secretion [32].

A hyperactive hypothalamic–pituitary–adrenal axis

A failure of the adrenal gland to suppress the secretion of cortisol to a dose of dexamethasone (also known as the dexamethasone suppression test) has been identified in about 50% of patients with major depressive disorders and has also been found in patients with TLE [80] and in animal models of epilepsy [81]. Furthermore, Kumar et al. demonstrated that corticosterone administration accelerated electrical amygdala kindling in female nonepileptic Wistar rats at 10–13 weeks of age [82].

High cortisol concentrations have a direct effect on serotonergic transmission, as shown by López et al. [83] in a study comparing basal plasma corticosteroids in rats subjected to chronic unpredictable stress to those of nonstressed rats. A high corticosterone blood level was associated with a decrease in $5\text{-}HT_{1A}$ mRNA binding in the hippocampus in the rats subjected to stress; of note, this effect was prevented with pretreatment with the tricyclic antidepressant drugs imipramine or desipramine. Furthermore, since $5\text{-}HT_{1A}$ receptor binding and its mRNA expression are under tonic inhibition by glucocorticoid receptor stimulation, reduction in $5\text{-}HT_{1A}$ receptor binding and its mRNA expression in depression may be caused by cortisol hypersecretion. This observation may explain the decreased $5\text{-}HT_{1A}$ receptor binding identified in PET studies of humans with DDs and epilepsy.

In experimental studies with rats and monkeys, cortisol has been found to be neurotoxic at high concentrations, causing (1) damage of hippocampal neurons, particularly CA3 pyramidal neurons, mediated by reduction of dendritic branching and loss of dendritic spines that are included in glutamatergic synaptic inputs; (2) decreased levels of brain-derived neurotrophic factor (BDNF) reversed by long-term administration of antidepressants; and (3) interference with neurogenesis of granule cells in the adult hippocampal dentate gyrus [84–86]. All of these effects result in structural changes in the dentate gyrus, pyramidal cell layer of hippocampus, amygdala, and temporal neocortex [84–87]. In the frontal lobes, high cortisol secretion has been associated with a decrease in glial cell numbers in subgenual, cingulated, and dorsolateral sections of the prefrontal cortex [88–92].

In humans with primary major depressive disorders, a hyperactive hypothalamic–pituitary–adrenal axis has been postulated as one of the operant pathogenic mechanisms mediating the atrophy of hippocampal formations and frontal lobes, including cingulate gyrus and orbitofrontal and dorsolateral cortex, as demonstrated by multiple investigators [93–96]. In fact, neuropathological consequences attributed to excessive cortisol have included (1) decreased glial densities and neuronal size in the cingulate gyrus; (2) decreased neuronal sizes and neuronal densities in layers II, III, and IV in the rostral orbitofrontal cortex, resulting in a decrease of cortical thickness; (3) a significant decrease of glial densities in cortical layers V and VI, associated with decreases in neuronal sizes in the caudal orbitofrontal cortex; and (4) a decrease of neuronal and glial density and size in all cortical layers of the dorsolateral prefrontal cortex [88–92]. Finally, elevated levels of glucocorticoids reduce astrocytes' activity and interfere with their function. In this manner, they may undermine neuronal and cortical function in major depressive disorder by causing the accumulation of excessive synaptic glutamate [97].

The impact of these data on seizure control can be appreciated from the following three studies. In the first study conducted in patients with TLE of mesial temporal lobe origin, Lin et al. identified decreased cortical thickness in temporal lateral and extratemporal cortex using voxel-based morphometric analyses of brain MRI studies [98]. The second study included 48 adults with treatment-resistant TLE (24 with and 24 without DD) and 96 healthy controls; patients with TLE with depression had a greater number of areas of gray matter volume loss than those without depression in temporal and frontal lobe regions bilaterally and in the left thalamus also using voxel-based morphometric analyses [99]. The third study included 165 patients with TLE done by the same group of investigators who found that gray matter atrophy in patients with treatment-resistant and remitting–relapsing epilepsy was more widespread than in patients who are seizure free [100]. Significant differences included cortical atrophy of bilateral periorbital cortex, cingulated gyrus, and temporal lobes. These findings may provide a possible explanation for the worse seizure control following pharmacotherapy and surgical treatment among patients with a lifetime history of DDs.

Clinical manifestations

As stated earlier, DDs in PWE can mimic the primary mood disorders described in the fourth edition (text revised) of the DSM-IV-TR (see also Chapter 3). Bipolar disorders also afflict PWE, but with a lower frequency than DD. Yet, as stated in this chapter's introduction, in up to 50% of mood disorders identified in PWE, the clinical characteristics fail to meet any of the DSM-IV-TR criteria.

The atypical clinical presentation of DDs in PWE has been recognized for a long time. Using *Diagnostic and Statistical Manual of Mental Disorders*, Third Edition, Revised (DSM-III-R) criteria, Mendez et al. studied the clinical semiology of 175 PWE and found that 22% of 96 patients with a depressive episode were classified as having atypical depression [101]. Kraepelin [102] and Bleuler [103] were the first authors to describe a pleomorphic pattern of symptoms, including affective symptoms consisting of prominent irritability intermixed with euphoric mood, fear, and symptoms of anxiety, as well as anergia, pain, and insomnia. Gastaut et al. [104] confirmed Kraepelin and Bleuler's observations, leading Blumer and Altshuler to coin the term "interictal dysphoric disorder" to refer to this type of depression in epilepsy [105]. Blumer and Altshuler described the chronic course of the disorder as having recurrent symptom-free periods and as responding well to low doses of antidepressant medication. Mula et al. confirmed Blumer and Altshuler's observations, but also concluded that this form of depression was not specific to epilepsy since it was also identified in patients with migraine [106].

Other investigators have been impressed by the pleomorphic presentation of DDs in epilepsy. Among 97 consecutive patients with refractory epilepsy and depressive episodes severe enough to merit pharmacotherapy, Kanner et al. found that 28 (29%) met DSM-IV criteria for major depressive disorder [9]. The remaining 69 patients (71%) failed to meet criteria for any of the DSM-IV categories and presented with a clinical symptomatology consisting of anhedonia (with or without hopelessness), fatigue, anxiety, irritability, poor frustration tolerance, and mood lability with bouts of crying. Some patients also reported changes in appetite and sleep patterns and problems with concentration. Most symptoms presented with a waxing and waning course, with repeated, interspersed symptom-free periods of one to several days duration. The semiology most resembled a dysthymic disorder, but the intermittent recurrence of symptom-free periods precluded DSM criteria for this condition. Kanner and colleagues referred to this form of depression as "dysthymic-like disorder of epilepsy."

Peri-ictal depressive episodes

In PWE, depressive, manic, and hypomanic episodes are categorized according to their temporal relation with seizure occurrence into peri-ictal (i.e., symptoms that precede, follow, or are the expression of the ictal activity) or interictal episodes (i.e., occur independently of seizure). The degree to which peri-ictal symptoms contribute to the overall clinical semiology of depression in PWE remains unknown because large studies characterizing their clinical manifestations have not been performed. Interictal depressive episodes are the most frequently recognized.

Peri-ictal depressive episodes consist of clusters of symptoms and episodes that usually last from a few hours to a few days. It is possible that peri-ictal symptoms account to some degree for the atypical manifestations of the DDs in PWE [18, 107–110].

Pre-ictal symptoms or episodes typically present as a dysphoric mood that precedes a seizure by several hours to days [107]; these symptoms increase in severity during the 24 hours prior to the seizure and remit postictally or persist for a few days after the seizure.

Postictal symptoms can be elusive because symptom-free periods of 1–5 days may exist between the seizure and onset of psychiatric symptoms. In a study of 100 consecutive patients with refractory epilepsy, Kanner et al. investigated the prevalence rate and clinical characteristics of postictal psychiatric symptoms during a 3-month period [18]. Forty-three patients experienced habitually (i.e., after more than 50% of their seizures) a median of five postictal symptoms of depression with a median duration of 24 hours (15). Twenty-five patients had a history of mood disorder and 11 of anxiety disorder. In addition, postictal suicidal ideation was identified in 13 patients; 10 of the 13 patients (77%) had a history of either major depression or bipolar disorder, and this association was highly significant. Among the 43 patients with postictal symptoms of depression, 27 (63%) had concurrent postictal symptoms of anxiety and 7 reported postictal psychotic symptoms.

In recent studies conducted by the current author, postictal phenomena were found to also result from an exacerbation of interictal symptoms of depression (Kanner et al., 2011, unpublished data). In fact, PWE with interictal depressive episodes may experience breakthrough depressive symptoms following seizures.

Comorbid anxiety symptoms in depression

A frequent comorbidity of mood and anxiety disorders has been identified in patients with and without epilepsy, with rates ranging between 50% and 80% in patients with primary mood disorders. Similar observations have been made in PWE, as indicated earlier [7]. Recognition and treatment of comorbid symptoms of anxiety is of the essence, as they may worsen the quality of life of depressed patients and significantly increase their risk of suicide. Thus, evaluation of mood disorders must include investigation of comorbid symptoms of anxiety and vice versa.

How to screen for DDs in the neurology clinic

Several screening instruments have been developed to identify symptoms of depression (see Chapter 7). A six-item screening instrument, the Neurological Disorders Depression Inventory for Epilepsy, was validated to screen for major depressive episodes in PWE [111]. This instrument has the advantage of being constructed specifically to minimize confounding symptoms that plague other instruments, such as somatic symptoms that may be the expression of a DD, of adverse events of AEDs, or of cognitive problems associated with epilepsy. Completion of the instrument takes less than 3 minutes. A score of >15 is suggestive of a major depressive episode and indicates that a more in-depth evaluation is necessary. Other self-rating screening instruments developed to identify symptoms of depression in the general population, such as the Beck Depression Inventory-II and the Center of Epidemiologic Studies–Depression, have also been validated to screen for symptoms of depression in PWE [112]. It should be emphasized that these instruments are *not diagnostic* of major depressive episodes or other mood disorders. Thus, an in-depth evaluation is necessary. Once the diagnosis of a mood disorder has been established by psychiatric evaluation, the self-rating screening instruments can be given at every visit to measure changes in symptom severity or document symptom remission.

As already discussed, comorbid anxiety disorders or symptoms of anxiety are a common occurrence, and their identification and effective treatment is of the essence. The seven-item Patient's Health Questionnaire Generalized Anxiety Disorder-7 (GAD-7) is an ideal self-rating instrument to screen for generalized anxiety disorder (GAD) [113]. It takes 2–3 minutes for patients to complete; a score of >10 is suggestive of a GAD.

DDs as an iatrogenic complication

Symptoms of depression and/or anxiety and depressive and anxiety episodes can result from the addition of AEDs with negative psychotropic properties (e.g., barbiturates, topiramate, levetiracetam, zonisamide, vigabatrin, and tiagabine) [28–31] and/or the discontinuation of AEDs with mood-stabilizing properties (e.g., valproic acid, carbamazepine, and lamotrigine) and/or anxiolytic properties (e.g., pregabalin, gabapentin) in patients with a prior history of a DD and/or anxiety disorder that have been kept in remission by the AED [114–118]. Patients with a personal or family psychiatric history are at increased risk of experiencing psychiatric adverse events.

Likewise, DDs are common following epilepsy surgery, in particular during the first 3–6 months after an anterotemporal lobectomy. Typically, symptoms tend to remit by 1 year, but in up to 15% of cases, symptoms of depression may persist despite various pharmacological and nonpharmacological interventions [20]. In a majority of cases, postsurgical depressive episodes may occur as an exacerbation in severity or recurrence of presurgical DD, but in up to 15%, these episodes represent a *de novo* depressive episode. Accordingly, it is of the essence to identify the existence of a lifetime history of DD in every surgical candidate and prepare the patient and family for the eventuality of symptom recurrence after surgery. In the experience of this author, the use of low dose SSRIs is effective in yielding a symptom remission in a significant number of patients.

Management of DDs in PWE

Despite the high prevalence of DDs in PWE, there are almost no controlled studies that have investigated the treatment of this psychiatric comorbidity in these patients. Accordingly, clinicians have had to use data from treatment paradigms of primary DD in the management of PWE. Yet, given the large percentage of patients with atypical forms of DD, whether these data are applicable to PWE is yet to be established in controlled studies. The reader is therefore referred to Chapters 2 and 8 of this book for detailed information regarding the treatment of primary DD.

Several principles need to be considered when treating PWE. First, before starting any treatment, it is of the essence to rule out the possibility that these episodes are the result of an iatrogenic process (see above). As in the case of primary DD, the aim of any type of treatment must be geared toward complete symptom remission because persistence of symptoms, even in the presence of improvement, is associated with a significant risk of recurrence of a major depressive disorder. The treatment of DD in PWE may consist of pharmacotherapy, psychotherapy, or a combination of both treatment modalities. Given the high comorbidity of DD and anxiety disorders, treatment of the latter must be incorporated into the overall treatment plan of the patient. Fortunately, most antidepressant drugs of the SSRI and SNRI families also have an anxiolytic therapeutic effect.

Pharmacotherapy

To date, there has been only one controlled study that compared the safety and efficacy of the SSRI sertraline with that of cognitive–behavior therapy (CBT) in a single-blind controlled study of 140 PWE with a major depressive episode [118]. Both treatments were equally effective, with symptom remission found in 60% of each treatment arm at the end of the study. Of note, there was no worsening in seizure frequency among patients randomized to sertraline.

In general, there is a consensus that SSRIs or SNRIs are the first line of therapy. The choice between SSRIs and SNRIs depends on the type of depressive episode: SNRIs are preferred for retarded depressive episodes (e.g., fatigue, slow thinking); otherwise, patients should be started on an SSRI. Among the six SSRI drugs, the choice must be based on (1) prior exposure and evidence of therapeutic profile (e.g., efficacy in DD and type of anxiety disorder), (2) potential pharmacokinetic and pharmacodynamic interactions with concurrent AEDs (see below), and (3) potential adverse event profile of the specific SSRI drug that could worsen underlying medical complications associated with the seizure disorder or other concurrent medical condition. For example, sexual adverse events have been associated with most SSRIs. Since sexual disturbances are identified in approximately 30% of PWE, an SNRI (e.g., duloxetine) may be chosen in a patient with a history of sexual disturbances.

Patients who continued to be symptomatic following a trial with an SSRI at optimal doses should be considered for a trial with an SNRI and vice versa. Referral to a psychiatrist should follow persistent symptoms despite two trials at optimal doses, one with an SSRI and one with an SNRI, as this is likely to represent a treatment-resistant form of depressive/anxiety disorder.

Is it safe to use antidepressant drugs in PWE?

Concerns of antidepressant drugs causing seizures constitute one of the most frequent obstacles to treatment of mood and anxiety disorders. Yet such concerns are based on several misconceptions. First, any suspicion of proconvulsant properties of antidepressant drugs must factor in the existence of the bidirectional relationship between epilepsy and depression, whereby not only are PWE at higher risk of developing depression, but patients with depression have a four- to sevenfold higher risk of developing epilepsy. Thus, the occurrence of a seizure in a depressed patient may be the expression of the natural course of the mood disorder and not of an adverse event of the antidepressant drug. There is a general consensus that antidepressant drugs can cause seizures at toxic doses, and in fact, most reported seizures were in cases of overdoses. On the other hand, four antidepressants have been found to significantly lower the risk of seizures in patients without epilepsy. These include maprotyline (incidence: 15.6%, in a dose-dependent manner), clomipramine (incidence: 1–12.2% in a dose-dependent manner), and bupropion (0.5–4.8% in a dose-dependent manner) [119–121].

Pharmacokinetic properties of AEDs and interaction with psychotropic drugs

From a pharmacokinetic standpoint, AEDs are divided among enzyme-inducing drugs of the cytochrome p450 (CYP) enzyme system. They include those considered as potent inducers (e.g., phenytoin, carbamazepine, phenobarbital primidone) and weak inducers (oxcarbazepine at doses >900 mg/day, topiramate at doses >400 mg/day, and rufinamide). Since the majority of antidepressant medications are substrates for one or more of the CYP isoenzymes, comedication with any of these AEDs is likely to increase their metabolism, resulting in lower serum concentrations and hampering their efficacy. Such is the case with sertraline, paroxetine, citalopram, and escitalopram [122]. Accordingly, the dose of these antidepressant drugs must be adjusted with the addition and/or discontinuation of one of these AEDs. In contrast to the enzyme-inducing drugs, the AED sodium valproate can inhibit certain CYP (2C9) and glucuronyltransferase enzymes, but no interaction with SSRIs or SNRIs have been reported.

On the other hand, several SSRIs can inhibit several CYP isoenzymes [122–124]. These include fluoxetine, which has been shown to inhibit CYP 3A4, CYP 2C9, CYP 2C19, CYP 2D6, and CYP 1A2, while its metabolite, norfluoxetine, has also been shown to inhibit CYP 2D6. Fluvoxamine is an inhibitor of CYP 1A2, 3A4, CYP 2C9, and 2C19. The most clinically relevant inhibition of SSRIs include those of CYP 3A4, CYP 2C9, and CYP 2C19 since they may lead to an increase of phenytoin and carbamazepine serum concentrations [122, 124]. Conversely, SSRIs with no or minimal inhibitory effects include citalopram and escitalopram, and it is believed that the SNRIs venlafaxine and duloxetine are unlikely to cause significant interactions with currently available AEDs [122].

Given that most of the second-generation AEDs do not induce or inhibit CYP-450 isoenzymes, they are unlikely to affect the metabolism of antidepressant drugs. On the other hand, there are limited clinical data on the effect of SSRIs on these AEDs.

Pharmacodynamic interactions between AEDs and antidepressants

Antidepressant drugs and AEDs have several adverse events that are similar in type. Accordingly, the combination of these two types of drugs could, at least theoretically, result in a potential worsening of these adverse events. Unfortunately, no data are available to document or refute this concern. Nonetheless, clinicians must caution their patients to report any worsening of the following adverse events when using AEDs and antidepressant drugs together:

1. *Worsening of sexual adverse events*, including decreased libido, anorgasmia, and sexual impotence, with the use of any SSRI and barbiturates in particular (phenobarbital and primidone), which can also be seen with other enzyme-inducing AEDs. This adverse event has been associated with the synthesis of the sex hormone-binding globulin, which binds the free fraction of sex hormones and limits their access to the central nervous system.
2. *Potentiation of weight gain* that can be caused by AEDs such as gabapentin, valproic acid, carbamazepine, pregabalin, and SSRIs, particularly sertraline and paroxetine.
3. *Potentiation of osteopenia and osteoporosis* between enzyme-inducing AEDs and SSRIs. Several population-based studies have suggested that exposure to SSRIs is associated with decreased bone mineral density and bone fractures [124–126]. One study found higher rates of bone loss at the hip for SSRI users, even after controlling for possible confounders such as depression [124]. In a Canadian population study, the adjusted OR for hip fracture was 2.4 (95% CI 2.0–2.7) for exposure to SSRIs compared with nonusers [125]. A third population-based study conducted in The Netherlands found the risk of nonvertebral fracture to be 2.35 (95% confidence interval, 1.32–4.18) for current users of SSRIs compared with nonusers of antidepressants, after adjustment for age, sex, lower-limb disability, and depression [126].

Nonpharmacological treatments

Cognitive behavior therapy has become one of the most frequently recommended types of psychotherapy in the treatment of primary DD. Gilliam et al. confirmed its efficacy in PWE [118]. While there are no controlled data on the efficacy of CBT and behavior therapy in anxiety disorders in PWE, these forms of therapy are known to be very effective in the treatment of primary anxiety disorders, particularly panic disorders with agoraphobia, phobias, and compulsions in obsessive–compulsive disorders. Often, patients may require the combination of pharmacotherapy and nonpharmacological interventions.

Should neurologists treat DDs in PWE?

In an ideal world, all PWE with comorbid depressive and anxiety disorders should be evaluated and treated by psychiatrists and mental health professionals. Unfortunately, access to these specialists is limited because of economic factors, as insurance coverage frequently does not include psychiatric services or offers only a limited number of visits per year. Thus, it is not unusual for neurologists to be the only source of treatment for patients with comorbid depression. When left untreated, primary major depressive episodes may persist for 6–24 months in 90–95% of cases, while symptoms may persist for more than 2 years in the remaining 5–10% patients. Thus, neurologists should be trained in the pharmacological management of major, dysthymic, and minor depressive episodes. On the other hand, referral to a psychiatrist should be considered in the following circumstances:

1. A depressive episode associated with suicidal ideation and/or attempts.
2. A major depressive episode with psychotic features, which represents 25% of major depressive episodes. In such cases, pharmacotherapy has to include antipsychotic and antidepressant drugs, and at times, electroshock therapy must be considered. Furthermore, the presence of psychotic symptomatology significantly increases suicidal risk.
3. Any major depressive or dysthymic episode that has failed to respond to two prior trials of SSRIs or SNRIs at optimal doses, as these may reflect treatment-resistant DD.
4. Bipolar disorder, since its management is fret with significantly lower therapeutic success and associated with potentially serious complications that are beyond the therapeutic skills of neurologists. The use

of antidepressant medication for a bipolar disorder can facilitate the development of manic and hypomanic episodes or of rapid cycling bipolar disorder (i.e., four or more depressive, manic, or hypomanic episodes in a 12-month period). The American Psychiatric Association guidelines for the treatment of acute depression in bipolar disease advise against an initial use of anti-depressant drugs [127]. Furthermore, bipolar disorder can begin with recurrent major depressive episodes before the first manic or hypomanic episode occurs. Accordingly, before prescribing antidepressant medica-tion, it is essential to inquire about a history of manic or hypomanic episodes as well as of a family history of bipolar disease.

Concluding remarks

DDs in PWE are a relatively frequent psychiatric comorbidity that often present with atypical clin-ical manifestations. Their timely recognition and treatment are of the essence to avert multiple complications, including the possibility of wors-ening the seizure disorder, increased suicidal risk, poor quality of life, poor tolerance to AEDs, and increased economic burden to the family and society. Research is necessary to establish the optimal treatment in PWE.

Illustrative case

The patient was a 28-year-old man with a 15-year history of partial complex seizures of left mesial temporal origin secondary to a dysembrioplastic neuroepithelioma. He had undergone one prior surgical procedure to resect the tumor, but con-tinued to have seizures after surgery with the same frequency. A postsurgical MRI revealed that the mesial structures had been left intact, and a residual tumor was also identified on MRI.

His seizures consisted of clusters of two to five complex partial seizures in a 24-hour period every 2–3 weeks and secondary generalized tonic–clonic seizures every 3–4 months.

A change in his personality had been noticed in the previous 6 years, consisting of a tendency to get easily frustrated when things did not go his way, mood lability without any reason, and recur-rent episodes of 3–4 days duration occurring

several times a month without any apparent trigger consisting of restlessness and constant worrying, early night insomnia and waking up in the middle of the night, loss of appetite, and a tendency to become withdrawn and isolated. Six to 10 episodes had occurred in the last 3 years and lasted between 6 weeks and 4 months.

One to 3 days after his seizure clusters, his symptoms of depression would worsen in sever-ity or tend to recur if he had been asymptomatic at the time of his seizures.

He had been treated with a course of an SSRI for a period of 3 months, which he discontinued because of sexual adverse events. He refused to accept any further trials with psychotropic medi-cation. His mother thought that his mood had improved significantly on the antidepressant. Of note, the SSRI did not prevent the occurrence of symptoms of depression after his clusters of seizures.

Because of his seizures, he had decided to stop working 4 years earlier. He underwent a second anterotemporal lobectomy to remove the mesial temporal structures and residual tumor. Postsurgically, he experienced only auras during the first 2 months. As of the third postsurgical month, he began experiencing complex partial seizures every 3–4 months, but not in clusters and primarily during sleep. Eight months after the surgical procedure he developed an episode that consisted of becoming withdrawn from everyone around him, refusing to leave the house, and claiming that the police were going to arrest him. He started responding to auditory hallucinations and took an overdose of his AED, which resulted in an inpatient admission.

> ### 💡 PEARLS TO TAKE HOME
>
> - DDs are the most frequent psychiatric comorbidity in PWE.
> - In a significant percentage of patients, DDs present with atypical clinical manifestations that fail to meet diagnostic criteria of DDs included in the *Diagnostic and Statistical Manual of Mental Disorders*.
> - There is a high comorbidity of symptoms of anxiety and anxiety disorders with DDs in PWE.

- DDs have a significant impact in the life of PWE because they are likely to worsen their quality of life, increase their suicidal risk, increase the economic burden on their family and society, and worsen their tolerance of AEDs.
- Patients with a DD are more likely to suffer from treatment-resistant epilepsy, while patients with TLE undergoing epilepsy surgery are less likely to achieve full remission of auras following epilepsy surgery.
- A bidirectional relationship exists between DD and epilepsy; that is, not only are PWE at an increased risk of suffering from a DD, but patients with a history of DD have a three- to sevenfold higher risk of developing epilepsy.
- The bidirectional relationship results from the existence of common pathogenic mechanisms operant in both disorders and explains the high comorbidity of the two conditions.
- There are very limited controlled data on the treatment of DD in PWE. Yet there is a consensus that the treatment modalities used in the management of primary DD can be applied to PWE.

References

1. Tellez-Zenteno JF, Patten SB, Jetté N, et al. Psychiatric comorbidity in epilepsy: a population-based analysis. *Epilepsia*, 48: 2336–2344, 2007.
2. American Psychiatric Association. *Diagnostic and Statistical Manuel of Mental Disorders—Forth Edition*. Washington, DC: American Psychiatric Press, 2000.
3. Forsgren L, Nystrom L. An incident case-referent study of epileptic seizures in adults. *Epilepsy Res*, 6: 66–81, 1990.
4. Hesdorffer DC, Hauser WA, Annegers JF, et al. Major depression is a risk factor for seizures in older adults. *Ann Neurol*, 47: 246–249, 2000.
5. Hesdorffer DC, Hauser WA, Ludvigsson P, et al. Depression and attempted suicide as risk factors for incident unprovoked seizures and epilepsy. *Ann Neurol*, 59: 35–41, 2006.
6. Kanner AM. Depression in epilepsy: prevalence, clinical semiology, pathogenic mechanisms and treatment. *Biol Psychiatry*, 54: 388–398, 2003.
7. Kanner AM, Barry JJ, Gilliam F, et al. Anxiety disorders, sub-syndromic depressive episodes and major depressive episodes: do they differ on their impact on the quality of life of patients with epilepsy? *Epilepsia*, 51: 1152–1158, 2010.
8. Wiegartz P, Seidenberg M, Woodard A, et al. Co-morbid psychiatric disorder in chronic epilepsy: recognition and etiology of depression. *Neurology*, 53, Suppl. 2: S3–S8, 1999.
9. Kanner AM, Kozak AM, Frey M. The use of sertraline in patients with epilepsy: is it safe? *Epilepsy Behav*, 1(2): 100–105, 2000.
10. Ettinger AB, Weisbrot DM, Nolan EE, et al. Symptoms of depression and anxiety in pediatric epilepsy patients. *Epilepsia*, 39(6): 595–599, 1998.
11. Hitiris N, Mohanraj R, Norrie J, et al. Predictors of pharmacoresistant epilepsy. *Epilepsy Res*, 75: 192–196, 2007.
12. Petrovski S, Szoeke CEI, Jones NC, et al. Neuropsychiatric symptomatology predicts seizure recurrence in newly treated patients. *Neurology*, 75: 1015–1021, 2010.
13. Kanner AM, Byrne R, Chicharro A, et al. A lifetime psychiatric history predicts a worse seizure outcome following temporal lobectomy. *Neurology*, 72: 793–799, 2009.
14. Anhoury S, Brown RJ, Krishnamoorthy ES, et al. Psychiatric outcome after temporal lobectomy: a predictive study. *Epilepsia*, 41: 1608–1615, 2000.
15. Christensen J, Vestergaard M, Mortensen P, et al. Epilepsy and risk of suicide: a population-based case-control study. *Lancet Neurol*, 6: 693–698, 2007.
16. Harris EC, Barraclough B. Suicide as an outcome for mental disorders: a meta-analysis. *Br J Psychiatry*, 170: 205–228, 1997.
17. Jones JE, Hermann BP, Barry JJ, et al. Rates and risk factors for suicide, suicidal ideation, and suicide attempts in chronic epilepsy. *Epilepsy Behav*, 4: S31–S38, 2003.
18. Kanner AM, Soto A, Gross-Kanner H. Prevalence and clinical characteristics of

postictal psychiatric symptoms in partial epilepsy. *Neurology*, 62: 708–713, 2004.

19. Fukuchi T, Kanemoto K, Kato M, et al. Death in epilepsy with special attention to suicide cases. *Epilepsy Res*, 51: 233–236, 2002.

20. Bladin PF. Psychosocial difficulties and outcome after temporal lobectomy. *Epilepsia*, 33(5): 898–907, 1992.

21. Dr. Katz memo and briefing document to PCNS and PD advisory board. June 12, 2008. Briefing document for the July 10, 2008 Advisory Committee to discuss antiepileptic drugs (AEDs) and suicidality. http://www.fda.gov/ohrms/dockets/ac/08/briefing/2008-4372b1-01-FDA-Katz.pdf

22. Hesdorffer DC, Kanner AM. The FDA alert on suicidality and antiepileptic drugs: fire or false alarm? *Epilepsia*, 50: 978–986, 2009.

23. Gibbons RD, Jur K, Brown CH, et al. Relationship between antiepileptic drugs and suicide attempts in patients with bipolar disorder. *Arch Gen Psychiatry*, 66: 1354–1360, 2009.

24. Olesen JB, Hansen PR, Erdal J, et al. Antiepileptic drugs and risk of suicide: a nationwide study. *Pharmacoepidemiol Drug Saf*, 19(5): 518–524, 2010.

25. Patorno E, Bohn RL, Wahl PM, et al. Anticonvulsant medications and the risk of suicide, attempted suicide, or violent death. *JAMA*, 303: 1401–1409, 2010.

26. VanCott AC, Cramer JA, Copeland LA, et al. Suicide-related behaviors in older patients with new anti-epileptic drug use: data from the VS hospital system. *BMC Med*, 8: 4, 2010.

27. Hesdorffer DC, Berg AT, Kanner AM. An update on antiepileptic drugs and suicide: do we know any more now? *Epilepsy Curr*, 10(6): 137–145, 2010.

28. Brent DA, Crumrine PK, Varma RR, et al. Phenobarbital treatment and major depressive disorder in children with epilepsy. *Pediatrics*, 80: 909–917, 1987.

29. Mula M, Sander JW. Suicidal ideation in epilepsy and levetiracetam therapy. *Epilepsy Behav*, 11: 130–132, 2007.

30. Mula M, Trimble MR, Yuen A, et al. Psychiatric adverse events during levetiracetam therapy. *Neurology*, 61: 704–706, 2003.

31. Trimble RM, RüSch N, Betts T, et al. Psychiatric symptoms after therapy with new antiepileptic drugs: psychopathological and seizure related variables. *Seizure*, 9: 249–254, 2000.

32. Nishikawa T, Scatton B. Evidence for a GABAeric inhibitory influence on serotonergic neurons originating from the dorsal raphe. *Brain Res*, 279: 325–329, 1983.

33. Lehrner J, Kalchmayr R, Serles W, et al. Health-related quality of life (HRQOL), activity of daily living (ADL) and depressive mood disorder in temporal lobe epilepsy patients. *Seizure*, 8(2): 88–92, 1999.

34. Perrine K, Hermann BP, Meador KJ, et al. The relationship of neuropsychological functioning to quality of life in epilepsy [see comments]. *Arch Neurol*, 52(10): 997–1003, 1995.

35. Gilliam F, Kuzniecky R, Faught E, et al. Patient-validated content of epilepsy-specific quality-of-life measurement. *Epilepsia*, 38(2): 233–236, 1997.

36. Cramer JA, Blum M, Reed M, et al. The influence of comorbid depression on quality of life for people with epilepsy. *Epilepsy Behav*, 4: 515–521, 2003.

37. Cramer JA, Blum D, Fanning K, et al. The impact of comorbid depression on health resource utilization in a community sample of people with epilepsy. *Epilepsy Behav*, 5: 337–342, 2004.

38. Kanner AM. Depression and epilepsy: how can we explain their bidirectional relation? *Epilepsia*, 52, Suppl. 1: 21–27, 2011.

39. Mazarati AM, Siddarth P, Baldwin RA, et al. Depression after status epilepticus: behavioural and biochemical deficits and effects of fluoxetine. *Brain*, 131: 2071–2083, 2008.

40. Salzberg M, Kumar G, Supit L, et al. Early postnatal stress confers enduring vulnerability to limbic epileptogenesis. *Epilepsia*, 48(11): 2079–2085, 2007.

41. Jones NC, Kumar G, O'Brien TJ, et al. Anxiolytic effects of rapid amygdala kindling, and the influence of early life experience in rats. *Behav Brain Res*, 203(1): 81–87, 2009.

42. Gilby KL, Sydserff S, Patey AM, et al. Postnatal epigenetic influences on seizure

susceptibility in seizure-prone versus seizure-resistant rat strains. *Behav Neurosci*, 123(2): 337–346, 2009.

43. Kanner AM. Depression and epilepsy: a review of multiple facets of their close relation. *Neurol Clin North America*, 27(4): 865–880, 2009.

44. Kanner AM. Depression and epilepsy: do glucocorticoids and glutamate explain their relationship? *Curr Neurol Neurosci Rep*, 9(4): 307–312, 2009.

45. Kanner AM. Mood disorder and epilepsy: a neurobiologic perspective of their relationship. *Dialogues Clin Neurosci*, 10(1): 39–45, 2008.

46. Kanner AM. Mood disorders in epilepsy: a complex relation with unexpected consequences. *Curr Opin Neurol*, 21(2): 190–194, 2008.

47. Jobe PC. Affective disorder and epilepsy comorbidity in the genetically epilepsy-prone-rat (GEPR). In: *Depression and Brain Dysfunction*, eds. F Gilliam, AM Kanner and YI Sheline. London: Taylor & Francis, pp. 121–157, 2006.

48. Jobe PC, Mishra PK, Browning RA, et al. Noradrenergic abnormalities in the genetically epilepsy-prone rat. *Brain Res Bull*, 35: 493–504, 1994.

49. Meldrum BS, Anlezark GM, Adam HK, et al. Anticonvulsant and proconvulsant properties of viloxazine hydrochloride: pharmacological and pharmacokinetic studies in rodents and the epileptic baboon. *Psychopharmacology (Berl)*, 76: 212–217, 1982.

50. Piette Y, Delaunois AL, De Shaepdryver AF, et al. Imipramine and electroshock threshold. *Arch Int Pharmacodyn Ther*, 144: 293–297, 1963.

51. Polc P, Schneeberger J, Haefely W. Effects of several centrally active drugs on the sleep wakefulness cycle of cats. *Neuropharmacology*, 18: 259–267, 1979.

52. Yanagita T, Wakasa Y, Kiyohara H. Drug-dependance potential of viloxazine hydrochloride tested in rhesus monkeys. *Pharmacol Biochem Behav*, 12: 155–161, 1980.

53. Robinson R, Drafts B, Fisher J. Fluoxetine increases GABAA receptor activity through a novel modulatory site. *J Pharmcol Exp Ther*, 304: 978–984, 2003.

54. Ye Z, Lu Y, Sun H, et al. Fluoxetine inhibition of glycine receptor activity in rat hippocampal neurons. *Brain Res*, 1239: 77–84, 2008.

55. Clinckers R, Smolders I, Meurs A, et al. Anticonvulsant action of hippocampal dopamine and serotonin is independently mediated by D2 and 5-HT1A receptors. *J Neurochem*, 89: 834–843, 2004.

56. Sargent PA, Kjaer KH, Bench CJ, et al. Brain serotonin 1A receptor binding measured by positron emission tomography with [11C] WAY-100635: effects of depression and antidepressant treatment. *Arch Gen Psychiatry*, 57: 174–180, 2000.

57. Toczek MT, Carson RE, Lang L, et al. PET imaging of 5-HT1A receptor binding in patients with temporal lobe epilepsy. *Neurology*, 60: 749–756, 2003.

58. Theodore WH, Giovacchini G, Bonwetsch R, et al. The effect of antiepileptic drugs on 5-HT-receptor binding measured by positron emission tomography. *Epilepsia*, 47(3): 499–503, 2006.

59. Hasler G, Bonwetsch R, Giovacchini G, et al. 5-HT(1A) receptor binding in temporal lobe epilepsy patients with and without major depression. *Biol Psychiatry*, 62(11): 1258–1264, 2007.

60. Favale E, Rubino V, Mainardi P, et al. The anticonvulsant effect of fluoxetine in humans. *Neurology*, 45: 1926, 1995.

61. Favale E, Audenino D, Cocito L, et al. The anticonvulsant effect of citalopram as an indirect evidence of serotonergic impairment in human epileptogenesis. *Seizure*, 12: 316–318, 2003.

62. Specchio LM, Iudice A, Specchio N, et al. Citalopram as treatment of depression in patients with epilepsy. *Clin Neuropharmacol*, 27(3): 133–136, 2004.

63. Alper KR, Schwartz KA, Kolts RL, et al. Seizure incidence in psychopharmacological clinical trials: an analysis of Food and Drug Administration (FDA) summary basis of approval reports. *Biol Psychiatry*, 62: 345–354, 2007.

64. Bonanno G, Giambelli R, Raiteri L, et al. Chronic antidepressants reduce

depolarization-evoked glutamate release and protein interactions favoring formation of SNARE complex in hippocampus. *J Neurosci*, 25: 3270–3279, 2005.

65. Kugaya A, Sanacora G. Beyond monoamines: glutamatergic function in mood disorders. *CNS Spectr*, 10(10): 808–819, 2005.

66. Zink M, Vollmayr B, Gebicke-Haerter PJ, et al. Reduced expression of glutamate transporters vGluT1, EAAT2 and EAAT4 in learned helpless rats, an animal model of depression. *Neuropharmacology*, 58(2): 465–473, 2010.

67. Zarate CA, Quiroz J, Payne J, et al. Modulators of the glutamatergic system: implications for the development of improved therapeutics in mood disorders. *Psychopharmacol Bull*, 36: 35–83, 2002.

68. Choudary PV, Molnar M, Evans SJ, et al. Altered cortical glutamatergic and GABAergic signal transmission with glial involvement in depression. *Proc Natl Acad Sci USA.*, 102: 15653–15658, 2005.

69. McCullumsmith RE, Meador-Woodruff JH. Striatal excitatory amino acid transporter transcript expression in schizophrenia, bipolar disorder, and major depressive disorder. *Neuropsychopharmacology*, 26: 368–375, 2002.

70. Capizzano AA, Jorge RE, Acion LC, et al. In vivo proton magnetic resonance spectroscopy in patients with mood disorders: a technically oriented review. *J Magn Reson Imaging*, 26(6): 1378–1389, 2007.

71. Walter M, Henning A, Grimm S, et al. The relationship between aberrant neuronal activation in the pregenual anterior cingulate, altered glutamatergic metabolism, and anhedonia in major depression. *Arch Gen Psychiatry*, 66(5): 478–486, 2009.

72. Machado-Vieira R, Salvadore G, Ibrahim LA, et al. Targeting glutamatergic signaling for the development of novel therapeutics for mood disorders. *Curr Pharm Des*, 15(14): 1595–1611, 2009.

73. Berman RM, Cappiello A, Anand A, et al. Antidepressant effects of ketamine in depressed patients. *Biol Psychiatry*, 47: 351–354, 2000.

74. Zarate CA, Jr, Singh JB, Carlson PJ, et al. A randomized trial of an N-methyl-D-aspartate antagonist in treatment-resistant major depression. *Arch Gen Psychiatry*, 63(8): 856–864, 2006.

75. Zarate CA, Jr, Quiroz JA, Singh JB, et al. An open-label trial of the glutamate-modulating agent riluzole in combination with lithium for the treatment of bipolar depression. *Biol Psychiatry*, 57: 430–432, 2005.

76. Sanacora G, Kendell SF, Levin Y, et al. Preliminary evidence of riluzole efficacy in antidepressant-treated patients with residual depressive symptoms. *Biol Psychiatry*, 61: 822–825, 2007.

77. Heckers S, Stone D, Walsh J, et al. Differential hippocampal expression of glutamic acid decarboxylase 65 and 67 messenger RNA in bipolar disorder and schizophrenia. *Arch Gen Psychiatry*, 59: 521–529, 2002.

78. Mason GF, Sanacora G, Hundal R, et al. Preliminary evidence of reduced cortical GABA synthesis rate in major depression. *Soc Neurosci*, 2001. Abstr 142.6.

79. Sanacora G, Mason GF, Rothman DL, et al. Increased occipital cortex GABA concentrations in depressed patients after therapy with selective serotonin reuptake inhibitors. *Am J Psychiatry*, 159: 663–665, 2002.

80. Zobel A, Wellmer J, Schulze-Rauschenbach S, et al. Impairment of inhibitory control of the hypothalamic pituitary adrenocortical system in epilepsy. *Eur Arch Psychiatry Clin Neurosci*, 254(5): 303–311, 2004.

81. Mazarati AM, Shin D, Kwon YS, et al. Elevated plasma corticosterone level and depressive behavior in experimental temporal lobe epilepsy. *Neurobiol Dis*, 34(3): 457–461, 2009.

82. Kumar G, Couper A, O'Brien TJ, et al. The acceleration of amygdala kindling epileptogenesis by chronic low-dose corticosterone involves both mineralocorticoid and glucocorticoid receptors. *Psychoneuroendocrinology*, 32(7): 834–842, 2007.

83. López JF, Chalmers DT, Little KY, et al. Regulation of serotonin1A, glucocorticoid, and mineralocorticoid receptor in rat and human hippocampus: implications for the neurobiology of depression. *Biol Psychiatry*, 43(8): 547–573, 1998.

84. Sapolsky RM. The possibility of neurotoxicity in the hippocampus in major depression: a primer on neuron death. *Biol Psychiatry*, 48(8): 755–765, 2000.

85. Sapolsky RM. Glucocorticoids and hippocampal atrophy in neuropsychiatric disorders. *Arch Gen Psychiatry*, 57: 925–935, 2000.

86. Shirayama Y, Chen AC, Nakagawa S, et al. Brain-derived neurotrophic factor produces antidepressant effects in behavioral models of depression. *J Neurosci*, 22(8): 3251–3261, 2002.

87. Bowley MP, Drevets WC, Ongur D, et al. Low glial numbers in the amygdala in major depressive disorder. *Biol Psychiatry*, 52: 404–412, 2002.

88. Öngür D, Drevets WC, Price JL. Glial reduction in the subgenual prefrontal cortex in mood disorders. *Proc Natl Acad Sci U S A*, 95: 13290–13295, 1998.

89. Rajkowska G, Miguel-Hidalgo JJ, Wei J, et al. Morphometric evidence for neuronal and glial prefrontal cell pathology in major depression. *Biol Psychiatry*, 45(9): 1085–1098, 1999.

90. Cotter DR, Pariante CM, Everall IP. Glial cell abnormalities in major psychiatric disorders: the evidence and implications. *Brain Res Bull*, 55: 585–595, 2001.

91. Cotter D, Mackay D, Landau S, et al. Reduced glial cell density and neuronal size in the anterior cingulate cortex in major depressive disorder. *Arch Gen Psychiatry*, 58: 545–553, 2001.

92. Cotter D, Mackay D, Chana G, et al. Reduced neuronal size and glial cell density in area 9 of the dorsolateral prefrontal cortex in subjects with major depressive disorder. *Cereb Cortex*, 12: 386–394, 2002.

93. Bremner JD, Narayan M, Anderson ER, et al. Hippocampal volume reduction in major depression. *Am J Psychiatry*, 157(1): 115–118, 2000.

94. Bremner JD, Vythilingam M, Vermetten E, et al. Reduced volume of orbitofrontal cortex in major depression. *Biol Psychiatry*, 51(4): 273–279, 2002.

95. Coffey CE. The role of structural brain imaging in ECT. *Psychopharmacol Bull*, 30(3): 477–483, 1994.

96. Sheline YI. Brain structural changes associated with depression. In: *Depression and Brain Dysfunction*, eds. F Gilliam, AM Kanner, YI Sheline. London: Taylor & Francis, pp. 85–104, 2006.

97. Crossin KL, Tai MH, Krushel LA, et al. Glucocorticoid receptor pathways are involved in the inhibition of astrocyte proliferation. *Proc Natl Acad Sci U S A.*, 94: 2687–2692, 1997.

98. Lin JJ, Salamon N, Lee AD, et al. Reduced neocortical thickness and complexity mapped in mesial temporal lobe epilepsy with hippocampal sclerosis. *Cereb Cortex*, 17: 2007–2018, 2007.

99. Salgado PC, Yasuda CL, Cendes F. Neuroimaging changes in mesial temporal lobe epilepsy are magnified in the presence of depression. *Epilepsy Behav*, 19: 422–427, 2010.

100. Bilevicius E, Yasuda CL, Silva MS, et al. Antiepileptic drug response in temporal lobe epilepsy: a clinical and MRI morphometry study. *Neurology*, 75(19): 1695–1701, 2010.

101. Mendez MF, Cummings J, Benson D, et al. Depression in epilepsy. Significance and phenomenology. *Arch Neurol*, 43: 766–770, 1986.

102. Kraepelin E. *Psychiatrie*, Vol. 3. Leipzig, Germany: Johann Ambrosius Barth, 1923.

103. Bleuler E. *Lehrbuch der Psychiatrie*, 8th ed. Berlin, Germany: Springer, 1949.

104. Gastaut H, Morin G, Lesèvre N. Étude du comportement des épileptiques psychomoteurs dans l'intervalle de leurs crises: les troubles de l'activité globale et de la sociabilité. *Ann Med Psychol (Paris)*, 113: 1–27, 1955.

105. Blumer D, Altshuler LL. Affective disorders. In: *Epilepsy: A Comprehensive Textbook*, Vol. II, eds. J Engel and TA Pedley. Philadelphia: Lippincott-Raven, pp. 2083–2099, 1998.

106. Mula M, Jauch R, Cavanna A, et al. Clinical and psychopathological definition of the interictal dysphoric disorder of epilepsy. *Epilepsia*, 49(4): 650–656, 2008.

107. Blanchet P, Frommer GP. Mood change preceding epileptic seizures. *J Nerv Ment Dis*, 174: 471–476, 1986.

108. Williams D. The structure of emotions reflected in epileptic experiences. *Brain*, 79: 29–67, 1956.

109. Weil A. Depressive reactions associated with temporal lobe uncinate seizures. *J Nerv Ment Dis*, 121: 505–510, 1955.

110. Daly D. Ictal affect. *Am J Psych*, 115: 97–108, 1958.

111. Gilliam FG, Barry JJ, Meador KJ, et al. Rapid detection of major depression in epilepsy: a multicenter study. *Lancet Neurology*, 5(5): 399–405, 2006.

112. Jones JE, Herman BP, Woodard JL, et al. Screening for major depression in epilepsy with common self-report depression inventories. *Epilepsia*, 46(5): 731–735, 2005.

113. Kroenke K, Spitzer RL, Williams JB, et al. Anxiety disorders in primary care: prevalence, impairment, comorbidity, and detection. *Ann Intern Med*, 146: 317–325, 2007.

114. Ettinger AB, Kustra RP, Hammer AE. Effect of lamotrigine on depressive symptoms in adult patients with epilepsy. *Epilepsy Behav*, 10(1): 148–154, 2007.

115. Fakhoury TA, Barry JJ, Mitchell Miller J, et al. Lamotrigine in patients with epilepsy and comorbid depressive symptoms. *Epilepsy Behav*, 10(1): 155–162, 2007.

116. Pande AC, Crockatt JG, Feltner DE, et al. Pregabalin in generalized anxiety disorder: a placebo-controlled trial. *Am J Psychiatry*, 160: 533–540, 2003.

117. Bech P. Dose-response relationship of pregabalin in patients with generalized anxiety disorder. A pooled analysis of four placebo-controlled trials. *Pharmacopsychiatry*, 40(4): 163–168, 2007.

118. Gilliam FG, Black KJ, Carter J, et al. Depression and health outcomes in epilepsy: a randomized trial. Presented at the 61st Annual Meeting of the American Academy of Neurology, 25 April–02 May 2009, Seattle, Washington, USA, http://www.abstracts2view.com/aan2009seattle/view.php?nu=AAN09L_S26.002&terms

119. Rosenstein D, Nelson J, Jacobs S. Seizures associated with antidepressants: a review. *J Clin Psych*, 54: 289–299, 1993.

120. Preskorn S, Fast G. Tricyclic antidepressant induced seizures and plasma drug concentration. *J Clin Psych*, 53: 160–162, 1992.

121. Davidson J. Seizures and bupropion: a review. *J Clin Psychiatry*, 50: 256–261, 1989.

122. Trimble MR, Mula M. Antiepileptic drug interactions in patients requiring psychiatric drug treatment. In: *Antiepileptic Drugs. Combination Therapy and Interactions*, eds. J Majkowski, B Bourgeois, P Patsalos, R Mattson. Cambridge, UK: Cambridge University Press, pp. 350–368, 2005.

123. Patsalos P, Perucca E. Clinically important drug interactions in epilepsy: interactions between antiepileptic drugs and other drugs. *Lancet Neurol*, 2: 473–481, 2003.

124. Haney EM, Warden SJ, Bliziotes MM. Effects of selective serotonin reuptake inhibitors on bone health in adults: time for recommendations about screening, prevention and management? *Bone*, 46(1): 13–17, 2010.

125. Diem SJ, Blackwell TL, Stone KL, et al. Use of antidepressants and rates of hip bone loss in older women: the study of osteoporotic fractures. *Arch Intern Med*, 167(12): 1240–1245, 2007.

126. Liu B, Anderson G, Mittmann N, et al. Use of selective serotonin-reuptake inhibitors or tricyclic antidepressants and risk of hip fractures in elderly people. *Lancet*, 351(9112): 1303–1307, 1998.

127. Hirschfield RMA, Bowden CL, Gitlin MJ, et al. Practice guideline for the treatment of patients with bipolar disorder. *Am J Psychiatry*, 159, Suppl. #4: 1–15, 2002.

Depression and Movement Disorders

Oliver Tüscher[1,2,3] and Ludger Tebartz van Elst[1]
[1]Section of Experimental Neuropsychiatry, Department of Psychiatry and Psychotherapy, University of Freiburg Medical Center, Freiburg, Germany
[2]Department of Neurology, University of Freiburg Medical Center, Freiburg, Germany
[3]Department of Psychiatry and Psychotherapy, University of Mainz Medical Center, Mainz, Germany

Introduction

Movement and mood disorders: wide range of etiopathogenetic entities

Virtually all movement disorders show some sort of behavioral symptoms [1, 2], most frequently mood disorder symptoms. Movement and mood disorders share common pathophysiological elements: both are disorders that involve the basal ganglia and their connections, at least to some extent [3]. Therefore, movement disorders have become model diseases for research into mood disorders, especially with the rise of modern functional neuroimaging and deep brain stimulation (DBS) techniques [4]. In addition, improved therapeutic options for motor symptoms, at least for Parkinson's disease (PD), has put behavioral symptoms back into focus since they are an important contributing factor to quality of life in movement disorders [5]. Consequently, movement disorders are re-recognized as neurobehavioral syndromes [1, 2, 6], even though the recognition of behavioral symptoms as an integral part of movement disorders dates back to their initial description [7]. This chapter aims to conceptualize movement and mood disorders as syndromal expressions of dysfunctional corticostriatothalamocortical neural circuits caused by a wide range of etiopathogenetic entities.

Depression in movement disorders: Parkinson's and Huntington's disease as paradigmatic entities

Movement disorders can be divided on a syndromal level into hypo- and hyperkinetic syndromes. Hypo- and hyperkinetic syndromes are caused by different etiologies, most of which can be classified as either so-called idiopathic (no known single cause; probably a mixture of genetic susceptibility and acquired changes) or primary genetic neurodegenerative diseases. The most prevalent hypokinetic syndrome is idiopathic PD. The classic but rare, monogenetically defined hyperkinetic syndrome is Huntington's disease (HD). Since most research has concentrated on these two conditions and the discussion of all entities of even rare movement disorders is beyond the scope of this chapter, we will focus on PD and HD as exemplary hypo- and hyperkinetic movement disorders.

Neurobehavioral symptoms in PD and HD: underdiagnosed and underestimated burden on patients and caregivers

PD is often characterized and still diagnosed only by its very visible and prominent motor symptoms. However, increased recognition of significant emotional dysfunction in PD has led to a

Depression in Neurologic Disorders: Diagnosis and Management, First Edition.
Edited by Andres M. Kanner.

reconceptualization of PD as a neurobehavioral syndrome [1, 6]. The effects of neurobehavioral nonmotor aspects of PD and the impact on the patient's [8] and caregivers' [9] quality of life have been increasingly recognized. Depression has been rated as a more important factor than motor disease severity or medication in quality of life assessments by patients with PD, caregivers, and physicians [5]. Nonetheless, a seminal study demonstrated that during routine office visits, neurologists failed to identify the presence of depression, anxiety, and fatigue in more than half of cases [10], indicating the need for better awareness of the presence of these symptoms. Recently, a randomized controlled trial showed that effective antidepressant treatment leads to an improvement of quality of life in these cases [11]. In patients with HD, behavioral abnormalities are traditionally better recognized but still receive comparably less attention than motor symptoms [12]. In sporadic cases of HD, behavior abnormalities also cause considerable diagnostic difficulties [13]. The often troubling impact of behavioral abnormalities on the quality of life of patients and caregivers [12] and the functional decline of patients with HD has only recently been systematically studied [14].

Depression in PD and HD

Prevalence, characteristics, and assessment of depression in PD and HD

Depressive symptoms are the most common neuropsychiatric symptoms affecting patients with PD, and prevalence figures have been estimated at 40–50% [15]. However, due to methodological flaws and the phenomenological overlap of some depressive and PD motor symptoms (e.g., hypomimia and psychomotor retardation), reported prevalence rates of depression in PD vary widely from approximately 3% to 90%. The largest systematic review on the prevalence of depression in PD reported clinically significant depressive symptoms in an average of 35% of cases, while according to *Diagnostic and Statistical Manual of Mental Disorders*, Fourth Edition (DSM–IV) criteria, major depressive disorders were found in 17%, minor depression in 22%, and dysthymia in 13% [16]. This suggests that the average prevalence of major depressive disorder in PD is not as high as generally assumed

[15]. Depression in PD is mostly of mild to moderate intensity, and the suicide rate is low, with the exception of suicides related to DBS. The latter are associated with presurgical depression and impulsivity and, presumably, with rapid reduction of dopaminergic medication following DBS [15].

Depression precedes the onset of motor symptoms in 2.5–37% of patients with PD [15, 17], potentially delaying proper diagnosis of the neurobehavioral movement disorder syndrome [17]. The course of depression in PD is characterized by two peaks: first, depression is common early in the course of PD, followed by a second peak in later stages [18]. There may also be a preponderance of severe depression in akinetic rigid compared with equivalent (akinetic rigid and tremor) forms of PD, possibly representing a subform of PD [19]. However, severity of motor symptoms does not correlate with frequency or severity of depression in PD [15, 18].

The clinical characteristics of depression in PD are primarily sadness, dysphoria, irritability, pessimism about the future, and suicidal ideation [20, 21]. The symptom profile differs slightly from primary depressive disorders by exhibiting less guilt, self-reproach, and feelings of failure. Also, there are fewer psychotic features (hallucinations and delusions; caveat: if those concurrently occur they are generally just secondary phenomena to dopaminergic medication), but there may be more anxiety [15, 21].

Assessment of depression in PD can be very challenging due to the overlap of PD and depressive symptoms. In fact, apathy or sleep disturbance, which otherwise may be regarded only as a symptom in primary depression, can be an independent feature of the neurobehavioral syndrome in PD [21, 22]. Another conceptual challenge is that most diagnostic instruments used for the diagnosis and severity assessment of depression include somatic symptoms which may be a symptom of the underlying neurologic disorder. These caveats have resulted in revised guidelines using common diagnostic instruments with inclusion of DSM-IV diagnostic criteria as well as of subsyndromal depression, specification of assessment timing with respect to motor states ("on"/"off" periods), and informant judgments [23, 24]. In addition, cut-off scores for PD have been established for some instruments like the Montgomery–Åsberg Depression Rating Scale (MADRS [14/15 points]) and the 17-item Hamilton Rating Scale for Depression (HAM-D17 [13/14 points]) [15, 21]. In addition, new PD-specific instruments for assessing depression have been devised, such as the non-motor symptom scale and questionnaire (NMSS and NMSQuest) or the revised Unified Parkinson's Disease Rating Scale (UPDRS) [25] and the Neuropsychiatric Inventory Questionnaire (NPI-Q) [26] (see also Chapter 4).

For HD, there are fewer data available regarding prevalence, assessment, and characteristics of depression. The largest study using a factor analysis of the Unified Huntington's Disease Rating Scale (UHDRS) identified depressive symptoms in 40% of individuals across all total functional capacity stages [27]. Interestingly, depressive symptoms decreased with increased severity of HD [27], underlining previous findings that depression in HD is not correlated with cognitive impairment, motor symptoms, or CAG repeat lengths [28]. An increased prevalence of depressive symptoms has recently been linked to presymptomatic HD gene carriers [29]. In contrast to PD, suicidal rates in HD are increased about fourfold compared with the general population. This has been attributed to the high rate of impulsive behaviors as one of the most prominent neurobehavioral features in HD [12]. Related to this, irritability is the most prominent and defining symptom of depression in HD [12, 30]. Assessment of depression and other neurobehavioral symptoms in HD is aided by the use of the Neuropsychiatric Inventory [26, 31].

Overlap with other affective and cognitive symptoms

There is a considerable overlap (60–90%) of depression with symptoms of anxiety (prevalence of approximately 35%) in PD [32]. Anxiety-like depression may precede motor symptoms [15, 21]. Apathy is another common co-occurring and probably independent neurobehavioral symptom in PD [21, 22]. Cognitive impairment occurs in approximately 30% of cases [15].

A similar situation can be found in HD. Along with depressive symptoms, the incidence of anxiety is also high [12, 31]. Irritability and other impulsive–aggressive symptoms are common

and often occur together with depression [12, 27, 30, 31].

Pathophysiology

Depressive symptoms in HD and PD: an intricate part of the behavioral syndrome, not just mere comorbidity

Depressive symptoms reflect a distinctive, PD-intrinsic disease process, rather than just an expected reaction to motor disability [15, 33]. This view is supported by the following factors: (1) a significantly higher prevalence of formally diagnosed depression in PD as compared with patients afflicted with equally debilitating diseases; (2) a different nonsomatic symptom pattern compared to primary depression; (3) the occurrence of depression preceding the onset of motor symptoms; (4) the specific course of depression in PD; and (5) the fact that there is only weak or no correlation between depression and motor symptom severity and duration [15, 18]. There is also no straightforward relationship between mood symptoms and the dopaminergic state [34] or the contribution of PD medications [35], although some anxiolytic and antidepressant effects have been shown [36].

In HD, earlier retrospective studies carried out before genetic testing became available also suggested that mood and anxiety changes often precede motor symptoms. Newer studies replicated the occurrence of depression with or following the onset of motor symptoms, arguing against purely reactive changes [12]. Increased depression frequency in presymptomatic HD gene carriers supports this notion [29]. These findings indicate that the occurrence of mood and anxiety symptoms in HD is a distinct part of the disease and not just a reactive or comorbid process [12].

In summary, mood and anxiety-related behavioral symptoms in HD and PD may be at least partially caused by the same pathological processes affecting the motor system in both diseases [12, 15]. However, unlike motor symptoms, not all patients with HD or PD develop mood symptoms, suggesting that degeneration of dopaminergic neurons of the substantia nigra in PD and of gamma-aminobutyric acid (GABA) ergic neurons in caudate and putamen in HD are important but not sufficient pathophysiological changes for the development of depression. Other contributing factors (environmental or genetic or both) may be necessary to add to the pathology causing mood-related behavioral symptoms.

Genetic basis of depression in PD and HD: contributing factors

Genetic factors in HD and PD can be divided into two classes: genes (mutations) that have been shown to be involved in the neurodegenerative process (familial disease forms) and genes that have been associated with and are thought to modify the disease.

In PD, so-called *PARK* genes have been shown to cause various forms of familial Parkinsonism as well as being susceptibility genes for sporadic PD [37]. With respect to mood and anxiety symptoms, a study of familial early-onset Parkinsonism with *Parkin* (*PARK2*) gene mutations found overt depression, anxiety, and obsessive–compulsive disorders [38].

HD is an autosomal dominant disease caused by the abnormal expansion (>39) of trinucleotide repeats (CAG) coding for glutamine at the N-terminus of the *huntingtin* protein. The physiological function of *huntingtin* remains to be determined. Psychiatric symptoms, including depression, seem not to be correlated with CAG repeat length [28], arguing against a simple relation to the disease-causing gene.

Many potential genetic associations have been studied with respect to their contribution to mood and anxiety disorders and PD [37]. However, there are no unequivocal results supporting dopamine or serotonin metabolism-related gene polymorphisms as risk factors for depression in PD or HD.

Insights into the neuroanatomy of HD and PD: neuroimaging studies

Structural and functional neuroimaging studies, especially radiotracer studies, have a firm role in clinical diagnostic and research applications in HD and PD [39, 40]. Functional magnetic resonance imaging (fMRI) was recently introduced into PD research and has already been successfully used in the characterization of the genetic risk in asymptomatic carriers of a single mutant *Parkin* allele [41]. A few fMRI studies have also investigated cognitive processing in overt and presymptomatic HD [30, 42–44].

Only two positron emission tomography (PET) imaging studies have related neuropsychiatric symptoms to brain changes in HD, and only one to mood symptoms [45]. That study compared early onset patients with HD, with or without depression, with normal controls and found reduced basal ganglia and cingulate metabolism in both patient groups. Interestingly, patients with HD with depression had lower orbitofrontal cortex metabolism than patients without depression [45]. Many more PET/single-photon emission computed tomography (SPECT) neuroimaging studies of psychiatric symptoms have been performed in PD. Clinically depressed [4, 46–49] and dysphoric [50] patients with PD demonstrated specific hypometabolism in mesial- and orbitofrontal regions, which represent key nodes in limbic striatal pathways. Recent PET/SPECT studies support the role of dopamine metabolism and signaling changes in depression and anxiety in PD [47–49] and in emotional processing [51]. Remy et al. explained depression-related dysfunction as a combination of dopaminergic and norepinephrinergic pathophysiology in the limbic system. Using a PET-ligand that binds to dopamine and norepinephrine reuptake sites, the authors detected decreased binding in the locus coeruleus and in the limbic system in patients with PD and depression compared with patients with PD and without depression [48].

Anatomical models in relation to pathological findings: PD and HD

Postmortem studies of PD neuropathology imply a sequential topographical degeneration of primarily monoaminergic cells. This process begins caudally in brainstem serotonergic raphe and noradrenergic locus coeruleus nuclei, advances into midbrain dopaminergic nuclei, and finally spreads into mesolimbic and neocortical regions [52]. The latter may correlate with premotor clinical symptoms such as depression [53]. This hypothesis is supported by some of the aforementioned imaging results. Also, findings of transcranial sonography related changes in echogenicity of brainstem serotonergic raphe nuclei to depression with and without PD and predicted later PD in depressed subjects through concurrent changes in midbrain substantia nigra [54].

The majority of such neuroanatomical hypotheses of affective symptoms in movement disorders build on the model of fronto–striato–limbic circuitry function in movement and mood disorders. The suggestion of parallel yet segregated frontal–subcortical circuit organization is a basic feature of this model [55]. However, current models favor open interconnected circuitries [56, 57], better explaining the co-occurrence of motor, cognitive, and behavioral dysfunctions and their varying symptom combinations.

In this framework, the anterior cingulate (or limbic) circuit, involving the ventral striatum, ventral pallidum, and anterior cingulate plus a putative subdivision of the medial orbitofrontal cortex and their extensive connections to the amygdala and other limbic structures, is of special importance with respect to behavioral symptoms [57].

The ventral striatum has been studied mainly in the context of motivational behavior and reward systems and is broadly conceived to mediate translation of emotionally relevant information into action [58]. A study of major depression demonstrated ventral striatum dysfunction in response to positive stimuli, suggesting a role in anhedonia [59].

The ventral striatum receives dopaminergic input primarily from the ventral tegmental area, which is adjacent to the substantia nigra in the midbrain and is clearly affected in PD [60], providing a plausible anatomic substrate for limbic system dysregulation in PD. Findings of deficient striatal regional cerebral blood flow (rCBF) response to reward [61]; of impaired amygdala activation to emotional stimuli, which is reversible with carbidopa–levodopa treatment [51]; and of reduced dopamine and noradrenaline transporter binding in patients with PD with depression versus patients with PD without depression in the different regions of this circuitry all support this model of neuro–motor–behavioral dysfunction in PD [48].

Less is known for HD. Neuropathological studies show that the ventral striatum is less affected in early stages of the disease. This may point to other critical sites of the frontal–subcortical circuits for the expression of behavioral symptoms [56]. The available data on depression in HD suggest a hypoactivity of the basal ganglia and the ventral striatum [45] as well as a disruption of normal emotion processing circuits underlying irritability in presymptomatic HD [30].

Therapy of depression in PD and HD

Despite the importance of depression in PD and HD, there are few studies on the treatment of depression in these movement disorders. This paucity of data means any recommendation on specific treatments of depression in movement disorders is more or less based on expert opinion, and most clinicians engage in a trial-and-error approach in the individual case, as will be exemplified in the case study presented later in this chapter.

Pharmacological and other somatic treatments

Dopaminergic (antiparkinsonian) medications have been suggested to improve depressive symptoms in patients with PD [21, 25]. Short-term changes in depressive mood and anxiety are correlated with intracerebral dopamine availability induced by levodopa administration, but there is no convincing long-term effect [21]. Dopamine agonists, especially those acting on mesolimbic D3 receptors, have been shown to be effective in the treatment of depression and anhedonia in open-label studies [25]. Pramipexol especially reduced depressive and motor symptoms [62], with results that were equal or even superior to sertralin [63] or pergolid [64]. Because of the established antidepressant activity of the monoamine oxidase inhibitors (MAOIs), trials with MAO-A and -B inhibitors were performed, in which the MAO-B inhibitor selegiline particularly showed some potential to reduce depressive symptoms [21].

Serotonergic and noradrenergic (antidepressant) medications have been evaluated in several trials, some of which were randomized controlled evaluations, mostly comparing tricyclic antidepressants (TCAs) and selective serotonin reuptake inhibitors (SSRIs) or norepinephrine reuptake inhibitors (SNRIs) with each other or to placebo [21, 65]. Meta-analyses suggest that SSRIs (possibly with the exception of sertraline) have no clear efficacy compared to placebo, while there is some evidence for the antidepressant efficacy of TCAs (amitriptyline/nortriptyline) [65]. This is in line with a recent randomized controlled trial showing a clear advantage of nortriptyline over paroxetine, which was not superior to placebo [66].

Given the neuroimaging and pharmacological findings, some authors suggest that depression in PD is primarily a problem of dopamine and noradrenaline imbalance [25] and that selective serotonin and norepinephrine reuptake inhibitors (SNRIs) such as venlafaxine may be a promising treatment alternative to TCAs [66]. And indeed, the latest and so far largest randomized, double-blind, placebo-controlled trial validated the SNRI venlafaxine (venlafaxine extended release) as an effective treatment of depression in PD [67]. However, in the same study paroxetine was superior to placebo and as effective as venlafaxine, adding paroxetine to the list of inconsistent findings concerning SSRI treatment for depression in PD [67].

Alternatively, transcranial repetitive magnetic stimulation (TMS) led to significant improvement of depression in several pilot studies [68]. In refractory cases, electroconvulsive therapy has been shown to be effective [69], although a critical meta-analysis did not support this notion [68].

There are no large studies on specific antidepressant treatment options for patients with HD. However, a recent case series ($n = 3$) evaluated aripiprazole, a new antipsychotic and partial D2 receptor agonist, for effects on motor, behavioral, and cognitive functions [70]. The authors measured depressive symptom severity and found an improvement after 2 months and 1 year of treatment [70]. Similarly, Brusa et al. compared aripiprazole to tetrabenazine, a dopamine depletory used to diminish hyperkinetic movements, in six patients and found a slight improvement in depressive symptoms with aripiprazole only [71]. The dopamine agonist pramipexole reduced depressive symptoms in a case of sporadic hypokinetic-rigid, Westphal variant of HD [72]. Aside from these anecdotal reports, expert opinion recommends a symptomatic treatment of symptoms in HD [12].

Psychotherapy and psychosocial treatment

In a pilot study of patients with PD, cognitive behavior therapy (CBT) has been shown to improve depressive symptoms and negative cognitions and increase the perception of social support [73]. In addition, caregivers were educated on issues of social support and response to patients' negative thoughts. Recently, the same group of investigators tested this type of CBT in a randomized-controlled trial against clinical monitoring only [74]. PD-tailored CBT was clearly superior to clinical monitoring and showed comparable effect sizes to antidepressant treatments [67, 74] thus providing an effective alternative treatment in moderate depression in PD. Other studies reported successful reductions in caregiver's distress via direct patient education programs on depression and anxiety [68]. Some limited evidence also points to positive effects of treatments such as music and physical therapy and exercise. Even thought the latter did not significantly change depression, a better physical functioning and quality of life could be shown [68].

New treatment approaches (DBS and cell replacement)

DBS has gained an increasing importance in the treatment of PD. Despite good effects on motor control, there are reports of psychiatric adverse effects, especially affective symptoms [75, 76]. Some authors see presurgical neuropsychiatric symptoms as a reason for the exclusion of affected patients from an otherwise very beneficial and often last-resort therapeutic approach, despite indications of potential beneficial DBS effects on neuropsychiatric symptoms [77]. However, a large multicenter study found DBS to be safe with respect to neuropsychiatric symptoms if patients were carefully selected before surgery [78].

Functional alterations in the prefrontostriatothalamoprefrontal circuits are commonly cited as the probable mechanism for significant psychotropic effects, both beneficial and detrimental, of DBS and other surgical therapies [76]. However, this model has not been validated. Interestingly, the occurrence of psychotropic effects is more prominent in subthalamic nucleus (STN) than in globus pallidus internus (GPi) DBS [75], pointing to the rich connectivity of the STN with the ventral striatum [79]. Local field potential measures during emotional processing in the STN of patients undergoing DBS surgery provided direct evidence for this limbic connectivity of the STN and/or passing white matter tracts [80]. Moreover, a case report investigating the depressive mood-inducing effect of a "marginally superior and lateral to the intended STN target" placed DBS electrode by means of fMRI showed brain activity patterns similar to those found in depression [81]. These differential, location-dependent effects of DBS point toward the intriguing potential of identifying possible target regions for the modulation of neurobehavioral symptoms not only in PD, but also in depression, anxiety, and obsessive–compulsive disorder [82].

The possible use of DBS in patients with HD is still open to discussion [83]. However, the focus of research is on cell replacement therapies, which are being validated in large multicenter studies [84]. Despite the small case numbers, unintended behavioral changes have been noted [85] and must be characterized further.

Conclusions and future development

From movement disorders to neurobehavioral syndromes: the need for conceptual development in neuropsychiatry

Depressive symptoms in PD and HD neurodegenerative movement disorders present with a complex mixture of "neurologic" and "psychiatric" symptoms, which need to be integrated into neurobehavioral syndromes. Therefore, a nosological reconceptualization as neuropsychiatric syndromes is warranted to facilitate a comprehensive diagnosis of the whole syndrome.

Difficult to see, difficult to diagnose: the need for accurate diagnosis

Classic "neurologic" and "psychiatric" symptoms may overlap or mask each other in individual patients. For example, it may be difficult to differentiate bradykinesia and hypomimia in the classic purely motor concept of PD from lack of drive and emotional emptiness in the context of the concept of major depression. Cognitive and emotional symptoms are easily overlooked when clinicians are not aware of these problems and do not actively inquire about them. Therefore, it is important to promote the concept of neurobehavioral syndromes because this ensures that behavioral aspects of basal ganglia disorders are not missed and will be treated. As mentioned earlier, the treatment of cognitive, affective, and motivational symptoms is often much more important with respect to quality of life than a minor reduction of motor symptoms. A unified neuropsychiatric diagnostic concept of basal ganglia disorders is therefore needed. Newly developed diagnostic tools such as NMSQuest and NPI are the first promising steps in this direction.

Difficult to measure, difficult to treat: the need for therapeutic efforts

Assessing and quantifying affective, cognitive, and motivational syndromes is another obstacle for the development of better treatment methods. On the other hand, this problem is very similar to assessing treatment methods in primary psychiatry and is therefore well resolvable. At the end of the day, it is probably the diagnostic and therapeutic routine of practicing physicians in this area that must be modified. In this context, a readiness to recognize behavioral symptoms as common and integral parts of basal ganglia disorders is the most important single step toward better diagnosis and treatment of depression in movement disorders.

Case study

Patient K.P. is a 75-year-old women presenting initially for diagnostic evaluation of her hypokinetic rigid syndrome. She suffered from slowing of the movements of her left arm and leg and numbness of her left arm and hand, including an alien limb-like feeling, postural instability (UPDRS motor score "off" 43 points, "on" 20 points), and cognitive (difficulties concentrating) and mild depressive symptoms (anhedonia, irritability, anxiety, and pessimism about the future). First motor symptoms occurred around age 73. First depressive symptoms (major depressive episode) and treatment (medication and psychotherapy) occurred around age 70. She worked as a physical therapist until age 60 and was divorced without children (at age 55). Comorbid conditions were diverticulitis, axonal polyneuropathy, and lower limb venous insufficiency. She took duloxetine (60 mg/day) but claimed that it had no effect. Diagnostic workup for the hypokinetic rigid syndrome included levodopa testing (positive), central motor and sensory eletrophysiological evaluation (negative), and MRI (moderate microvascular disease, no other pathological findings). A diagnosis of idiopathic PD and depression was made (differential diagnosis atypical PD, e.g., cortico-basal degeneration). Medication was changed to ropinirole (0.75 mg/day) and mirtazapine (15 mg/day) and escitaloprame (10 mg/day). On a follow-up visit after 6 months, motor symptoms were stable and depressive symptoms were subjectively slightly improved. Another 6 months later, depressive symptoms were aggravated, and antidepressant medication was changed back to duloxetine. PD motor symptoms had deteriorated only slightly (UPDRS "on" 25 points). Because of the ongoing worries of the patient and the alien limb symptoms in combination with newly developed bladder dysfunction and gait worsening, an iodobenzamide–SPECT and 18-2-fluoro-2-deoxy-D-glucose–PET were performed without clear conclusive results. Formal neuropsychological testing was also inconclusive. Due to the development of lower limb edema, ropinirole was changed to carbergoline. After another 6 months, the patient was hospitalized initially in a neurologic ward and later in a psychiatric ward. PD motor symptoms had not changed significantly, but depressive symptoms had worsened and now fulfilled diagnostic criteria for a major depressive episode including apathy. A new modification of antidepressant medication (venlafaxine 112.5 mg/day) and cognitive–behavioral therapy led to substantial improvement of the depression.

In hindsight, PD motor symptoms only changed slightly but were distorted by the pessimistic view and the apathy of the worsening depression. Nonetheless, several PD-related medication changes and diagnostic measures were undertaken before effective multimodal antidepressive therapy could improve the patient's situation.

PEARLS TO TAKE HOME

- Movement and mood disorders may be viewed as syndromal expressions of neuropsychiatric diseases, all affecting corticostriatothalamocortical neural circuits caused by a wide range of etiopathogenetic entities.
- PD (hypokinetic, idiopathic neurodegeneration) and HD (hyperkinetic, primary genetic neurodegeneration) represent a continuum of movement disorders as paradigmatic entities.
- Neurobehavioral symptoms in PD and HD are underdiagnosed, and the burden on patients and caregivers is underestimated.
- Depression has the highest prevalence among neurobehavioral symptoms in movement disorders.
- Depressive symptoms often overlap with and are masked by motor symptoms or other neurobehavioral symptoms.
- The pattern of depressive symptoms in movement disorders is subtly different from primary depression.
- Depression in PD and HD overlaps with anxiety, apathy, and irritability.
- Depressive symptoms in PD and HD are an intricate part of the biology of the behavioral syndrome, not just mere comorbidities or reactions to severe medical conditions.
- Genetic variation probably contributes to development of depression in PD and HD, but so far there are no clear relations to transmitter systems.
- Neuroimaging has provided evidence of frontolimbic dysfunction in depression in PD and HD.
- Reduction in dopaminergic and noradrenergic neurotransmission probably plays a critical pathogenetic role.
- Treatment of depression is guided by individual empirical treatment attempts. PD-tailored CBT is an effective treatment for moderate depression in PD. Current pharmacological evidence supports treatment attempts with dopamine agonists, SNRIs (venlafaxine) and TCAs (nortriptyline) with inconsistent efficacy for SSRIs (paroxetine, sertraline) in PD. In HD, aripirazole may be an alternative to classic antidepressants.

References

1. Bédard M-A, Agid Y, Chouinard S, et al., eds. *Mental and Behavioral Dysfunction in Movement Disorders.* Totowa, NJ: Humana Press, Inc., 2003.

2. Anderson KE, Weiner WJ, Lang AE. *Behavioral Neurology of Movement Disorders*, 2nd ed. Philadelphia: Lippincott Williams & Wilkins, 2005.

3. Lauterbach EC. Mood disorders and the globus pallidus. In: *Mental and Behavioral Dysfunction in Movement Disorders*, eds. M-A Bédard, Y Agid, S Chouinard, S Fahn, A Korczyn, P Lespérance. Totowa, NJ: Humana Press, Inc., pp. 305–320, 2003.

4. Mayberg HS, Starkstein SE, Sadzot B, et al. Selective hypometabolism in the inferior frontal lobe in depressed patients with Parkinson's disease. *Ann Neurol*, 28(1): 57–64, 1990.

5. GPDSSC. Factors impacting on quality of life in Parkinson's disease: results from an international survey. Global Parkinson's Disease Survey Steering Committee. *Mov Disord*, 17(1): 60–67, 2002.

6. Agid Y, Arnulf I, Bejjani P, et al. Parkinson's disease is a neuropsychiatric disorder. *Adv Neurol*, 91: 365–370, 2003.

7. Goetz CG. Historical issues in the study of behavioral dysfunction in movement disorders. In: *Mental and Behavioral Dysfunction in Movement Disorders*, eds. M-A Bédard, Y Agid, S Chouinard, S Fahn, A Korczyn, P Lespérance. Totowa, NJ: Humana Press, Inc., pp. 3–9, 2003.

8. Thanvi BR, Munshi SK, Vijaykumar N, et al. Neuropsychiatric non-motor aspects of Parkinson's disease. *Postgrad Med J*, 79(936): 561–565, 2003.

9. Aarsland D, Larsen JP, Karlsen K, et al. Mental symptoms in Parkinson's disease are important contributors to caregiver distress. *Int J Geriatr Psychiatry*, 14(10): 866–874, 1999.

10. Shulman LM, Taback RL, Rabinstein AA, et al. Non-recognition of depression and other non-motor symptoms in Parkinson's disease. *Parkinsonism Relat Disord*, 8(3): 193–197, 2002.

11. Menza M, Dobkin RD, Marin H, et al. The impact of treatment of depression on quality of life, disability and relapse in patients with Parkinson's disease. *Mov Disord*, 24(9): 1325–1332, 2009.

12. Anderson KE, Marshall FJ. Behavioral symptoms associated with Huntington's disease. *Adv Neurol*, 96: 197–208, 2005.

13. Tost H, Wendt CS, Schmitt A, et al. Huntington's disease: phenomenological diversity of a neuropsychiatric condition that challenges traditional concepts in neurology and psychiatry. *Am J Psychiatry*, 161(1): 28–34, 2004.

14. Hamilton JM, Salmon DP, Corey-Bloom J, et al. Behavioural abnormalities contribute to functional decline in Huntington's disease. *J Neurol Neurosurg Psychiatry*, 74(1): 120–122, 2003.

15. Mentis MJ, Delalot D. Depression in Parkinson's disease. *Adv Neurol*, 96: 26–41, 2005.

16. Reijnders JS, Ehrt U, Weber WE, et al. A systematic review of prevalence studies of depression in Parkinson's disease. *Mov Disord*, 23(2): 183–189; quiz 313, 2008.

17. O'Sullivan SS, Williams DR, Gallagher DA, et al. Nonmotor symptoms as presenting complaints in Parkinson's disease: a clinicopathological study. *Mov Disord*, 23(1): 101–106, 2008.

18. Tolosa E, Gaig C, Santamaria J, et al. Non-motor symptoms in the early stages of Parkinson's disease. In: *Non-Motor Symptoms of Parkinson's Disease*, eds. KR Chaudhuri, E Tolosa, A Scchapira, W Poewe. Oxford: Oxford University Press, pp. 19–36, 2009.

19. Starkstein SE, Petracca G, Chemerinski E, et al. Depression in classic versus akinetic-rigid Parkinson's disease. *Mov Disord*, 13(1): 29–33, 1998.

20. Cummings JL. Depression and Parkinson's disease: a review. *Am J Psychiatry.*, 149(4): 443–454, 1992.

21. Kostic VS, Stefanova E, Dragasevic N, et al. Diagnosis and treatment of depression in Parkinson's disease. In: *Mental and Behavioral Dysfunction in Movement Disorders*, eds. M-A Bédard, Y Agid, S Chouinard, S Fahn, A Korczyn, P Lespérance. Totowa, NJ: Humana Press, Inc., pp. 351–368, 2003.

22. Levy ML, Cummings JL, Fairbanks LA, et al. Apathy is not depression. *J Neuropsychiatry Clin Neurosci*, 10(3): 314–319, 1998.

23. Marsh L, McDonald WM, Cummings J, et al. Provisional diagnostic criteria for depression in Parkinson's disease: report of an NINDS/NIMH Work Group. *Mov Disord*, 21(2): 148–158, 2006.

24. Starkstein SE, Merello M, Jorge R, et al. A validation study of depressive syndromes in Parkinson's disease. *Mov Disord*, 23(4): 538–546, 2008.

25. Chaudhuri KR, Schapira AH. Non-motor symptoms of Parkinson's disease: dopaminergic pathophysiology and treatment. *Lancet Neurol*, 8(5): 464–474, 2009.

26. Kaufer DI, Cummings JL, Ketchel P, et al. Validation of the NPI-Q, a brief clinical form of the Neuropsychiatric Inventory. *J Neuropsychiatry Clin Neurosci*, 12(2): 233–239, 2000.

27. Paulsen JS, Nehl C, Ferneyhough Hoth K, et al. Depression and stages of Huntington's disease. *J Neuropsychiatry Clin Neurosci*, 17(4): 496–502, 2005.

28. Zappacosta B, Monza D, Meoni C, et al. Psychiatric symptoms do not correlate with cognitive decline, motor symptoms, or CAG repeat length in Huntington's disease. *Arch Neurol*, 53(6): 493–497, 1996.

29. van Duijn E, Kingma EM, Timman R, et al. Cross-sectional study on prevalences of psychiatric disorders in mutation carriers of Huntington's disease compared with mutation-negative first-degree relatives. *J Clin Psychiatry*, 69(11): 1804–1810, 2008.

30. Klöppel S, Stonnington CM, Petrovic P, et al. Irritability in pre-clinical Huntington's disease. *Neuropsychologia*, 48: 549–557, 2010.

31. Paulsen JS, Ready RE, Hamilton JM, et al. Neuropsychiatric aspects of Huntington's disease. *J Neurol Neurosurg Psychiatry*, 71(3): 310–314, 2001.

32. Richard IH. Anxiety disorders in Parkinson's disease. *Adv Neurol*, 96: 42–55, 2005.

33. McDonald WM, Richard IH, DeLong MR. Prevalence, etiology, and treatment of depression in Parkinson's disease. *Biol Psychiatry*, 54(3): 363–375, 2003.

34. Lauterbach EC. The neuropsychiatry of Parkinson's disease and related disorders. *Psychiatr Clin North Am*, 27(4): 801–825, 2004.

35. Schiffer RB. Anxiety disorders in Parkinson's disease: insights into the neurobiology of neurosis. *J Psychosom Res*, 47(6): 505–508, 1999.

36. Lemke MR, Brecht HM, Koester J, et al. Anhedonia, depression, and motor functioning in Parkinson's disease during treatment with pramipexole. *J Neuropsychiatry Clin Neurosci*, 17(2): 214–220, 2005.

37. Gasser T. Overview of the genetics of parkinsonism. *Adv Neurol*, 91: 143–152, 2003.

38. Wu RM, Shan DE, Sun CM, et al. Clinical, 18F-dopa PET, and genetic analysis of an ethnic Chinese kindred with early-onset parkinsonism and parkin gene mutations. *Mov Disord*, 17(4): 670–675, 2002.

39. Carbon M, Edwards C, Eidelberg D. Functional brain imaging in Parkinson's disease. *Adv Neurol*, 91: 175–181, 2003.

40. Brooks DJ, Andrews T. Imaging Huntington's disease. In: *Huntington's Disease*, 3rd ed. eds. G Bates, PS Harper, L Jones. Oxford: Oxford University Press, pp. 95–110, 2002.

41. Buhmann C, Binkofski F, Klein C, et al. Motor reorganization in asymptomatic carriers of a single mutant Parkin allele: a human model for presymptomatic parkinsonism. *Brain*, 128(Pt 10): 2281–2290, 2005.

42. Paulsen JS, Zimbelman JL, Hinton SC, et al. fMRI biomarker of early neuronal dysfunction in presymptomatic Huntington's disease. *AJNR Am J Neuroradiol*, 25(10): 1715–1721, 2004.

43. Clark VP, Lai S, Deckel AW. Altered functional MRI responses in Huntington's disease. *Neuroreport*, 13(5): 703–706, 2002.

44. Aron AR, Schlaghecken F, Fletcher PC, et al. Inhibition of subliminally primed responses is mediated by the caudate and thalamus: evidence from functional MRI and Huntington's disease. *Brain*, 126(Pt 3): 713–723, 2003.

45. Mayberg HS, Starkstein SE, Peyser CE, et al. Paralimbic frontal lobe hypometabolism in depression associated with Huntington's disease. *Neurology*, 42(9): 1791–1797, 1992.

46. Mayberg HS, Solomon DH. Depression in Parkinson's disease: a biochemical and organic viewpoint. *Adv Neurol*, 65: 49–60, 1995.

47. Weintraub D, Newberg AB, Cary MS, et al. Striatal dopamine transporter imaging correlates with anxiety and depression symptoms in Parkinson's disease. *J Nucl Med*, 46(2): 227–232, 2005.

48. Remy P, Doder M, Lees A, et al. Depression in Parkinson's disease: loss of dopamine and noradrenaline innervation in the limbic system. *Brain*, 128(Pt 6): 1314–1322, 2005.

49. Black KJ, Hershey T, Hartlein JM, et al. Levodopa challenge neuroimaging of levodopa-related mood fluctuations in Parkinson's disease. *Neuropsychopharmacology*, 30(3): 590–601, 2005.

50. Mentis MJ, McIntosh AR, Perrine K, et al. Relationships among the metabolic patterns that correlate with mnemonic, visuospatial, and mood symptoms in Parkinson's disease. *Am J Psychiatry*, 159(5): 746–754, 2002.

51. Tessitore A, Hariri AR, Fera F, et al. Dopamine modulates the response of the human amygdala: a study in Parkinson's disease. *J Neurosci*, 22(20): 9099–9103, 2002.

52. Braak H, Del Tredici K, Rub U, et al. Staging of brain pathology related to sporadic Parkinson's disease. *Neurobiol Aging*, 24: 197–211, 2003.

53. Wolters E, Braak H. Parkinson's disease: premotor clinico-pathological correlations. *J Neural Transm Suppl*, (70): 309–319, 2006.

54. Walter U, Hoeppner J, Prudente-Morrissey L, et al. Parkinson's disease-like midbrain sonography abnormalities are frequent in depressive disorders. *Brain*, 130(Pt 7): 1799–1807, 2007.

55. Alexander GE, DeLong MR, Strick PL. Parallel organization of functionally segregated circuits linking basal ganglia and cortex. *Annu Rev Neurosci*, 9: 357–381, 1986.

56. Joel D. Open interconnected model of basal ganglia-thalamocortical circuitry and its relevance to the clinical syndrome of Huntington's disease. *Mov Disord*, 16(3): 407–423, 2001.

57. Tekin S, Cummings JL. Frontal-subcortical neuronal circuits and clinical neuropsychiatry: an update. *J Psychosom Res*, 53(2): 647–654, 2002.

58. Heimer L. A new anatomical framework for neuropsychiatric disorders and drug abuse. *Am J Psychiatry*, 160(10): 1726–1739, 2003.

59. Epstein J, Pan H, Kocsis J, et al. Lack of ventral striatal response to positive stimuli in depressed versus normal subjects. *Am J Psychiatry*, 163: 1784–1790, 2006.

60. Storch A, Ludolph AC, Schwarz J. Dopamine transporter: involvement in selective dopaminergic neurotoxicity and degeneration. *J Neural Transm*, 111(10–11): 1267–1286, 2004.

61. Kunig G, Leenders KL, Martin-Solch C, et al. Reduced reward processing in the brains of Parkinsonian patients. *Neuroreport*, 11(17): 3681–3687, 2000.

62. Lemke MR, Brecht HM, Koester J, et al. Effects of the dopamine agonist pramipexole on depression, anhedonia and motor functioning in Parkinson's disease. *J Neurol Sci*, 248(1–2): 266–270, 2006.

63. Barone P, Scarzella L, Marconi R, et al. Pramipexole versus sertraline in the treatment of depression in Parkinson's disease: a national multicenter parallel-group randomized study. *J Neurol*, 253(5): 601–607, 2006.

64. Rektorova I, Rektor I, Bares M, et al. Pramipexole and pergolide in the treatment of depression in Parkinson's disease: a national multicentre prospective randomized study. *Eur J Neurol*, 10(4): 399–406, 2003.

65. Aarsland D, Marsh L, Schrag A. Neuropsychiatric symptoms in Parkinson's disease. *Mov Disord*, 24(15): 2175–2186, 2009.

66. Menza M, Dobkin RD, Marin H, et al. A controlled trial of antidepressants in patients with Parkinson disease and depression. *Neurology*, 72(10): 886–892, 2009.

67. Richard IH, McDermott MP, Kurlan R, et al. A randomized, double-blind, placebo-controlled trial of antidepressants in Parkinson disease. *Neurology*, 78(16): 1229–1236, 2012.

68. Gallagher DA, Schrag A. Depression, anxiety and apathy in Parkinson's disease. In: *Nonmotor Symptoms of Parkinson's Disease*, eds. KR Chaudhuri, E Tolosa, A Scchapira, W Poewe. Oxford: Oxford University Press, pp. 107–120, 2009.

69. Moellentine C, Rummans T, Ahlskog JE, et al. Effectiveness of ECT in patients with parkinsonism. *J Neuropsychiatry Clin Neurosci*, 10(2): 187–193, 1998.

70. Ciammola A, Sassone J, Colciago C, et al. Aripiprazole in the treatment of Huntington's disease: a case series. *Neuropsychiatr Dis Treat*, 5: 1–4, 2009.

71. Brusa L, Orlacchio A, Moschella V, et al. Treatment of the symptoms of Huntington's disease: preliminary results comparing aripiprazole and tetrabenazine. *Mov Disord*, 24(1): 126–129, 2009.

72. Bonelli RM, Niederwieser G, Diez J, et al. Pramipexole ameliorates neurologic and psychiatric symptoms in a Westphal variant of Huntington's disease. *Clin Neuropharmacol*, 25(1): 58–60, 2002.

73. Dobkin RD, Allen LA, Menza M. Cognitive-behavioral therapy for depression in Parkinson's disease: a pilot study. *Mov Disord*, 22(7): 946–952, 2007.

74. Dobkin RD, Menza M, Allen LA, et al. Cognitive-behavioral therapy for depression in Parkinson's disease: a randomized, controlled trial. *Am J Psychiatry*, 168(10): 1066–1074, 2011.

75. Rodriguez-Oroz MC, Obeso JA, Lang AE, et al. Bilateral deep brain stimulation in Parkinson's disease: a multicentre study with 4 years follow-up. *Brain*, 128(Pt 10): 2240–2249, 2005.

76. Burn DJ, Troster AI. Neuropsychiatric complications of medical and surgical therapies for Parkinson's disease. *J Geriatr Psychiatry Neurol*, 17(3): 172–180, 2004.

77. Funkiewiez A, Ardouin C, Krack P, et al. Acute psychotropic effects of bilateral subthalamic nucleus stimulation and levodopa in Parkinson's disease. *Mov Disord*, 18(5): 524–530, 2003.

78. Witt K, Daniels C, Reiff J, et al. Neuropsychological and psychiatric changes after deep brain stimulation for Parkinson's disease: a randomised, multicentre study. *Lancet Neurol*, 7(7): 605–614, 2008.

79. Groenewegen HJ, Wright CI, Uylings HB. The anatomical relationships of the prefrontal cortex with limbic structures and the basal ganglia. *J Psychopharmacol*, 11(2): 99–106, 1997.

80. Kuhn AA, Hariz MI, Silberstein P, et al. Activation of the subthalamic region during emotional processing in Parkinson disease. *Neurology*, 65(5): 707–713, 2005.

81. Stefurak T, Mikulis D, Mayberg H, et al. Deep brain stimulation for Parkinson's disease dissociates mood and motor circuits: a functional MRI case study. *Mov Disord*, 18(12): 1508–1516, 2003.

82. Schlaepfer TE, Lieb K. Deep brain stimulation for treatment of refractory depression. *Lancet*, 366(9495): 1420–1422, 2005.

83. Moro E, Lang AE, Strafella AP, et al. Bilateral globus pallidus stimulation for Huntington's disease. *Ann Neurol*, 56(2): 290–294, 2004.

84. Peschanski M, Bachoud-Levi AC, Hantraye P. Integrating fetal neural transplants into a therapeutic strategy: the example of Huntington's disease. *Brain*, 127(Pt 6): 1219–1228, 2004.

85. Dunnett SB, Rosser AE. Cell therapy in Huntington's disease. *NeuroRx*, 1(4): 394–405, 2004.

Depression and Multiple Sclerosis

Dana J. Serafin,[1] Deborah M. Weisbrot,[2] and Alan B. Ettinger[3]

[1]Department of Neurology, Stony Brook University Medical Center, Stony Brook, NY, USA
[2]Department of Psychiatry and Behavioral Sciences, Stony Brook University Medical Center, Stony Brook, NY, USA
[3]Neurological Surgery P.C., Lake Success, NY, USA

Introduction

Individuals who have been diagnosed with multiple sclerosis (MS) face an ongoing struggle to maintain their independence and dignity in the face of this chronic, disabling illness. Until recently, the emphasis for neurologists has been on mastering the complexities of the diagnosis and treatment of this condition. However, no less important is the profound impact that MS may have on an individual's mood and overall quality of life. This disorder, with its remitting and relapsing qualities, generally progressive nature, potentially detrimental impacts on cognitive functioning, fatigue, and mood, takes the patient and his or her family on an emotional rollercoaster that can last for generations. This chapter will review different aspects of depression in MS, including an exploration of the neuropathological underpinnings, and discuss clinical assessment of mood and treatment interventions when depression is present in the MS patient.

Multiple sclerosis: general overview

MS is a chronic inflammatory demyelinating disorder of the central nervous system (CNS) [1, 2] whose etiology is unknown but may represent the effects of both genetic and environmental factors. Demyelination may affect the white matter tracts of the cerebral hemispheres, brain-stem, spinal cord, cerebellum, and optic nerves. Symptoms associated with MS include weakness of one or more extremities, ataxia, vision loss, bladder and bowel malfunction, fatigue, and mood changes [3, 4]. There is a higher prevalence of MS in individuals under 40 years of age and in females, who make up about 80% of relapsing–remitting multiple sclerosis (RRMS) and about half of primary progressive multiple sclerosis (PPMS) [5]. The majority of persons diagnosed with MS (60%) initially begin with RRMS, in which exacerbations, or relapses, of symptoms are followed by recovery periods. RRMS begins with a single mono- or multifocal demyelinating episode, that is, clinically isolated syndrome (CIS). RRMS generally progresses to secondary progressive multiple sclerosis (SPMS), which is characterized by a steady worsening of symptoms, sometimes including occasional flare-ups [6]. The later stage of MS takes the form of PPMS, which is characterized by a steady progression of disease symptoms from the time of onset, representing about 12% of patients with MS [6, 7].

Although much is known about the symptoms and prevalence of MS, little is known regarding its cause. There is strong evidence for environmental and genetics factors in the etiology of MS, and it is probable that both play a role. Hereditary propensity is indicated by increased risk in siblings and more so in twins with a diagnosis

Depression in Neurologic Disorders: Diagnosis and Management, First Edition.
Edited by Andres M. Kanner.
© 2012 Blackwell Publishing Ltd. Published 2012 by Blackwell Publishing Ltd.

[8, 9]. Epidemiologic studies have distinguished relationships between prevalence of disease and geographical location as well as migration patterns. The prevalence of MS varies considerably throughout the world, with the highest rates in northern Europe, Southern Australia, Canada, and the United States [10, 11]. MS is rare in Asia as well as in regions of temperate climates since MS prevalence increases with latitude north and south of the equator [12]. Furthermore, a person's risk of getting MS changes if he or she migrates to an area of higher or lower prevalence [13]. Many have suggested this is due to sunlight exposure increasing vitamin D levels [14]. Finally, there is additional research proposing infections as the cause of MS [15, 16]. Many theories exist; however, the cause of MS and of autoimmune diseases in general remains unknown.

Although the general assessment of disability in MS heavily weighs motor function and ambulation and less heavily weighs pain and fatigue [17], there are a wide range of neuropsychiatric comorbidities, including cognitive impairment, anxiety, and depression [18, 19]. The diagnosis of MS can have a profound effect on the social and psychological aspects of a patient's quality of life. This is partly due to the diagnosis of a chronic illness, but also because MS most commonly affects young adults and has an extremely unpredictable nature [20]. However, depression in MS may be more complicated than simply being a reactive phenomenon to incurring a debilitating disorder; structural, immunological, and neurochemical abnormalities in MS also play an important role.

According to the World Health Organization, five of the 10 leading causes of worldwide disability are psychiatric conditions, including unipolar depression, substance abuse, bipolar disorder, schizophrenia, and obsessive–compulsive disorder. In the general population, a family practitioner can expect one in four patients to have an active psychiatric disorder; for adult neurologists, that number jumps to 4 in 10 [21]. The National Comorbidity Survey administered a structural psychiatric interview to a representative national sample in the United States and found, according to *Diagnostic and Statistical Manual of Mental Disorders*, Third Edition, Revised (DSM-III-R) criteria, that 50% of respond-

ents reported at least one lifetime disorder and 17% reported a history of major depressive episode (MDE) in their lifetime. About one in every five respondents reported a lifetime history of at least one affective disorder; alcohol dependence and anxiety disorder were among the other most common psychiatric symptoms found. More than half of all lifetime disorders occurred in 14% of the population with a history of three or more comorbid disorders [22]. The notable Australian Survey of Mental Health and Well-Being of Adults (SMHWB) found 6% of individuals aged 18 years and over suffer from depression [23]. These statistics provide a reference point for the comparison of rates of depression in MS.

Symptoms and signs of depression in MS

Major depression, or major depressive disorder (MDD), is a mental disorder characterized by the presence of symptoms such as sad mood, loss of interest in usual activities, sleeping problems, fatigue, irritability, reduced appetite, negative self-image, reduced concentration, and suicidal thoughts [24]. Less frequently, some individuals with major depressive symptoms also have psychotic symptoms, such as delusions or hallucinations. Many somatic MS symptoms, such as fatigue, reduced concentration, irritability, and suicidal thoughts [18, 19] overlap with depression and can cause confusion when assessing the presence of depression. One issue is that measures of depression in this population may be inflated, or conversely, the depressive symptoms may be assumed to be a symptom of MS, leaving the depression undiagnosed. Clinicians sometimes assume that any individual who is dealing with a severe, chronic, neurologic condition such as MS will naturally be depressed. Consequently, opportunities are missed to identify the presence of a treatable psychiatric condition.

Bipolar disorder is a complex psychiatric condition in which depressed mood alternates with manic and/or hypomanic episodes. The estimated prevalence of bipolar disorder is 1% worldwide [25]. Rates of bipolar disorder, or at least bipolar symptoms, are elevated in MS, with prevalence rates ranging from 2% to 13% among different epidemiologic studies [26], although few formal studies exist. Bipolar disorder must be distinguished from manic-like symptoms that may occur as a result of steroid administration for MS, which can cause euphoria, increased energy, and diminished sleep [27]. Recently, it has also become common to informally and incorrectly apply the term "bipolar" to individuals who have frequent mood swings or who have high levels of anger. This is quite different from the actual diagnosis of a bipolar disorder and can be indicative of a number of other psychiatric diagnoses. When obtaining a family psychiatric history, it is important to clarify whether formal diagnoses and symptoms of bipolar disorder were actually present or whether the term is being applied more informally.

Along with the presence of very severe depression, which is indicative of an MDE, it is also important for clinicians to recognize the presence of dysthymic disorder [24]. Dysthymic disorder is sometimes referred to as "chronic depression," in which the symptoms are described as less severe than in an MDE but can fluctuate in intensity. The essential symptom in dysthymic disorder is the presence of depressed feelings for a majority of the time over at least 2 years. Disturbances in sleep or appetite and low self-esteem are typical of the clinical presentation, and the disorder can precede or follow the development of a full-blown MDE. Dysthymic disorder can exist unrecognized and untreated for such a long period of time that the individual may conclude that a depressed mood is a part of his or her personality [24].

Pseudobulbar affect

Pseuobulbar affect, informally termed "emotional incontinence," is characterized by sudden and uncontrolled emotional displays that are unrelated to the true emotions experienced by the patient. For example, a slight stimulus may induce bouts of prolonged laughter or crying [28, 29]. This condition, although often treated with antidepressants, is common in advanced MS and must be distinguished from true depression or bipolar disorder [29]. Patients with pseudobulbar affect can often identify and describe their overt emotional reactions as much more intense than their actual emotional state. In contrast to the heightened emotional presentation of pseudobulbar affect, disorders such as MS that heavily affect subcortical regions may cause an abulic state characterized by minimal initiative and apathy [28]. This is another condition that should be distinguished from a true depressive disorder.

Prevalence of depression in MS

The relationship between depression and MS has been recognized and studied for many years [30, 31], with most studies showing high rates of depression in the MS population. In one study, administration of a psychiatric interview of 221 patients with MS attending an MS clinic in Vancouver revealed that 34.4% of patients had a current or lifetime diagnosis of depression, with 50.3% of patients estimated to have a cumulative risk for depression by age 59 [32]. Another Canadian study combining self-report measures with psychiatric interviews of 100 consecutive MS clinic patients reported a 42% lifetime prevalence of major depression [26]. Through the use of a structured psychiatric interview, along with standardized rating scales, Minden et al. determined that 54% of the 50 enrolled MS study patients met research diagnostic criteria for major depression at least once since they were diagnosed, and 14% of this group met criteria prior to their diagnosis [33]. In a more recent study, Schiffer found that up to 65% of MS clinic patients reported depressive symptoms. This higher rate emphasizes the importance of recognizing subthreshold depressive symptoms that do not necessarily meet criteria for DSM-based depressive disorder [21]. These substantial depression rates are likely to be higher than what would be anticipated in community-based populations since tertiary centers tend to attract more severe cases.

There are far fewer population-based studies of depression in MS, yet the frequencies of depression here are also notable. One population-based study examined 115,071 patients aged 18 years and older using a predictive depression scale from a Community Health Survey, the Composite International Diagnostic Interview Short Form for Major Depression. Of the 322 participants with MS, the 12-month prevalence rate was found to be 25.7% as compared with only 8.9% in those without MS [34]. In a mail survey of a large community sample, 739 patients with MS completed the self-Expanded Disability Status Scale (EDSS) and the Center for Epidemiologic Studies Depression Scale (CES-D). The EDSS is a method of quantifying disability in MS and takes into account eight functional systems [35]. Symptoms of clinical depression were found in 41.8% of the subjects, while 29.1% had moderate to severe depression. Additional findings showed that depressive symptoms increased with greater disease severity (higher EDSS) and shorter disease duration [18]. In a cross-sectional populated-based study in Norway, it was shown that the frequency of symptoms of depression and anxiety doubled and tripled, respectively, in patients with MS compared to the general Norwegian population [36].

Understanding why depression is so prevalent in MS is a challenging and complex task. To conclude that it is simply the result of the burden of a neurologic disorder does not suffice because there are other, more disabling neurologic disorders in which depression is infrequent, such as amyotrophic lateral sclerosis [37]. While many studies of patients with MS from specialty centers report high rates of depression—sometimes exceeding rates of depression reported in other chronic and progressive disorders [26, 38–40]—comparative rates should be interpreted with caution since these disorders are not usually studied in a controlled fashion, matching each disorder's population on a range of variables such as duration and severity of disease.

Although a wealth of information exists regarding depression in adult patients with MS, little is known about the nature and severity of psychiatric comorbidity in pediatric MS. A study of 23 children aged 6–17 years with demyelinating disorders of the CNS including MS, acute disseminated encephalomyelitis, CIS, neuromyelitis optica, and recurrent optic neuritis was conducted at an MS specialty center. Disability was judged by the EDSS, and patients were assessed and diagnosed with a semistructured interview, the Schedule for Affective Disorders and Schizophrenia, present and lifetime version, and several self-report measures. Results showed that nearly half (11/23) of the patients met criteria for at least one psychiatric diagnosis, and 7 of these 11 patients had an MS diagnosis.

Additionally, 74% of all patients expressed at least one worry or concern during the psychiatric interview. Given the high rates presented here, the study suggests that clinicians should screen for psychiatric comorbidity in pediatric demyelinating disorders and lays the groundwork for larger prospective studies to be performed in the future [41].

Relationship of MS severity to depression

While it is intuitive that depression rates and severity would follow linearly with the severity of deficits and impairment in MS, this has not been uniformly seen. This disparity between depression and degree of impairment contributes to the argument that depression is driven significantly by biological forces. The location of lesions in patients with MS and their impact upon limbic circuits may be a more compelling cause of depression than the patient's bodily deficits. One notable study found an association of depression with major cognitive impairment, social stress, and quality of life, but surprisingly not with any degree of neurologic impairment or disability [42, 43]. Most studies, however, have found at least a rough correlation of decreased physical functioning with depression. One such study found that increased anxiety and depression in patients led to a greater correlation between worse scores on the EDSS and quality of life decrements [44]. Another study of 50 MS participants from an MS outpatient facility found that Beck Depression Inventory (BDI) scores and risk for MDD increased with disease severity and physical disability. BDI scores did increase with disease duration, but this correlation was not significant after controlling for age and gender [45]. Although these findings are comparable to several studies [46–48], they are not supported by others, which report a higher rate of depression during the first period of diagnosis [18] and in patients under 35 years of age [49].

In a study of 115 Parisian patients recruited through specialty associations and MS clinics, 58% were disabled, 66.7% had an EDSS score >4, and 48% used a wheelchair on a full- or part-time basis. Depression and sociodemographic factors were collected through questionnaires filled out at the patients' homes during a visit with a psychology student. The EDSS was determined by their neurologist and mailed in. The results showed that the functional status (by EDSS), anxiety, alexithymia (inability to express feelings in words), and social support were the most effective predicting factors of depression in MS. Anxiety and functional status showed the strongest correlation, while alexithymia and social support had an indirect correlation [50]. Although significant correlations were found with these predictors and depression, the total sample was generally not depressed, with only 25% showing symptoms of depression and only 5% with severe depressive symptoms. Additionally, as the authors point out, the high correlation between depression and alexithymia could be due to overlapping symptoms endorsement, especially on items asking about difficulty in identifying and expressing one's own feelings [50].

Of note, many of the studies finding positive correlations used the EDSS to evaluate disability [35]. Although the EDSS is the most commonly used physical disability scale in MS, some authors have questioned its sensitivity [51, 52]. In one study of 172 patients with MS, depressive symptoms were reported significantly more frequently than in the general population, with 25.7% of patients with MS reporting symptoms versus 10.6% of controls ($p < 0.001$). However, there was no significant difference in the EDSS scores between patients with clinically significant symptoms of anxiety and depression, judged by the Hospital Anxiety and Depression scale [53], and patients who did not express these symptoms [54].

An interesting study of 136 patients with MS compared RRMS and PPMS and found that although the EDSS was higher in PPMS than RRMS (6.5 and 5.0, respectively), the lifetime prevalence of major depression was 26.4% in the RRMS group and only 10% in the PPMS group. The authors theorized that this was due to the later age of onset in PPMS, which allows for well-established social support [52, 55]. Another possibility is the coping level of patients with PPMS and their acceptance of the disease, as opposed to the devastation of changes in condition during relapses in RRMS. In a sample of 166 patients, exacerbations in illness drastically increased patients' level of uncertainty and increased their depression as seen by a significant correlation between depression scores and current exacerbations in illness ($r = 0.31$, $p = 0.001$) [56].

Aspects of age and gender in MS-associated depression

Rates of MS are higher in women and individuals over the age of 40. Depression itself is more common in women [57, 58]. Due to this skewed prevalence, research on rates of depression across age and gender in MS are contradictory. It has been reported that patients diagnosed with MS under age 35 were significantly more likely to report a history of MDD than those over 35. Included in the group with higher reported depression were women and those who had a family history of MS [49]. Women with MS were seen to have a significantly higher prevalence of depression than men. Of the 99 women participating in the previously cited study of 164 patients, 28% had major depression, while only 8% of the men met criteria for major depression [49]. Similar findings regarding gender and depression and anxiety were seen in other studies [45, 59]. To explain the increased prevalence of depression in women with MS, one study showed that women with MS report decreased social support and higher social demands of the illness [5]; however, no comparison between males with MS was attempted in this study.

There have been several studies that found no significant difference in depression across genders [18, 36] and in fact have used this point as evidence that the MS disease process, as opposed to the emotional reaction to a diagnosis of a chronic illness, is a direct source of depression [60]. The difficulty here is that if depression is more prevalent in females in the general population, then why would that not be the case in MS? One study admits to a possible sample bias in that the males in the study had a significantly higher EDSS and therefore greater severity of disease [18]. An earlier study, which also reported no difference in depression across genders in MS, proposed that hormonal or biological factors in women with MS may explain this disparity [61].

Several community-based and tertiary center studies have found that older patients with MS report fewer depressive symptoms than younger patients [52, 62]. These findings coincide with another study that found lower rates of depression in patients with a longer duration of disease [18]. One possible reason for this is the stressful and unpredictable nature of first being diagnosed with and then dealing with the disease. Older patients with MS have had the time to cope with their disease and to develop social support, strategies which younger patients may not have learned yet. Additionally, younger patients with MS may feel they have more to lose in terms of starting a career or a family.

Potential etiologies of depression in MS

As mentioned earlier, the idea that depression in MS arises as a reactive phenomenon to incurring such a chronic and debilitating disorder does not explain the higher prevalence of depression in MS compared to many other chronic disorders [34]. Furthermore, the presumptive link between all chronic illness and depression fails to explain the compelling associations of depression with the structural and inflammatory factors inherent to MS.

While psychosocial factors [42, 63, 64], issues with coping [65, 66], and pessimistic outlook [67, 68] undoubtedly play a major role in depression in MS, other factors such as immune dysregulation [69] and the development of brain lesions [47, 70] are likely to be important factors. However, MS has unique features compared to some other diseases, such as its unpredictable and variable course, which can make adjustment to this disorder particularly challenging. Interventions designed to help patients combat feelings of demoralization may reduce or prevent many of the symptoms associated with depression, such as a sense of hopelessness [27].

Correlations between CNS injury and depression, as revealed by neuroimaging studies, have been seen in a number of neurologic conditions, such as stroke [71], head trauma [72], and epilepsy [73]. Lateralization (often dominant hemisphere) and specific localizations (e.g., temporal lobe) of the lesion have often correlated with

higher rates of depression as well. While it is clear that cerebral predominant MS is much more associated with depression than spinal cord MS [47, 74, 75], studies of lateralization and localization of cerebral regions of demyelination have had conflicting results.

In a study of 95 patients with MS, 97 patients with rheumatoid disease, and 110 healthy subjects, participants underwent a 1.5-Tesla MRI as well as assessments of disability, independence, cognitive performances, and depression and anxiety. A DSM-IV-based diagnosis of major depression occurred in 18.9% of patients with MS. Depression was correlated with right frontal lesion load, decreased right temporal brain volume, decreased total temporal brain volume, and diminished right hemisphere brain volume [47].

Conversely, in a study of 45 patients with MS, seven patients ranked as severely depressed by the BDI. Worse BDI scores correlated with lesion load of the left arcuate fasciculus region, of which these lesions were only a small part of the total lesions. No correlation was found with depression and lesions in the frontotemporal white matter or the total lesion area, an observation comparable to those of several other studies [76]. Variations in the assessment of depression severity among different studies may be one of many explanations for variability in results.

In a study of 62 patients meeting McDonald Criteria for MS diagnosis [77], subjects with depression (by BDI) had smaller, normal appearing white matter (NAWM) volume in the left superior frontal region and greater hypointense lesion volume in the right medial inferior frontal region. Diffusion tensor imaging showed significantly higher mean diffusivity in the left anterior temporal lobe normal appearing gray matter (NAGM) of the group with depression. Additionally, the fractional anisotropy was reduced in the NAWM of the left anterior temporal lobe in the group with depression. These data, in addition to lesion and atrophy data, explain 34.8% of the depression variance, which leads to the following conclusion: depression in MS is correlated with decreased brain volume and brain atrophy in the frontal and temporal brain regions, and reduction in NAWM volume is highly correlated with depression [78].

A study of 10 patients with MS with depression found a significant effect of depression on perfusion asymmetries in the limbic cortex compared with 10 MS patients without depression. Perfusion asymmetries in the limbic cortex correlated significantly with depression scores, as measured by the Beck and Hamilton scales. The authors suggest that depression in MS could be "induced by a disconnection between subcortical and cortical areas involved in the function of the limbic system" [79]. Irrespective of distinct localizations, neuroimaging studies emphasize the role of structural abnormalities in MS and argue strongly for biologic pathogenesis of depression in MS.

A recent study of high resolution MRI among 29 patients with RRMS found that the subset with depression had smaller dentate gyrus subregion hippocampal volumes [80]. These data are compatible with studies in the general population with primary depression [81] and the epilepsy population [82]. The results are particularly intriguing because, when placed in the context of other studies, they suggest that the hippocampal region may serve as a common pathway for causation or effect of depression [80].

Immunological aspects of depression in MS

There are many intriguing commonalities among the immunological abnormalities of MS and depression, suggesting that there may be an immunological contribution to depressive symptoms in this disorder. For example, primary depression has been associated with diminished natural killer B, T-helper, and suppressor–cytotoxic T cells [83] and increased proinflammatory cytokines (regulatory proteins released by immune system cells that mediate the generation of immune responses). Administration of antidepressants in primary depression has been associated with a reduction in cytokine levels. Furthermore, stress, which is intimately associated with depression, can affect cytokine levels [27].

High rates of depression in MS (a hallmark inflammatory disease) lead to speculation that inflammation itself may play a role in the pathogenesis of depression in this disorder [84]. For example, interferon (IFN)-γ, the cytokine generated by the T-helper cells, may play a role in MS [85] and has been found in elevated concentrations in individuals with depression. While it remains unclear whether depression is an epiphenomenon of the inflammatory changes that occur in MS, future studies of these relationships may be of substantial value in furthering our understanding of the pathogenesis of depression in general as well as offer another avenue of treatment for this important comorbidity of MS.

Basic assessment of depression in MS

Not every MS patient needs to be referred for psychiatric evaluation. However, the underrecognition of depression in MS is a reality, which means that there are many individuals whose depression is going untreated. Clinicians need to do a basic assessment of psychiatric symptoms, and then, if there are concerns about depression or any other psychiatric symptoms (e.g., anxiety, mania, psychosis, or cognitive difficulties), consultation with a psychiatrist should be considered. The diagnosis of depression in MS is a complex and challenging one; the psychiatrist must be well informed about the nature of depressive symptoms in this disorder, including the role that disease-modifying medications could be playing in exacerbating depression. There may be patients who have subsyndromal symptoms of depression who nonetheless need to be treated for this condition even if they do not meet formal criteria for a diagnosis of an MDE or another depressive disorder such as dysthymic disorder, in which chronic symptoms of depression may be present for months or years.

Every initial psychiatric assessment involves gathering information with regard to a wide range of psychiatric symptoms. For example, symptoms of anxiety are often present in individuals with depression. In MS, problems with cognitive difficulties can play a critical role. It is important to inquire about the patient's understanding of the nature and prognosis of his or her condition. Whenever possible, the assessment of psychiatric symptoms should involve not only the patient, but also a close family member who knows the patient well. Patients often have complex reasons for denying depressive symptoms and other difficulties, whereas a family member may be more revealing. Furthermore, the family's response to the patient's neurologic disorder may be playing a critical role in the patient's depressive symptoms.

Asking patients about MS and depression

Given the high prevalence of symptoms of depression in patients with MS, clinicians should always inquire about the presence of such symptoms. Taking the time to ask a few questions about a patient's mood symptoms can be invaluable. In the section below, we have provided a set of questions that can be used as a model to screen for depression. These questions represent only one aspect of a full psychiatric assessment, which should elicit information on all types of psychiatric symptoms [86].

Asking about MS

1. Can you tell me about your understanding of MS and your particular condition?
2. Can you tell me how having MS has changed your daily life?
3. How has MS changed your life with your spouse/parents/friends?
4. How has MS changed your life at work/ school?
5. Do you think that you (and your parents/ spouse/family/friends) have accepted that you have MS?

Asking about depression

1. Are you having difficulty finding pleasure in activities you used to enjoy?
2. Do you have to push yourself now to do things that you used to enjoy in the past?
3. Do people get on your nerves for things that never used to bother you before?
4. Do you have little tolerance for people?
5. Do you notice that your mood changes without any apparent reason? For example, one day you are happy, and without any reason you get moody, cranky, and cannot enjoy anything the next day?
6. Do you feel so bad that you feel completely hopeless?
7. Do you feel that there is nothing you can do to feel better about yourself?
8. Do you find yourself crying for things that never made you cry before?
9. Do you sometimes wish you were dead?
10. Do you think about ways of harming yourself?

Screening inventories for depression in MS

Given the substantial rates of mood disorders in MS and the potential opportunity to successfully treat another disabling comorbidity, screening for depression is a compelling but often neglected aspect of the evaluation of patients with MS. Such assessments may receive low priority among the overwhelming numbers of other neurologic and systemic complications of MS, such as paresthesias, visual deficits, cognitive difficulties, and bladder impairments. There are a number of self-report scales that can enhance efficiency in the evaluation of depression and related comorbidities and may help detect symptoms that are not clear from responses to verbal queries from the clinician. For example, the previously mentioned CES-D is a 20-item depression inventory, with 0 being the least depressed and 60 being the most depressed [87]; generally, a score of 16 or higher is defined as clinically significant [18, 87, 88]. The CES-D is commonly used in research studies of depression in MS. Another popular depression screening tool is the BDI, a 21-item self-report rating inventory [89].

Some argue that symptoms of MS or its treatments may be spuriously endorsed in some depression screening tools, and thus that screening measures would pick up fewer false positives by focusing predominantly on mood symptoms. In epilepsy, a similar concern led to the development of the Neurologic Disorders Depression Inventory for Epilepsy [90]. In MS, tools with higher specificity, such as the Chicago Multiscale Depression Inventory [91] or the highly efficient BDI-Fast Screen [46], have been recently used.

Screening measures for comorbidities that often impact depression include the Multiple Sclerosis Severity Score, which measures speed of disability accumulation by relating an individual patient's disease course and duration to a large patient sample [92]. The Fatigue Severity Scale is a nine-item scale, with 1 being the least fatigued and 7 being the most fatigued [93]. The EDSS was described earlier in this chapter [35].

Suicidality in MS

Given the high rates of depression in MS, suicide risk is also of major concern. In fact, the statistics on suicide rates in patients with MS are staggering, with suicide rates estimated to be several times higher than in the general population [94]. A study of patients from two separate MS clinics looked at etiologies of 119 deaths within a patient sample from 1972 to 1988. While 56 deaths were attributable to MS complications, of the remaining 63 patients, 18 (28.6%) committed suicide, a rate 7.5 times higher than in an age-matched general population. The remaining deaths were caused by malignancy (30.2%), acute myocardial infarction (20.6%), stroke (5.9%), and miscellaneous causes (9.5%) [95]. A Danish study also reported a high prevalence of suicide in patients with MS as compared with the general population, with the highest risk in younger male patients [96]. When 140 consecutive patients from an MS clinic in Canada were assessed for suicidal ideation, a 28.6% lifetime prevalence of suicide was detected, with 6.4% having made an actual suicide attempt. Severe depression, alcohol problems, and living alone characterized 85% of the suicidal intent cases. Additionally, two-thirds of the patients with major depression were not being treated for their depression [40, 97]. Men, patients newly diagnosed with MS, and patients who received their diagnosis before the age of 30 may be at a particularly elevated risk of suicide [98].

In a nationwide investigation in Scandinavia, the risk of death by suicide for patients with MS was assessed using records kept at the Danish Multiple Sclerosis Registry (DMSR) and the Danish National Register of Cause of Death. The investigation covered all patients with MS registered with the DSMR with an onset of the disease within the period 1953–1985, or for whom MS was diagnosed in the same period. Fifty-three of the 5525 cases in the onset cohort group committed suicide. Using the figures from the population death statistics by adjustment to number of subjects, duration of observation, sex, age, and calendar year at the start of observation, the expected number of suicides was calculated to be nearly 29. The cumulative lifetime risk of suicide

from onset of MS, using an actuarial method of calculation, was 1.95%. The standardized mortality ratio (SMR) of suicide in MS was 1.83. The SMR was highest for males, patients with onset of MS before the age of 30, and those diagnosed before the age of 40. The SMR was highest within the first 5 years after diagnosis [96]. Identification of patients with suicidal ideation warrants urgent psychiatric evaluation. The aforementioned studies suggest that early detection of depression and suicidal ideation is crucial in the population. Proper recognition could lead to antidepressant interventions, which may ultimately be life saving [99].

Fatigue, depression, and MS

Fatigue has often been reported as the most frequent and disabling symptom in MS [100, 101]. Fatigue is also a common symptom of depression; therefore, distinguishing fatigue as a symptom of the demyelinating disease versus a symptom of depression can be challenging. Fatigue symptoms may predict subsequent manifestations of depression and vice versa [102]. A number of other symptoms of depression, such as lack of motivation and sleep disturbance, can also overlap with fatigue [103, 104]. However, recognizing fatigue and depression as distinct entities is very important because treatments may vary. Furthermore, treatment of depression may or may not improve fatigue symptoms. One study of fatigue and depression eliminated overlapping items between the two symptoms from the depression scale, only to leave those questions associated with mood aberration. The results showed that fatigue still had a highly significant correlation with the depressive mood symptoms ($p < 0.001$) [105]. The same study performed a regression analysis to control for education and disability and found that depressed mood persisted as a significant predictor of fatigue, and the correlation between the two remained highly significant ($r = 0.38$) [105].

Effects of MS-associated cognitive deficits on depression

Anecdotal experience and numerous studies have demonstrated the common occurrence of cognitive impairments in MS, with a prevalence rate of over 40% [106–108]. The most commonly recognized cognitive impairments in MS include memory dysfunction, particularly deficits in working, semantic, and episodic memory, as well as in complex attention, information processing speed, and executive functions [19]. Language and attention span are generally spared [109]. Cognitive impairments in combination with depression can be devastating for a patient's level of function, which in turn could contribute to depressive symptoms.

Although impaired cognitive functioning and depression are both major symptoms in MS, there has been conflicting research as to whether impaired cognition is directly etiologic for depression. A study of 106 patients with MS found 29.3% of patients to be cognitively impaired, and impaired cognition to be significantly correlated with anxiety, depression, fatigue, and quality of life [110]. However, the low number of impaired individuals, and more importantly, the mild impairment seen, could contribute to a misrepresented correlation between this impaired group and depression. Furthermore, when controlling for quality of life, the correlation with depression and cognitive impairment was no longer significant, causing some confusion as to this relationship. In a study of 63 patients with RRMS and PPMS, approximately 30% showed moderate to severe depression on the BDI, while about 70% had only mild depression or were not depressed at all and 37% showed cognitive impairment in sustained attention, concentration, and verbal memory. However, no correlation was found between cognitive impairment and BDI scores [109], a result that is consistent with other similar studies [111].

Cognitive impairments may also be related to depression through its adverse impact on coping strategies. One study of 44 parents with MS used the coping index (CI) and a neurocognitive battery to determine this relationship. It was found that successful coping with the disease (high CI) correlated with fewer depressive symptoms, a higher level of complex attention, and a lower premorbid verbal intelligence. While such studies demonstrate association rather than causality, these relationships suggest that cognitive impairments may raise the risk of depression through their effects on coping [112].

A study of negative affect and cognitive impairment examined a cohort of 38 patients with MS, excluding those meeting criteria for major depression but including cases with milder forms of depressive symptomatology. Negative affect and symptoms of depression consistently predicted decreased cognition over a 1-year period. This study not only shows that there is a link between cognitive impairment and depressive symptoms, but also that patients without clinical depression but with a negative affect can experience adverse consequences [113]. The disparities in the conflicting studies could be due to the use of a different neuropsychological battery, participant bias, variability in the severity and duration of the disease, some overlapping symptoms of depression, and quality of life. Furthermore, looking at cognitive impairments in a global fashion may dilute relationships that do exist between very specific cognitive deficits and depression [48]. Clarification of the relationship between cognitive impairment and depression deserves further study since the identification of specific cognitive problems would enable the clinician to identify patients at higher risk for depression.

Adverse effect of disease-modifying treatments on depression in MS

As previously mentioned, there are several stages of MS, and the majority of the treatments currently available are targeted at RRMS or CIS, though some are also approved for SPMS. The first-line agents are immunomodulators, consisting mainly of interferon-β (IFN-β) and glatiramer acetate. IFN-β can be found in three different forms: IFN-β-1a intramuscular (IM) weekly injections (Avonex, Biogen Idec, Weston, MA) [114, 115], IFN-β-1a three times per week subcutaneous injections (Rebif, Pfizer, New York) [116], and IFN-β-1b (Betaseron, Bayer HealthCare, Leverkusen, Germany) every other day subcutaneous injections [117]. In 1993, IFN-β-1b became the first immunomodulatory therapy approved for the treatment of RRMS [117, 118]. Glatiramer acetate (Copaxone, Teva Pharmaceutical Industries Ltd., Petah Tikva, Israel) is a synthetic amino acid polymer that was approved for treatment of RRMS in 1997 [119]. Monoclonal antibody natalizumab (Tysabri, Biogen Idec) is an example of a second-line therapy for MS [120]. Tysabri has been shown to provide some drastic benefits to patients; however, there is a slight risk of a deadly brain infection, progressive multifocal leukoencephalopathy, along with other infections, which causes physicians to prescribe it with extreme caution and only as a second-line therapy [121].

The most common adverse reactions with the use of IFN-βs are lymphopenia, injection site reactions, asthenia, flu-like symptoms, headache, pain, and elevated liver enzymes. Soon after the introduction of the beta interferons, reports arose of patients who had received this treatment experiencing heightened depression [122–124] or even attempting suicide [125]. Depression was also reported to be higher among recipients of Avonex as compared to controls in a major trial [126]. However, later analysis of earlier reports of IFN-associated depression found that studies implementing more rigorous validated depression measures did not yield a higher rate of depression in the IFN group [127]. Furthermore, subsequent trials, such as the Secondary Progressive Efficacy Trial of Rebif in Multiple Sclerosis (SPECTRIMS), found no difference in depression in IFN recipients [128]. Subsequent studies have suggested that depression and suicidality formerly attributed to IFN treatments were actually more closely related to pretreatment depression [129, 130]. Therefore, the current thinking then is that interferons should not be withheld out of fear of exacerbating depression or inducing suicidal thoughts. On the other hand, there may be individual patients in whom treatment with an IFN-β appears to be associated with increased depression. In such cases, glatiramer acetate may be an alternative, particularly because it enhances production of brain-derived neurotrophic factor [131], which in turn may have theoretical benefits in depression [132].

Currently there are no black box warnings for either IFN-β-1a or IFN-β-1b. The prescribing information for IFN-β-1b does report three suicides and eight suicide attempts in four randomized controlled trials (1532 patients) compared with four attempted suicides in the placebo groups of these trials with 952 subjects [133]. In 2003, the Food and Drug Administration (FDA) released postmarketing reports of suicide and suicidal ideation for IFN-β-1a; however, no black box warnings were issued.

During MS exacerbations, steroids, which are associated with a wide variety of potential mood-altering effects, may be utilized. Depression and irritability symptoms in particular are a commonly encountered adverse effect of steroids, although as mentioned earlier, euphoric states and mood swings may also be induced, sometimes to the point of a "steroid psychosis."

Effects of depression on MS treatment adherence

Adherence with MS treatment recommendations is an ongoing challenge for clinicians managing patients with MS. The hassle and cost of using injection treatment is especially difficult. Depression can adversely impact treatment adherence. In a multicenter observational survey study, 798 MS patients from 17 neurology clinics completed three waves of online surveys consisting of the Multiple Sclerosis Quality of Life-54 Instrument (MSQOL-54), the BDI, the Herth Hope Index, and a self-report adherence survey regarding injection behavior. Adherent patients had more favorable scores on the BDI compared with those encountered in nonadherent patients. Adherent patients also had higher scores on most of the physical and emotional sections of the MSQOL-54. While respondent bias may have influenced the results, striking differences between adherent and nonadherent groups suggest that these were genuine correlations [134]. Treating depression appears to improve adherence [135] and is thus another reason why screening for depression is so important.

Clinical management of depression in MS

While treating primary depression can be difficult, treating depression in patients with MS proves to be even more of a challenge. Studies have shown that effectively treating depressed patients with MS can lead to improved quality of life, functionality, self-esteem, and even compliance with MS treatment [65, 136, 137]. In contrast, untreated depression in MS may become more severe over time [138]. For many reasons, perhaps including the clinician's focus on other issues afflicting the patient as well as the patient's failure to recognize or ask for assistance for depression symptoms, depression is often inadequately treated in the MS population [137, 139]. In one study [140], 495 patients with MS completed the Functional Assessment Screening Questionnaire Revised, the General Information Multiple Sclerosis questionnaire, and the CES-D via mail survey. About 60% of participants demonstrated significant depressive symptoms (>16 on the CES-D) over the 2-year period. Among the patients with clinical depression, only 26.2% reported receiving treatment after being encouraged to do so by phase 2 of the study. Another interesting issue is that the majority of those patients who sought treatment for depression had only consulted their general practitioner and did not seek, nor were they referred to, any specialized help such as psychology or counseling. The authors noted that this is a serious issue because of the risk of side effects and other treatments that have proven to be effective in patients with MS [140].

Psychopharmacologic approaches to MS-related depression

Considering the very high frequency of depression in MS, it is surprising that there is a paucity of large sample studies and even fewer large gold standard randomized trials assessing the efficacy and side effects of specific antidepressant agents in MS [141]. One commonly cited controlled trial of antidepressants in MS showed beneficial effects of the tricyclic agent desiprimine [142]. Another small controlled trial found superiority of sertraline or cognitive–behavioral therapy (CBT) over placebo in treating depression [143]. Another small trial [144] found paroxetine to be superior to placebo, but intention-to-treat analysis substantially narrowed the difference between improvements in the treatment versus placebo groups. Otherwise, there are few randomized studies of the diverse choices of selective serotonin reuptake inhibitors (SSRIs) or serotonin norepinephrine reuptake inhibitors (SNRIs) in MS. Most of the literature on this subject comprises case reports and small case series. For example, among 12 patients who received fluoxetine (Prozac, Eli Lilly and Company, Indianapolis, IN) over 3 months, 10 improved as measured by the Clinical Global Impression scale, while minimal side effects were evident [145]. Another study of 10 patients with MS who received the monoamine oxidase inhibitor moclobemide also showed improvements, although this class of drugs is not generally used as a first-line agent in depression [146, 147]. When 60 patients with MS with depression were administered the SSRI sertraline (Zoloft, Pfizer) [146], depression in association with fatigue was significantly improved.

In the absence of abundant randomized trials of antidepressants in MS, good clinical judgment would dictate the selection of agents that would be most likely to be efficacious while avoiding exacerbations of the kinds of deficits that are common in MS. Earlier generation antidepressant agents (e.g., tricyclic antidepressants) are occasionally still used as a treatment for depression. In MS, however, caution should be taken in their use because of potential anticholinergic effects, which could worsen bowel and bladder impairments as well as cognition. On the other hand, they may be useful for some types of bladder dysfunction, such as detrusor spasm. Furthermore, tricyclic antidepressants such as desipramine or the SSRI paroxetine can be beneficial for their sedative and appetite-stimulating effects for patients with MS suffering from insomnia or weight loss. Tricyclic antidepressants or the SNRI duloxetine may also be useful to treat pain associated with MS.

Generally, SSRIs are better tolerated, especially those with less tendency for drug interactions such as citalopram or escitalopram. However, some SSRIs may cause or exacerbate preexisting fatigue or sexual dysfunction. In these cases, alternative agents such as bupropion or an SNRI (e.g., venlafaxine) may be more optimal.

Psychotherapeutic treatment modalities for depression in MS

Other traditional approaches to depression can also be used as primary or supplementary approaches to the treatment of depression in MS. Psychotherapy-related options, including individual exploratory and supportive psychotherapy, support groups, counseling, and CBT, can be considered. Social support techniques alone are unlikely to be sufficient [148]. In a study of 63 patients with MS with moderate depression, participants received 16 weeks of supportive expressive group therapy, CBT, and sertraline. While decreased symptoms of depression were evident, the contributions of each specific modality could not be discerned [149, 150]. Subsequent studies have suggested that CBT, which uses goal-oriented procedures to focus on coping skills, is more efficacious than insight-oriented therapy for depression in MS [151]. In a small study that compared CBT to sertraline, greater efficacy was found for the CBT group. A study of telephone-based CBT was also reported to be effective. As is the case with the treatment of MS-related depression with antidepressants, further study of psychotherapeutic interventions in MS is clearly needed.

Quality of life in MS

The experience of having MS, with all of its symptoms and difficulties, can have a profound effect on an individual's sense of well-being, happiness, and overall quality of life. Until recently, clinicians have been taught to focus on clinical and MRI measures of MS rather than on measurements of quality of life. The World Health Organization defines quality of life as individuals' perception of their position in life in the context of the culture and value systems in which they live and in relation to their goals, expectations, standards, and concerns [152]. Health-related quality of life represents the functional effect of an illness and its therapy as it is perceived by the patient [153]. Most patients with MS live with their illness for many decades and struggle with an extensive range of symptoms and difficulties during that time; therefore, it is not surprising that there would be relationships between quality of life measures and mood. A longitudinal study of patients with MS and CIS recruited from an MS specialty center found that depression was highly correlated with a number of health-related quality of life measures. More specifically, significance was seen with the Mental Health Inventory, the Mental Component Summary Score of the Short Form, and the Modified Fatigue Impact Scale [111].

Future directions in the study of MS-related depression

Further understanding of the clinical correlations between depression in MS and other variables, such as levels of cognitive impairment, physical disability, fatigue, and pain are needed. Future studies should study the relationships between depression and the inflammatory changes that occur in MS. Further advances in knowledge of how to treat depression when it occurs in MS are critical. Clinicians treating patients with MS must be more extensively trained regarding practical assessments of depression and suicidal ideation in these patients. There are significant gaps in our knowledge of how to treat depression when it occurs in MS. The relationship between disease-modifying medications, MS, depression, and suicidal behavior needs to be further clarified. The existing clinical studies on treating depression in MS with SSRIs, other antidepressant medications, and psychotherapy are quite limited and almost all have small sample sizes. There is a great need for large, multicenter placebo-controlled trials of antidepressants and psychotherapy in MS. Further study of the psychiatric aspects of pediatric MS is also needed. Early interventions could potentially decrease the severe impact that depression has on the quality of life in patients with MS.

Case study

MW is a 40-year-old woman who has had diagnosis of RRMS for the preceding 5 years, characterized by episodes of optic neuritis, paraparesis, appendicular ataxia, and bladder dysfunction. She is married and is a full-time homemaker with two children, aged 4 and 7. Each attack has left her with some degree of accruing permanent deficits. When she has met with the neurologist in the past, she has always appeared upbeat and insisted that she's "hanging in there" when asked about her emotional state. On the current visit to the neurologist, the patient's husband revealed his observation that she seemed to be much more withdrawn and emotionally detached over the past few months. In her response to the neurologist's inquiries, the patient revealed that she has recently experienced much more difficulty falling asleep, with episodic awakenings. She also reported diminished appetite with substantially reduced daily oral intake and weight loss. Upon further inquiry, she revealed that she had been experiencing much more pessimism about her prognosis, saying, "I've been thinking a lot about life and death recently." She also said she now experienced minimal pleasure when playing with her children and that her lack of energy and enjoyment of family life had been a strain on her marriage. The neurologist asked her specifically about suicidal thoughts, which she denied.

The patient was immediately referred to a psychiatrist. This led to further clarification of her depressive symptoms and confirmed a diagnosis of an MDE. The psychiatrist did not feel that she was acutely suicidal. She recommended a trial of antidepressants along with a trial of individual psychotherapy. Due to the concern about her decreased appetite and weight loss, the psychiatrist selected paroxetine, ultimately titrated up to a dosage of 30 mg per day. The psychiatrist also recommended that she begin to attend an MS support group and encouraged her to ask her husband to attend some of the therapy sessions with her, which he did. With the help of her psychiatrist, the patient also generated a list of questions on her mind about her MS symptoms and treatment that she could bring to her next meeting with her neurologist. With the weekly psychotherapy sessions and antidepressant regimen, she demonstrated gradual but significant improvements in her mood.

💡 PEARLS TO TAKE HOME

- Patients with MS have high rates of depression, suicidal ideation, and completed suicide. It is essential to check for the presence of suicidal ideation and behaviors in all patients with MS.
- Cognitive impairment may be significantly related to depression, anxiety, and quality of life in MS.
- Symptoms of fatigue, which are common in MS, may mask underlying depression.
- The presence of depressive symptoms in patients with MS should lead to a referral for psychiatric consultation.
- Psychotherapeutic options are important to consider, including a range of psychotherapeutic options as well as patient support groups. However, psychotherapy alone may not be sufficient.
- SSRI antidepressants are generally well tolerated, although some agents can cause or exacerbate preexisting fatigue or sexual dysfunction.

- Untreated depression can negatively impact upon MS treatment adherence.
- Psychiatric intervention should begin as early as possible as this could potentially decrease the severe impact that depression has on quality of life in patients with MS.

References

1. Schumacher GAM, Beebe G, Kibler RF, et al. Problems of experimental trials of therapy in multiple sclerosis: report by the panel on the evaluation of experimental trials of therapy in multiple sclerosis. *Ann N Y Acad Sci*, 122: 552–568, 1965.
2. Poser CM, Brinar VV. Diagnostic criteria for multiple sclerosis: an historical review. *Clin Neurol Neurosurg*, 106(3): 147–158, 2004.
3. Schapiro RT. Managing symptoms of multiple sclerosis. *Neurol Clin*, 23(1): 177–187, vii, 2005.
4. Svendsen KB, Jensen TS, Hansen HJ, et al. Sensory function and quality of life in patients with multiple sclerosis and pain. *Pain*, 114(3): 473–481, 2005.
5. Beal CC, Stuifbergen A. Loneliness in women with multiple sclerosis. *Rehabil Nurs*, 32(4): 165–171, 2007.
6. Kantarci OH, Weinshenker BG. Natural history of multiple sclerosis. *Neurol Clin*, 23(1): 17–38, v, 2005.
7. Kantarci O, Siva A, Eraksoy M, et al. Survival and predictors of disability in Turkish MS patients. Turkish Multiple Sclerosis Study Group (TUMSSG). *Neurology*, 51(3): 765–772, 1998.
8. Ebers GC, Sadovnick AD, Risch NJ. A genetic basis for familial aggregation in multiple sclerosis. Canadian Collaborative Study Group. *Nature*, 377(6545): 150–151, 1995.
9. Sadovnick AD, Armstrong H, Rice GP, et al. A population-based study of multiple sclerosis in twins: update. *Ann Neurol*, 33(3): 281–285, 1993.
10. Kurtzke JF. Multiple sclerosis: changing times. *Neuroepidemiology*, 10(1): 1–8, 1991.
11. Rosati G, Aiello I, Pirastru MI, et al. Epidemiology of multiple sclerosis in Northwestern Sardinia: further evidence for higher frequency in Sardinians compared to other

Italians. *Neuroepidemiology*, 15(1): 10–19, 1996.

12. Kurtzke JF. MS epidemiology world wide. One view of current status. *Acta Neurol Scand Suppl*, 161: 23–33, 1995.

13. Gale CR, Martyn CN. Migrant studies in multiple sclerosis. *Prog Neurobiol*, 47(4-5): 425–448, 1995.

14. Ascherio A, Munger KL. Environmental risk factors for multiple sclerosis. Part II: noninfectious factors. *Ann Neurol*, 61(6): 504–513, 2007.

15. Gilden DH. Infectious causes of multiple sclerosis. *Lancet Neurol*, 4(3): 195–202, 2005.

16. Ascherio A, Munger KL. Environmental risk factors for multiple sclerosis. Part I: the role of infection. *Ann Neurol*, 61(4): 288–299, 2007.

17. Beiske AG, Pedersen ED, Czujko B, et al. Pain and sensory complaints in multiple sclerosis. *Eur J Neurol*, 11(7): 479–482, 2004.

18. Chwastiak L, Ehde DM, Gibbons LE, et al. Depressive symptoms and severity of illness in multiple sclerosis: epidemiologic study of a large community sample. *Am J Psychiatry*, 159(11): 1862–1868, 2002.

19. Huijbregts SC, Kalkers NF, de Sonneville LM, et al. Cognitive impairment and decline in different MS subtypes. *J Neurol Sci*, 245(1–2): 187–194, 2006.

20. Mullins L, Cote MP, Fuemmeler BF, et al. Illness intrusiveness, uncertainty and distress in individuals with multiple sclerosis. *Rehabil Psychol*, 46(2): 139–153, 2001.

21. Schiffer RB. Depression in neurological practice: diagnosis, treatment, implications. *Semin Neurol*, 29(3): 220–233, 2009.

22. Kessler RC, McGonagle KA, Zhao S, et al. Lifetime and 12-month prevalence of DSM-III-R psychiatric disorders in the United States. Results from the National Comorbidity Survey. *Arch Gen Psychiatry*, 51(1): 8–19, 1994.

23. Reavley NJ, Jorm AF, Cvetkovski S, et al. National Depression and Anxiety Indices for Australia. *Aust N Z J Psychiatry*, 45(9): 780–787, 2011.

24. American Psychiatric Association. *Diagnostic and Statistical Manual of Mental Disorders DSM-IV-TR, (Fourth Edition (Text Revision) ed.)*. Washington, DC: American Psychiatric Publishing, Inc., 2000.

25. Belmaker RH. Bipolar disorder. *N Engl J Med*, 351(5): 476–486, 2004.

26. Joffe RT, Lippert GP, Gray TA, et al. Mood disorder and multiple sclerosis. *Arch Neurol*, 44(4): 376–378, 1987.

27. Kaplin A, Carroll K. Multiple sclerosis. In: *Psychiatric Aspects of Neurologic Diseases. Practical Approaches to Patient Care*, eds. C Lyketsos, PV Rabins, JR Lipsey, PR Slavney. New York: Oxford University Press, pp. 132–157, 2008.

28. Dark FL, McGrath JJ, Ron MA. Pathological laughing and crying. *Aust N Z J Psychiatry*, 30(4): 472–479, 1996.

29. Feinstein A, Feinstein K, Gray T, et al. Prevalence and neurobehavioral correlates of pathological laughing and crying in multiple sclerosis. *Arch Neurol*, 54(9): 1116–1121, 1997.

30. Whitlock FA, Siskind MM. Depression as a major symptom of multiple sclerosis. *J Neurol Neurosurg Psychiatry*, 43(10): 861–865, 1980.

31. Schubert DS, Foliart RH. Increased depression in multiple sclerosis patients. A meta-analysis. *Psychosomatics*, 34(2): 124–130, 1993.

32. Sadovnick AD, Remick RA, Allen J, et al. Depression and multiple sclerosis. *Neurology*, 46(3): 628–632, 1996.

33. Minden SL, Orav J, Reich P. Depression in multiple sclerosis. *Gen Hosp Psychiatry*, 9(6): 426–434, 1987.

34. Patten SB, Beck CA, Williams JV, et al. Major depression in multiple sclerosis: a population-based perspective. *Neurology*, 61(11): 1524–1527, 2003.

35. Kurtzke JF. Rating neurologic impairment in multiple sclerosis: an expanded disability status scale (EDSS). *Neurology*, 33(11): 1444–1452, 1983.

36. Beiske AG, Svensson E, Sandanger I, et al. Depression and anxiety amongst multiple sclerosis patients. *Eur J Neurol*, 15(3): 239–245, 2008.

37. Rabkin JG, Albert SM, Del Bene ML, et al. Prevalence of depressive disorders and change over time in late-stage ALS. *Neurology*, 65(1): 62–67, 2005.

38. Ron MA, Logsdail SJ. Psychiatric morbidity in multiple sclerosis: a clinical and MRI study. *Psychol Med*, 19(4): 887–895, 1989.

39. Silverstone PH. Prevalence of psychiatric disorders in medical inpatients. *J Nerv Ment Dis*, 184(1): 43–51, 1996.

40. Siegert RJ, Abernethy DA. Depression in multiple sclerosis: a review. *J Neurol Neurosurg Psychiatry*, 76(4): 469–475, 2005.

41. Weisbrot DM, Ettinger AB, Gadow KD, et al. Psychiatric comorbidity in pediatric patients with demyelinating disorders. *J Child Neurol*, 25(2): 192–202, 2010.

42. Gilchrist AC, Creed FH. Depression, cognitive impairment and social stress in multiple sclerosis. *J Psychosom Res*, 38(3): 193–201, 1994.

43. Lobentanz IS, Asenbaum S, Vass K, et al. Factors influencing quality of life in multiple sclerosis patients: disability, depressive mood, fatigue and sleep quality. *Acta Neurol Scand*, 110(1): 6–13, 2004.

44. Janssens AC, van Doorn PA, de Boer JB, et al. Anxiety and depression influence the relation between disability status and quality of life in multiple sclerosis. *Mult Scler*, 9(4): 397–403, 2003.

45. Galeazzi GM, Ferrari S, Giaroli G, et al. Psychiatric disorders and depression in multiple sclerosis outpatients: impact of disability and interferon beta therapy. *Neurol Sci*, 26(4): 255–262, 2005.

46. Feinstein A, Feinstein K. Depression associated with multiple sclerosis. Looking beyond diagnosis to symptom expression. *J Affect Disord*, 66(2–3): 193–198, 2001.

47. Zorzon M, de Masi R, Nasuelli D, et al. Depression and anxiety in multiple sclerosis. A clinical and MRI study in 95 subjects. *J Neurol*, 248(5): 416–421, 2001.

48. Arnett PA, Higginson CI, Voss WD, et al. Depressed mood in multiple sclerosis: relationship to capacity-demanding memory and attentional functioning. *Neuropsychology*, 13(3): 434–446, 1999.

49. Patten SB, Metz LM, Reimer MA. Biopsychosocial correlates of lifetime major depression in a multiple sclerosis population. *Mult Scler*, 6(2): 115–120, 2000.

50. Gay MC, Vrignaud P, Garitte C, et al. Predictors of depression in multiple sclerosis patients. *Acta Neurol Scand*, 121(3): 161–170, 2010.

51. Schwartz CE, Coulthard-Morris L, Zeng Q, et al. Measuring self-efficacy in people with multiple sclerosis: a validation study. *Arch Phys Med Rehabil*, 77(4): 394–398, 1996.

52. Beal CC, Stuifbergen AK, Brown A. Depression in multiple sclerosis: a longitudinal analysis. *Arch Psychiatr Nurs*, 21(4): 181–191, 2007.

53. Zigmond AS, Snaith R. The Hospital Anxiety and Depression scale. *Acta Psychiatr Scand*, 67(6): 361–370, 1983.

54. Dahl OP, Stordal E, Lydersen S, et al. Anxiety and depression in multiple sclerosis. A comparative population-based study in Nord-Trondelag County, Norway. *Mult Scler*, 15(12): 1495–1501, 2009.

55. Zabad RK, Patten SB, Metz LM. The association of depression with disease course in multiple sclerosis. *Neurology*, 64(2): 359–360, 2005.

56. Kroencke DC, Denney DR, Lynch SG. Depression during exacerbations in multiple sclerosis: the importance of uncertainty. *Mult Scler*, 7(4): 237–242, 2001.

57. Kessler RC, McGonagle KA, Swartz M, et al. Sex and depression in the National Comorbidity Survey. I: lifetime prevalence, chronicity and recurrence. *J Affect Disord*, 29(2–3): 85–96, 1993.

58. Weissman MM, Bland RC, Canino GJ, et al. Cross-national epidemiology of major depression and bipolar disorder. *JAMA*, 276(4): 293–299, 1996.

59. Korostil M, Feinstein A. Anxiety disorders and their clinical correlates in multiple sclerosis patients. *Mult Scler*, 13(1): 67–72, 2007.

60. Okiishi CG, Paradiso S, Robinson RG, et al. Gender differences in depression associated with neurologic illness: clinical correlates and pharmacologic response. *J Gend Specif Med*, 4(2): 65–72, 2001.

61. Moller A, Wiedemann G, Rohde U, et al. Correlates of cognitive impairment and depressive mood disorder in multiple sclerosis. *Acta Psychiatr Scand*, 89(2): 117–121, 1994.

62. Kneebone II, Dunmore EC, Evans E. Symptoms of depression in older adults with multiple sclerosis (MS): comparison with a matched sample of younger adults. *Aging Ment Health*, 7(3): 182–185, 2003.

63. Barnwell AM, Kavanagh DJ. Prediction of psychological adjustment to multiple sclerosis. *Soc Sci Med*, 45(3): 411–418, 1997.

64. Gulick EE. Correlates of quality of life among persons with multiple sclerosis. *Nurs Res*, 46(6): 305–311, 1997.

65. Mohr DC, Goodkin DE, Gatto N, et al. Depression, coping and level of neurological impairment in multiple sclerosis. *Mult Scler*, 3(4): 254–258, 1997.

66. Arnett PA, Higginson CI, Voss WD, et al. Relationship between coping, cognitive dysfunction and depression in multiple sclerosis. *Clin Neuropsychol*, 16(3): 341–355, 2002.

67. Janssens AC, van Doorn PA, de Boer JB, et al. Perception of prognostic risk in patients with multiple sclerosis: the relationship with anxiety, depression, and disease-related distress. *J Clin Epidemiol*, 57(2): 180–186, 2004.

68. Jopson NM, Moss-Morris R. The role of illness severity and illness representations in adjusting to multiple sclerosis. *J Psychosom Res*, 54(6): 503–511; discussion 513–514, 2003.

69. Fassbender K, Schmidt R, Mossner R, et al. Mood disorders and dysfunction of the hypothalamic-pituitary-adrenal axis in multiple sclerosis: association with cerebral inflammation. *Arch Neurol*, 55(1): 66–72, 1998.

70. Honer WG, Hurwitz T, Li DK, et al. Temporal lobe involvement in multiple sclerosis patients with psychiatric disorders. *Arch Neurol*, 44(2): 187–190, 1987.

71. Lyketsos CG, Treisman GJ, Lipsey JR, et al. Does stroke cause depression? *J Neuropsychiatry Clin Neurosci*, 10(1): 103–107, 1998.

72. Jorge RE, Starkstein SE. Pathophysiologic aspects of major depression following traumatic brain injury. *J Head Trauma Rehabil*, 20(6): 475–487, 2005.

73. Altshuler LL, Devinsky O, Post RM, et al. Depression, anxiety, and temporal lobe epilepsy. Laterality of focus and symptoms. *Arch Neurol*, 47(3): 284–288, 1990.

74. Rabins PV, Brooks BR, O'Donnell P, et al. Structural brain correlates of emotional disorder in multiple sclerosis. *Brain*, 109(Pt 4): 585–597, 1986.

75. Schiffer RB, Caine ED, Bamford KA, et al. Depressive episodes in patients with multiple sclerosis. *Am J Psychiatry*, 140(11): 1498–1500, 1983.

76. Pujol J, Bello J, Deus J, et al. Lesions in the left arcuate fasciculus region and depressive symptoms in multiple sclerosis. *Neurology*, 49(4): 1105–1110, 1997.

77. McDonald WI, Compston A, Edan G, et al. Recommended diagnostic criteria for multiple sclerosis: guidelines from the International Panel on the diagnosis of multiple sclerosis. *Ann Neurol*, 50(1): 121–127, 2001.

78. Feinstein A, O'Connor P, Akbar N, et al. Diffusion tensor imaging abnormalities in depressed multiple sclerosis patients. *Mult Scler*, 16(2): 189–196, 2010.

79. Sabatini U, Pozzilli C, Pantano P, et al. Involvement of the limbic system in multiple sclerosis patients with depressive disorders. *Biol Psychiatry*, 39(11): 970–975, 1996.

80. Stefan MG, Kyle CK, Mary-Frances OC, et al. Smaller cornu ammonis 2–3/dentate gyrus volumes and elevated cortisol in multiple sclerosis patients with depressive symptoms. *Biol Psychiatry*, 68(6): 553–559, 2010.

81. Sheline YI, Wang PW, Gado MH, et al. Hippocampal atrophy in recurrent major depression. *Proc Natl Acad Sci U S A*, 93(9): 3908–3913, 1996.

82. Gilliam FG, Maton BM, Martin RC, et al. Hippocampal 1H-MRSI correlates with severity of depression symptoms in temporal lobe epilepsy. *Neurology*, 68(5): 364–368, 2007.

83. Kaufman D, Smuckler DJ. Multiple sclerosis. In: *Psychosomatic Medicine*, eds. M Blumenfeld and J Strain. Philadelphia: Lippincott Williams & Wilkins, 2006.

84. Stefan MG, Michael RI. Depression and immunity: inflammation and depressive symptoms in multiple sclerosis. *Immunol Allergy Clin North Am*, 29(2): 309–320, 2009.

85. Cohen S, Herbert TB. Health psychology: psychological factors and physical disease

from the perspective of human psychoneu-roimmunology. *Annu Rev Psychol*, 47: 113–142, 1996.

86. Kanner AM, Weisbrot DM. Psychiatric evaluation of the adult and pediatric patient with epilepsy: a practical approach for the "nonpsychiatrist". In: *Psychiatric Issues in Epilepsy: A Practical Guide to Diagnosis and Treatment*, 2nd ed. eds. AB Ettinger and AM Kanner. Philadelphia: Williams & Wilkins, pp. 119–132, 2007.

87. Radloff L. The CESD scale, a self-report depression scale for research in the general population. *J Appl Psychol Meas*, 1: 385–401, 1977.

88. Patten SB, Lavorato DH, Metz LM, et al. Clinical correlates of CES-D depressive symptom ratings in an MS population. *Gen Hosp Psychiatry*, 27(6): 439–445, 2005.

89. Beck AT, Ward CH, Mendelson M, et al. An inventory for measuring depression. *Arch Gen Psychiatry*, 4: 561–571, 1961.

90. Gilliam FG, Barry JJ, Hermann BP, et al. Rapid detection of major depression in epilepsy: a multicentre study. *Lancet Neurol*, 5(5): 399–405, 2006.

91. Smith MM, Arnett PA. Factors related to employment status changes in individuals with multiple sclerosis. *Mult Scler*, 11(5): 602–609, 2005.

92. Roxburgh RH, Seaman SR, Masterman T, et al. Multiple Sclerosis Severity Score: using disability and disease duration to rate disease severity. *Neurology*, 64(7): 1144–1151, 2005.

93. Krupp LB, LaRocca NG, Muir-Nash J, et al. The fatigue severity scale. Application to patients with multiple sclerosis and systemic lupus erythematosus. *Arch Neurol*, 46(10): 1121–1123, 1989.

94. Feinstein A. Neuropsychiatric syndromes associated with multiple sclerosis. *J Neurol*, 254, Suppl. 2: II73–II76, 2007.

95. Sadovnick AD, Eisen K, Ebers GC, et al. Cause of death in patients attending multiple sclerosis clinics. *Neurology*, 41(8): 1193–1196, 1991.

96. Stenager EN, Stenager E, Koch-Henriksen N, et al. Suicide and multiple sclerosis: an epidemiological investigation. *J Neurol Neurosurg Psychiatry*, 55(7): 542–545, 1992.

97. Feinstein A, Roy P, Lobaugh N, et al. Structural brain abnormalities in multiple sclerosis patients with major depression. *Neurology*, 62(4): 586–590, 2004.

98. Stenager EN, Koch-Henriksen N, Stenager E, et al. Risk factors for suicide in multiple sclerosis. *Psychother Psychosom*, 65(2): 86–90, 1996.

99. Wallin MT, Wilken JA, Turner AP, et al. Depression and multiple sclerosis: review of a lethal combination. *J Rehabil Res Dev*, 43(1): 45–62, 2006.

100. Minden SL, Frankel D, Hadden L, et al. The Sonya Slifka Longitudinal Multiple Sclerosis Study: methods and sample characteristics. *Mult Scler*, 12(1): 24–38, 2006.

101. Krupp LB, Alvarez LA, LaRocca NG, et al. Fatigue in multiple sclerosis. *Arch Neurol*, 45(4): 435–437, 1988.

102. Brown RF, Valpiani EM, Tennant CC, et al. Longitudinal assessment of anxiety, depression, and fatigue in people with multiple sclerosis. *Psychol Psychother*, 82(Pt 1): 41–56, 2009.

103. Schwartz CE, Coulthard-Morris L, Zeng Q, et al. Psychosocial correlates of fatigue in multiple sclerosis. *Arch Phys Med Rehabil*, 77(2): 165–170, 1996.

104. Sauter C, Zebenholzer K, Hisakawa J, et al. A longitudinal study on effects of a six-week course for energy conservation for multiple sclerosis patients. *Mult Scler*, 14(4): 500–505, 2008.

105. Kroencke DC, Lynch SG, Denney DR, et al. Fatigue in multiple sclerosis: relationship to depression, disability, and disease pattern. *Mult Scler*, 6(2): 131–136, 2000.

106. Rao SM, Leo GJ, Bernardin L, et al. Cognitive dysfunction in multiple sclerosis. I. Frequency, patterns, and prediction. *Neurology*, 41(5): 685–691, 1991.

107. Rao SM, Leo GJ, Ellington L, et al. Cognitive dysfunction in multiple sclerosis. II. Impact on employment and social functioning. *Neurology*, 41(5): 692–696, 1991.

108. McIntosh-Michaelis SA, Roberts MH, Wilkinson SM, et al. The prevalence of cognitive impairment in a community survey of multiple sclerosis. *Br J Clin Psychol*, 30(Pt 4): 333–348, 1991.

109. Goretti B, Portaccio E, Zipoli V, et al. Impact of cognitive impairment on coping strategies in multiple sclerosis. *Clin Neurol Neurosurg*, 112(2): 127–130, 2010.

110. Simioni S, Ruffieux C, Bruggimann L, et al. Cognition, mood and fatigue in patients in the early stage of multiple sclerosis. *Swiss Med Wkly*, 137(35–36): 496–501, 2007.

111. Glanz BI, Healy BC, Rintell DJ, et al. The association between cognitive impairment and quality of life in patients with early multiple sclerosis. *J Neurol Sci*, 290(1–2): 75–79, 2010.

112. Ehrensperger MM, Grether A, Romer G, et al. Neuropsychological dysfunction, depression, physical disability, and coping processes in families with a parent affected by multiple sclerosis. *Mult Scler*, 14(8): 1106–1112, 2008.

113. Christodoulou C, Melville P, Scherl WF, et al. Negative affect predicts subsequent cognitive change in multiple sclerosis. *J Int Neuropsychol Soc*, 15(1): 53–61, 2009.

114. Rudick RA, Goodkin DE, Jacobs LD, et al. Impact of interferon beta-1a on neurologic disability in relapsing multiple sclerosis. The Multiple Sclerosis Collaborative Research Group (MSCRG). *Neurology*, 49(2): 358–363, 1997.

115. Simon JH, Jacobs LD, Campion M, et al. Magnetic resonance studies of intramuscular interferon beta-1a for relapsing multiple sclerosis. The Multiple Sclerosis Collaborative Research Group. *Ann Neurol*, 43(1): 79–87, 1998.

116. Panitch H, Goodin DS, Francis G, et al. Randomized, comparative study of interferon beta-1a treatment regimens in MS: the EVIDENCE Trial. *Neurology*, 59(10): 1496–1506, 2002.

117. Group, T.I.M.S.S. Interferon beta-1b is effective in relapsing-remitting multiple sclerosis. I. Clinical results of a multicenter, randomized, double-blind, placebo-controlled trial. *Neurology*, 43(4): 662–667, 1993.

118. Paty DW, Li DK. Interferon beta-1b is effective in relapsing-remitting multiple sclerosis. II. MRI analysis results of a multicenter, randomized, double-blind, placebo-controlled trial. UBC MS/MRI Study Group and the IFNB Multiple Sclerosis Study Group. *Neurology*, 43(4): 662–667, 1993.

119. Ollendorf DA, Jilinskaia E, Oleen-Burkey M. Clinical and economic impact of glatiramer acetate versus beta interferon therapy among patients with multiple sclerosis in a managed care population. *J Manag Care Pharm*, 8(6): 469–476, 2002.

120. Rudick RA, Polman CH. Current approaches to the identification and management of breakthrough disease in patients with multiple sclerosis. *Lancet Neurol*, 8(6): 545–559, 2009.

121. Berger JR, Houff S. Opportunistic infections and other risks with newer multiple sclerosis therapies. *Ann Neurol*, 65(4): 367–377, 2009.

122. Mohr DC, Likosky W, Boudewyn AC, et al. Side effect profile and adherence to in the treatment of multiple sclerosis with interferon beta-1a. *Mult Scler*, 4(6): 487–489, 1998.

123. Mohr DC, Goodkin DE, Likosky W, et al. Therapeutic expectations of patients with multiple sclerosis upon initiating interferon beta-1b: relationship to adherence to treatment. *Mult Scler*, 2(5): 222–226, 1996.

124. Neilley LK, Goodin DS, Goodkin DE, et al. Side effect profile of interferon beta-1b in MS: results of an open label trial. *Neurology*, 46(2): 552–554, 1996.

125. Klapper M. Letter to the editor. *Neurology*, 44: 188, 1994.

126. Jacobs LD, Beck RW, Simon JH, et al. Intramuscular interferon beta-1a therapy initiated during a first demyelinating event in multiple sclerosis. CHAMPS Study Group. *N Engl J Med*, 343(13): 898–904, 2000.

127. Sobel RM, Lotkowski S, Mandel S. Update on depression in neurologic illness: stroke, epilepsy, and multiple sclerosis. *Curr Psychiatry Rep*, 7(5): 396–403, 2005.

128. Patten SB, Metz LM. Interferon beta1a and depression in secondary progressive MS: data from the SPECTRIMS Trial. *Neurology*, 59(5): 744–746, 2002.

129. Feinstein A, O'Connor P, Feinstein K. Multiple sclerosis, interferon beta-1b and depression A prospective investigation. *J Neurol*, 249(7): 815–820, 2002.

130. Mohr DC, Likosky W, Dwyer P, et al. Course of depression during the initiation of

interferon beta-1a treatment for multiple sclerosis. *Arch Neurol*, 56(10): 1263–1265, 1999.

131. Blanco Y, Moral EA, Costa M, et al. Effect of glatiramer acetate (Copaxone) on the immunophenotypic and cytokine profile and BDNF production in multiple sclerosis: a longitudinal study. *Neurosci Lett*, 406(3): 270–275, 2006.

132. Russo-Neustadt AA, Beard RC, Huang YM, et al. Physical activity and antidepressant treatment potentiate the expression of specific brain-derived neurotrophic factor transcripts in the rat hippocampus. *Neuroscience*, 101(2): 305–312, 2000.

133. Interferon beta-1a (Betaseron®). Prescribing information. Bayer Healthcare. Montiville, NY February 2009, assessed from http://berlex.bayerhealthcare.com/html/products/pi/Betaseron_PI.pdf on July 22, 2010.

134. Treadaway K, Cutter G, Salter A, et al. Factors that influence adherence with disease-modifying therapy in MS. *J Neurol*, 256(4): 568–576, 2009.

135. Ziemssen T. Multiple sclerosis beyond EDSS: depression and fatigue. *J Neurol Sci*, 277, Suppl. 1: S37–S41, 2009.

136. Thomas PW, Thomas S, Hillier C, et al. Psychological interventions for multiple sclerosis. *Cochrane Database Syst Rev*, (1): CD004431, 2006.

137. Mohr DC, Goodkin DE, Likosky W, et al. Treatment of depression improves adherence to interferon beta-1b therapy for multiple sclerosis. *Arch Neurol*, 54(5): 531–533, 1997.

138. Mohr D, Goodkin DE. Treatment of depression in multiple sclerosis: review and meta-analysis. *Clin Psychol: Sci Pract*, 6: 1–9, 1999.

139. Feinstein A. An examination of suicidal intent in patients with multiple sclerosis. *Neurology*, 59(5): 674–678, 2002.

140. Sollom AC, Kneebone II. Treatment of depression in people who have multiple sclerosis. *Mult Scler*, 13(5): 632–635, 2007.

141. Gill D, Hatcher S. Antidepressants for depression in medical illness. *Cochrane Database Syst Rev*, (4): CD001312, 2000.

142. Schiffer RB, Wineman NM. Antidepressant pharmacotherapy of depression associated with multiple sclerosis. *Am J Psychiatry*, 147(11): 1493–1497, 1990.

143. Mohr DC, Boudewyn AC, Goodkin DE, et al. Comparative outcomes for individual cognitive-behavior therapy, supportive-expressive group psychotherapy, and sertraline for the treatment of depression in multiple sclerosis. *J Consult Clin Psychol*, 69(6): 942–949, 2001.

144. Ehde DM, Kraft GH, Chwastiak L, et al. Efficacy of paroxetine in treating major depressive disorder in persons with multiple sclerosis. *Gen Hosp Psychiatry*, 30(1): 40–48, 2008.

145. Barak Y, Achiron A, Shoshani D, et al. Fluoxetine treatment of depression in patients suffering from multiple sclerosis. *Hum Psychopharmacol*, 13: 63–67, 1997.

146. Stahl SM. *Essential Psychopharmacology: The Prescriber's Guide*. New York: Cambridge Press, 2006.

147. Barak Y, Ur E, Achiron A. Moclobemide treatment in multiple sclerosis patients with comorbid depression: an open-label safety trial. *J Neuropsychiatry Clin Neurosci*, 11(2): 271–273, 1999.

148. Uccelli M, Mohr M, Battaglia M, et al. Peer support groups in multiple sclerosis: current effectiveness and future directions. *Mult Scler*, 10(1): 80–84, 2004.

149. Spiegal DM, Classen C. *Group Psychotherapy for Cancer Patients*. New York: Basic Books, 2000.

150. Mohr DC, Classen C, and Barrera M Jr, et al. The relationship between social support, depression and treatment for depression in people with multiple sclerosis. *Psychol Med*, 34(3): 533–541, 2004.

151. Tesar N, Baumhackl U, Kopp M, et al. Effects of psychological group therapy in patients with multiple sclerosis. *Acta Neurol Scand*, 107(6): 394–399, 2003.

152. World Health Organization. WHOQOL: measuring quality of life. 2007, Accessed from http://www.who.int/mentalhealth/media/68.pdf on August, 7 2010.

153. Schipper HM, Clinch JJ, Olweny CLM. Quality of life studies: definitions and conceptual issues. In: *Quality of Life and Pharmacoeconomics in Clinical Trials*, ed. B Spilker. Philadelphia: Lippincott-Raven, pp. 11–23, 1996.

Depression and Alzheimer's Disease

Pablo Richly,[1,2] Facundo Manes,[1,2] and Julián Bustin[1,2]
[1]Institute of Cognitive Neurology (INECO), Buenos Aires, Argentina
[2]Institute of Neuroscience, Favaloro University, Buenos Aires, Argentina

Introduction

Alzheimer's disease (AD) is the most prevalent type of dementia and has a devastating impact on patients' and families' quality of life. The risk of developing AD increases with age and reaches nearly 50% by age 85. AD exacts not only a massive emotional burden, but also an economic toll on individuals and society. In 2010, AD and other dementias cost US$604 billion worldwide. If dementia were a country, it would be the world's 18th largest economy. As the population of the world ages, it is estimated that AD will become one of the most important problems in public health. In the United States alone, the cost of AD and other dementias is projected to increase from US$172 billion in 2010 to US$1.08 trillion in 2050 [1].

In addition to cognitive and functional impairment, behavioral and neuropsychiatric symptoms are frequently observed in patients with AD. In clinical practice, dementia of Alzheimer type is diagnosed when there are cognitive and/or behavioral (neuropsychiatric) symptoms that interfere with the ability to function at work or at instrumental activities of daily living and that represent a decline from previous levels of functioning and performing and are not explained by delirium or major psychiatric disorders. The cognitive or behavioral impairment involves a minimum of two of the following domains:

- *Impaired ability to acquire and remember new information.* This includes repetitive questions or conversations, misplacing personal belongings, forgetting events or appointments, and getting lost on a familiar route.
- *Impaired reasoning and handling of complex tasks, poor judgment.* This includes poor understanding of safety risks, inability to manage finances, poor decision-making ability, and inability to plan complex or sequential activities
- *Impaired visuospatial abilities.* These include inability to recognize faces or common objects or to find objects in direct view despite good acuity, inability to operate simple implements, or orient clothing to the body.
- *Impaired language functions (speaking, reading, or writing).* These include difficulty thinking of common words while speaking, hesitations; speech, spelling, and writing errors.
- *Changes in personality, behavior, or comportment.* These include uncharacteristic

Depression in Neurologic Disorders: Diagnosis and Management, First Edition.
Edited by Andres M. Kanner.

mood fluctuations such as agitation, impaired motivation, initiative, apathy, loss of drive, social withdrawal, decreased interest in previous activities, loss of empathy, compulsive or obsessive behaviors, and socially unacceptable behaviors [2].

AD will affect each patient differently. However, in all patients, AD is a progressive disorder. Memory loss is often the first sign of AD, with short-term memory impacted before long-term memory. The patient may forget a name or misplace objects. Forgetting words and names of objects begins to produce language problems. These cognitive deficits affect judgment. The patient exhibits denial and anxiety and may start to withdraw from social situations. As the disease progresses, memory problems worsen. The ability to recall new information hampers the ability to learn. Memory problems may affect familiar information, such as telephone numbers and the names of family members. Personality and emotional changes can manifest themselves in a variety of ways: delusions (false beliefs), obsession (persistent idea or feeling), increasing anxiety, and aggression. The patient eventually cannot survive without some assistance as the ability to perform activities of daily living is increasingly diminished. In the latter stages of the disease, verbal abilities are greatly compromised or lost entirely. There may be a loss of psychomotor skills, which are physical activities dependent on mental processes. In severe cases, the motor disturbances may render patients immobile and bedridden. The patient may become incontinent and unable to feed himself.

In 1910, Emil Kraepelin named the syndrome and pathology described by Alois Alzheimer after him [3]. Even after more than a century of scientific and clinical research later, the physiopathology of this neurodegenerative illness has still not been fully uncovered. Two hallmark pathologic features of the brains of patients with AD are extracellular neuritic plaques and intracellular neurofibrillary tangles. The formation of neuritic plaques is linked to the abnormal processing of amyloid precursor protein. Neurofibrillary tangles result from the abnormal phosphorylation of the tau protein in axons [4]. However, the presence of these lesions is not necessarily asso-

ciated with the clinical manifestation of AD. The pivotal Nun Study showed that many of the nuns had a brain autopsy positive for AD but never developed the symptoms of the illness, while others had the same amount of neuritic plaques and neurofibrillary tangles plus vascular lesions and developed AD. The same study also confirmed that cardiovascular illnesses are closely related to AD. The more brain vascular lesions, the greater the risk of developing AD [5]. There are many risk factors associated with AD. By far, the most important factor is advancing age. There are other unmodifiable risk factors such as family history and, related to this, the presence of certain genes (APOE-e4, amyloid precursor protein, presenilin 1, and presenilin 2). However, there are also modifiable risk factors such as head trauma and vascular disease [4]. The latter is becoming a very important aspect of disease prevention, similar to what has happened with heart disease.

AD is diagnosed through a combination of the following methods:

- History-taking from the patient and a knowledgeable informant
- Objective cognitive assessment using either a "bedside" mental status examination or neuropsychological testing
- A general neurologic and physical examination, which should be performed on all patients presenting with dementia and is a critical step for ruling out asymmetric neurologic findings
- Investigations such as blood tests, brain imaging, and lumbar puncture

Despite the advances since its first description, AD remains underdiagnosed. According to the Alzheimer's Association, there are up to 50% of people with dementia in the United States who have not received a diagnosis [6]. A survey in six European countries showed that the average time from when AD symptoms are noticed until a doctor consultation is made is 47 weeks [7]. The insidious and different forms of initial presentation and the lack of one test to confirm the diagnosis are important contributors to these figures. Therefore, after 27 years, new criteria have been established by the National Institute on Aging and the Alzheimer's Association to try to encourage early diagnosis of the disease by incorporating innovations in clinical, imaging, and laboratory assessment [2]. These new criteria also emphasize the importance of neuropsychiatric symptoms as a core aspect of the disease's manifestations.

Although the exact prevalence of behavioral symptoms in AD varies according to the population studied, stage of illness, and assessment method used, they are known to affect a large proportion of patients. For example, it has been estimated that certain behavioral symptoms (e.g., depression, irritability, agitation, and aggression) may affect up to 80% of patients with AD. Once present, behavioral symptoms tend to worsen as the disease progresses and cause considerable stress among caregivers. Depression is by far the most frequent type of comorbid psychiatric disorder [8]. Depression and cognitive impairment are both common in old age and frequently occur together. The relationship between depression and dementia may be due to four factors: (1) depression may be an initial manifestation of the neurodegenerative process; (2) depression may be the cause of the neurodegenerative process; (3) depression may be a reaction to cognitive decline; and (4) both depression and dementia may result from a common process. This chapter will describe the epidemiologic features of depression in AD, its clinical manifestations, and the available data on potential pathogenic mechanism, diagnosis, and treatment.

Prevalence of depression in AD

Of all psychiatric syndromes that may occur in AD, depression is the most common. However, it is not as prevalent in AD as in vascular dementia, Lewy body dementia, and Parkinson's disease dementia [9]. There is a high variation in the estimations of the prevalence of depression in patients with AD. This is due to multiple methodological factors in epidemiologic studies, such as diagnostic criteria, rating scales used, and sample selection. For example, Vilalta-Franch et al. [10] applied different diagnostic criteria to the same group of patients with dementia of Alzheimer's type and found significant differences in the estimated prevalence of depression: International Classification of Diseases, Tenth

Edition (ICD-10), 4.9%; Cambridge Examination for Mental Disorders (CAMDEX) criteria, 9.8%; *Diagnostic and Statistical Manual of Mental Disorders*, Fourth Edition (DSM-IV), 13.4%; Provisional Diagnostic Criteria for Depression of Alzheimer's disease, 27.4%; and Neuropsychiatric Inventory depression subscale, 43.7%. In spite of these factors, an approximate prevalence of depression in patients with AD has been estimated to be in the range of 30–50%, presenting as major or minor depression with the lowest rates in the community samples [11].

Impact of depression in AD

Clinically, it is extremely important to diagnose depression in patients with AD. Depression has a negative impact at various levels. Comorbid depression is associated with greater impairment in activities of daily living, earlier placement in a nursing home, and increased mortality risk. It is also associated with a faster decline in cognitive functions and poorer quality of life. Finally, depression increases stress and psychological morbidity of the AD patient's caregiver and family [11].

Clinical manifestations and diagnosis of depression in AD

Despite the high prevalence and important impact of depression in AD, it is difficult to diagnose depression in a clinical or research setting. It is particularly challenging to make an adequate diagnosis in patients with moderate to severe dementia. There are many reasons for this. Some of the core "biological" symptoms of depression (altered activity, energy, libido, appetite, and sleep) are also frequently altered in AD without any evidence of changed mood [9]. Symptoms of depression could also overlap with apathy, which is one of the most common neuropsychiatric symptoms in AD. Older patients with depression tend to complain about somatic symptoms and deny feeling sad or fail to acknowledge a lack of interest or pleasure in activities. This tendency is captured in the concept of "depression without sadness" [12]. However, in DSM-IV or ICD-10 criteria for depression, depressed mood and diminished interest or pleasure are two core criteria, and somatic complaints are not included. In addition, patients with AD and depression are often unable to verbally express different symptoms since this requires relatively unimpaired cognitive functions (language, executive function, abstract thinking, episodic memory, etc.) commonly affected in AD. Finally, there is a general consensus that depression in dementia is less severe than in patients without dementia, with specific symptoms often failing to meet DSM-IV or ICD-10 criteria of a discrete mood disorder [8].

In order to tackle these limitations and facilitate the diagnosis of depression in AD, the National Institute of Mental Health (NIMH) published the Provisional Diagnostic Criteria for Depression of Alzheimer's Disease [13]:

A. Three (or more) of the following symptoms have been present during the same 2-week period and represent a change from previous functioning. Do not include symptoms that, in your judgment, are clearly due to a medical condition other than AD or are a direct result of non-mood-related dementia symptoms (e.g., loss of weight due to difficulties with food intake).
   1. Clinically significant depressed mood (e.g., depressed, sad, hopeless, discouraged, tearful)
   2. Decreased positive affect or pleasure in response to social contacts and usual activities (either 1 or 2 are required)
   3. Disruption in appetite
   4. Disruption in sleep
   5. Psychomotor changes (e.g., agitation or retardation)
   6. Fatigue or loss of energy
   7. Feelings of worthlessness, hopelessness, or excessive or inappropriate guilt
   8. Diminished ability to think or concentrate
   9. Recurrent thoughts of death, suicidal ideation, plan, or attempt
   10. Social isolation or withdrawal
   11. Irritability
B. All criteria met for Dementia of the Alzheimer's Type (DSM-IV-TR). The symptoms are not better accounted for by other conditions, such as major depressive disorder, bipolar disorder, bereavement, schizophrenia, schizoaffective disorder, psychosis

of AD, anxiety disorders, or substance-related disorder.
C. The symptoms are not due to the direct physiological effects of substance use (e.g., a drug of abuse or a medication).
D. The symptoms cause clinically significant distress or disruption in functioning.

Despite representing an important improvement for the diagnosis of depression in AD, these specific criteria still fail to reflect the importance of somatic complaints and "depression without sadness." There are also doubts about the refinement of these criteria to distinguish among major and minor depression, dysthymia, and adjustment disorder in AD.

Finally, the majority of studies concur that dysphoria, loss of interest, indecisiveness, and diminished ability to concentrate but with limited depressive ideation are the most common symptoms of depression in AD [14].

Semistructured or structured interviews

In addition to the NIMH criteria, semistructured or structured interviews can also be used in the diagnosis of depression in AD. The following have been validated for depression in AD:

• Structured Clinical Interview for DSM-IV Axis I Disorders (SCID-I).
• National Institute of Mental Health Provisional Diagnostic Criteria for Depression of Alzheimer's disease (NIMH-dAD).

These interviews allow a detailed assessment of depressive symptoms. However, they are time consuming, making them very difficult to use in clinical practice and even in some research settings.

Screening instruments for depression in AD

A number of screening scales are used for detection of depressive symptoms in patients with AD. These scales can be classified into three groups:

1. Developed to identify depressive symptoms in the general population
   • Beck Depression Inventory (BDI)
   • Hamilton Rating Scale for Depression (HAM-D)

- Geriatric Depression Scale (GDS)
- Center for Epidemiological Studies Depression Scale (CES-D)
- Montgomery–Åsberg Depression Rating Scale (MADRS)
- Zung Self-Rating Depression Scale

2. Developed to identify neuropsychiatric symptoms in patients with dementia
   - Behavioral Pathology in Alzheimer's Disease Rating Scale (BEHAVE-AD)
   - The Neuropsychiatric Inventory (NPI)
   - The Neuropsychiatric Inventory–Clinician Rating Scale (NPI-C)
   - Consortium to Establish a Registry for Alzheimer's Disease Behavior Rating Scale for Dementia (CERAD-BRSD)
   - Columbia University Scale for Psychopathology in Alzheimer's Disease (CUSPAD)
   - Dementia Signs and Symptoms Scale (DSS)

3. Developed to detect depressive symptoms in patients with dementia
   - Cornell Scale for Depression in Dementia (CSDD)
   - Dementia Mood Assessment Scale (DMAS)

Despite not being designed specifically for depression in AD, many of the instruments in the first and second group have become popular because they are easy to use in clinical practice and have a high sensitivity. However, given the complexity of the diagnosis of depression in AD, it is better to use scales specifically designed and validated for this group of patients. A widely used scale is the CSDD. It is based on information obtained from the patient, the caregiver, and the clinician's own observations. In AD, patients' awareness about their symptoms may be reduced; therefore, the score resulting from a self-administered scale for depression may be lower than that obtained by a scale administered by a trained professional. At the same time, caregivers' perceptions of the presence of depressive symptoms may be influenced by their emotional state. For example, a caregiver who is looking after a relative and feeling stressed may overestimate the depressive symptoms of the patient. The CSDD reduces this bias by requiring health

professionals to interview the patient and the informant and integrate this information with their own clinical assessment.

Subtypes of depression in AD

There are at least four subtypes of depressive episodes in patients with dementia [14]:

- *Emotional reaction to cognitive deficits.* This refers specifically to the psychological impact of acknowledging having AD.
- *Recurrence of early and midlife major and minor depressive disorder.* Simply, the recurrence of depression while having AD.
- *Vascular disease associated with AD causing depressive symptoms.* This subtype is related to the vascular depression hypothesis, which proposes that vascular brain disease may predispose to, precipitate, or perpetuate late-life depression. Up to 50% of patients diagnosed with AD have a significant presence of vascular brain injury. Therefore, vascular depression may partly explain the interaction between depression and AD [15, 16].
- *Neurodegenerative process of AD causing depressive symptoms.* There is evidence of a relationship between the neuropathology of AD and the development of depression. Depression in AD has been associated with different neurochemical abnormalities, including loss of noradrenergic cells in the locus ceruleus and loss of doral raphe serotoninergic nuclei. This loss could be due to apoptotic processes that occur in AD. There is also a possibility of shared susceptibility genes for both illnesses [13].

In order to better understand depression in AD, clinicians should consider two subtypes for each depressive episode.

Natural course of depression in AD

There is little agreement regarding the natural course of depression in AD because depressive symptoms tend to fluctuate over time. However, there is some evidence that depression tends to occur early in the illness and becomes increasingly common in moderate dementia, whereas its prevalence tends to decrease later in severe dementia [11]. Left untreated, major depression in AD may last for about 12 months, whereas minor depression has a shorter course [14].

Differential diagnosis

Apathy and pathological affect are two important symptoms/syndromes in AD that are sometimes confused with depression. These are particularly problematic for the differential diagnosis of depression in AD because they can be present in patients with AD both with and without depression.

Apathy

Apathy is a very common symptom/syndrome in patients with AD, presenting in around 36–80% of patients with AD. It usually appears early in the course of AD and persists during the course of the illness [17]. Apathy is characterized by a lack of motivation or interests that results in social withdrawal and a reduction in daily activities. Lack of emotional responsiveness is an important characteristic of apathy. Clinically, dysphoric symptoms (sadness, feelings of guilt, self-criticism, helplessness, hopelessness, tearfulness, sadness, anxiety, agitation) could help to distinguish depression from apathy [14].

Table 14.1 shows the differential symptoms of patients with AD presenting with symptoms indicative of apathy or depression or apathy and depression.

Pathological affect

Pathological affect is usually described as sudden episodes of crying that cannot be contained by the patient. When this syndrome appears in patients with a congruent emotional state, it is referred to as "affective or emotional lability"; if it appears in patients with an incongruent emotional state or without any particular reason, it is called "unmotivated or pathological crying" [11]. Patients with pathological affective display crying show a significantly higher frequency of major and minor depression than patients with no pathological affect. Therefore, some authors suggest that pathological affect crying in AD may be a marker of underlying depression. However, in spite of its frequency in patients with depression in AD, pathological affect is not a core symptom and is also a differential diagnosis [14]. In order to make an appropriate differential diagnosis with depression in AD, it is particularly useful to assess for other core symptoms of depression in AD (depressed mood, anhedonia, hopelessness, etc.) immediately after an episode of crying.

The complex relationship between depression and AD

Different approaches can lead to different interpretations of the relationship between depression and AD. Depression could be considered a risk factor for AD, a prodromal or early symptom of AD, a consequence of AD, or a differential diagnosis of AD.

Depression as a risk factor of AD

Patients with a history of depression, and particularly those with late-onset depressive disorders, have an increased risk of developing AD [18]. Some studies have found an increased risk of dementia even when depression occurred 10 years before the development of AD. This association is even stronger in recurrent depressive disorder cases. One possible explanation for this association is the catalyzing effect of the

Table 14.1 Differential symptoms in apathy and depression

Symptoms Indicative of Apathy	Shared Symptoms	Symptoms Indicative of Depression
Reduced emotional response	Reduced interest	Dysphoria
Indifference	Psychomotor retardation	Suicidal ideation
	Fatigue/hypersomnia	Self-criticism
	Low insight	Feelings of guilt
	Reduced sociability	Hopelessness

Adapted from Landes et al. [17].

inflammatory process associated with late-onset depressive disorder on the underlying physiopathology AD [16].

Depression as a prodrome of AD

There is growing evidence supporting the hypothesis that depressive symptoms could also be the initial manifestation of AD rather than a risk factor. A recent and important study of identical twins supports this hypothesis [19]. Therefore, some researchers suggest that late-onset depressive disorder, mild cognitive impairment, and dementia may be part of a continuum [20]. In addition, the interaction between depression and AD is made evident by the higher presence of beta-amyloid neuritic plaques and neurofibrillary tangles in the hippocampi of patients with AD with a history of depression. This is mainly observed in patients who are depressed when diagnosed with dementia. These findings have led to the study of a subtype of depression that could specifically represent this transition to dementia: amyloid-associated depression [21]. In these cases, higher biomarkers of deposits of beta-amyloid protein (e.g., low levels of Aβ42 in cerebrospinal fluid) as well as higher cognitive impairment are observed relative to other patients with depression.

In summary, it seems that the time elapsed between the last depressive episode and the onset of AD is a key factor. If the depression occurred only a few years before, it is likely that the altered mood was a prodromal feature of AD and not a risk factor for dementia; on the other hand, if the depressive episode occurred many years before the development of dementia, it is more difficult to envisage a prodrome lasting this long [9]. That said, there is also growing evidence that the prodromal phase of AD can last for many years [4]. Therefore, there is still no definite answer for this debate.

Depression as a differential diagnosis of AD

Depressive pseudodementia does not appear as a diagnosis in most worldwide psychiatric classifications such as DSM-IV or ICD-10. However, the term "depressive pseudodementia" is still frequently used and relevant in clinical practice. Depressive pseudodementia is characterized by a major depressive disorder in which subjective and/or objective cognitive impairment is the main motivation to seek help from a health professional. Depressive pseudodementia can sometimes be misdiagnosed as a case of dementia. It usually exhibits a subacute onset and evolves quickly, and its functional impact is disproportionately high relative to its cognitive impairment. The following signs and symptoms are a useful approach for the differential diagnosis of depressive pseudodementia [22, 23]:

- *Interview.* This includes repetitive complaints about amnestic and/or somatic problems, repetitive complaints about personal performance, psychomotor retardation, absence of sundowning symptoms and matinal pole, and fulfills criteria for major depressive disorder.
- *Cognitive assessment.* This includes dysexecutive profile, slow information processing, cognitive inconsistencies during the assessment, and good performance with cueing in memory tests.
- *Brain imaging.* This includes the absence of or mild hippocampal atrophy and absence of or mild generalized cortical atrophy.

Treatment of depression in AD

The treatment of depression in AD must be prescribed in conjunction with the treatment of dementia as a whole, and the caregiver must also be incorporated into the different treatment strategies. It is important to exclude any medical disorders or medications that could be precipitating, predisposing, or maintaining any symptoms of depression. Finally, it is important to establish target symptoms and monitor their response regularly [9].

Pharmacological treatment

The goal of pharmacological treatment for depression is remission rather than response. Patients that do not achieve remission in depression tend to recur more frequently. Depression studies in the general population have found that patients with moderate to severe depression are more likely to respond to antidepressants compared to placebo. However, the evidence for the efficacy of antidepressant treatment compared to placebo in mild depression, minor depression, and dysthymia is less strong [24]. In AD depression, there is an important debate regarding the efficacy and safety of antidepressant treatments. Some studies have found evidence that antidepressants are efficacious and well tolerated in this group of patients. Unfortunately, the most recent meta-analysis was more cautious [25]. In addition, the Health Technology Assessment Study into the Use of Antidepressants for Depression in Dementia (HTA-SADD) trial published after this meta-analysis was also negative. This was the most important trial for depression in AD so far. It was a multicenter, randomized, double-blind, placebo-controlled trial of the clinical effectives of sertraline or mirtazapine for depression in dementia. A total of 326 participants were randomized. The authors did not find statistically significant differences in depression scores between groups, but did find more adverse reactions and serious adverse events with sertraline or mirtazapine compared to placebo. However, importantly, there was a clear improvement in depressive symptomatology in all groups [26]. Nevertheless, there are still many individual cases in which antidepressants are necessary. Due to the physiological changes of old age, it is always important to start slow and titrate up slowly while checking for potential adverse effects. Given the lack of convincing data on efficacy with any of the antidepressant drug family, the first choice must be based on safety, tolerance, and potential pharmacokinetic interactions with other drugs. Therefore, selective serotonin reuptake inhibitor (SSRI) antidepressants are the first-choice medications [8]. Sertraline, citalopram, and escitalopram are the SSRIs with fewer pharmacokinetic interactions. Table 14.2 provides information regarding different types of SSRI suitable for treating patients with AD.

If there is a partial response after 4 weeks of maximum dose, it is clinically reasonable to wait for up to 8 more weeks for a full response. However, if there is no response after 4 weeks at a maximum dose or the response is still partial after 12 weeks, it is suggested to switch medications to another SSRI or another pharmacological group [8].

There are no controlled studies in patients with AD regarding the commonly used selective serotonin norepinephrine reuptake inhibitors (SNRIs) venlafaxine or duloxetine, regarding the noradrenergic and dopaminergic reuptake inhibitor bupropion, or involving atypical antidepressants such as trazodone or melatoninergic agonists such as agomelatine. Finally, tricyclic antidepressants are, in general, worse tolerated, with anticholinergic side effects. There is some evidence supporting the potential benefits of acetilcholinesterase inhibitors (ACHIs) in depressive symptoms of AD [28]. The improvement in mood symptoms seems to be independent of the effect of ACHI on cognition.

Nonpharmacological treatments

Given the modest efficacy of pharmacological interventions in depression in AD, nonpharmacological treatments are extremely relevant. There is some evidence, although limited, that psychosocial interventions such as cognitive/emotion-oriented interventions, behavior techniques, and exercise can improve the mood of patients with dementia. Positive effects were most frequently found in persons with mild to moderate AD living in the community. For people with dementia living in an institution, positive effects were found most frequently in subgroups of moderate to severe dementia, severe to very severe dementia, and in the subgroup with behavioral problems. Music therapy, multisensory stimulation, light therapy, and cognitive stimulation can also have potential benefits on depressive symptoms in patients with AD with depressive symptoms [29]. Finally, electroconvulsive therapy (ECT) could also be considered as a therapeutic option in patients with AD with depression. There is evidence of a beneficial effect on affective and cognitive symptoms. However, delirium is a frequent complication of ECT in patients with AD [30].

Avenues for future research

There are many areas that are ripe for future research. For example, is there a specific type of depression that is more likely to signal the development of dementia (e.g., late onset, accompanied by white matter changes)? The difference between dysphoria and major depression needs to be explored along with the specific clinical features of depression/dementia. The impact of

Table 14.2 Dosage and side effect profile of main SSRI

Drug	Starting Dose (mg/day)	Average Daily Dose (mg/day)	Main Side Effects	Main Differences
Sertraline	25	50–150	Nausea, vomiting, dyspepsia, abdominal pain, diarrhea, headache, sexual dysfunction, risk of gastric bleeding, inappropriate antidiuretic hormone (ADH) secretion	Very few pharmacokinetic interactions
Fluoxetine	10	20	Nausea, vomiting, dyspepsia, abdominal pain, diarrhea, headache, sexual dysfunction, risk of gastric bleeding, inappropriate ADH secretion, insomnia, and agitation	Very long half-life and more activating properties
Escitalopram	5	10	Nausea, vomiting, dyspepsia, abdominal pain, diarrhea, headache, sexual dysfunction, risk of gastric bleeding, inappropriate ADH secretion	Very few pharmacokinetic interactions
Paroxetine	10	20	Nausea, vomiting, dyspepsia, abdominal pain, diarrhea, headache, sexual dysfunction, risk of gastric bleeding, inappropriate ADH secretion, sedation, and anticholinergic effects	More sedation and anticholinergic effects
Citalopram	10	20–40	Nausea, vomiting, dyspepsia, abdominal pain, diarrhea, headache, sexual dysfunction, risk of gastric bleeding, inappropriate ADH secretion	Very few pharmacokinetic interactions

Adapted from Baldwin [27].

depression treatment on cognitive outcome has not been systemically explored and deserves study. Finally, the specific pathoanatomic features that are characteristic of depression/dementia need to be investigated. It is only through the discovery of these mechanisms that specific and rational treatment strategies for these clinical problems will be developed.

Summary

Late life depression can be a prodrome of dementia. Depression occurs frequently in dementia and has a negative impact at multiple levels on patients and caregivers. Therefore, it is extremely important to make an early diagnosis in order to start an adequate treatment and reduce the impact of depression in patients with AD. The diagnosis of depression in dementia is a challenge that can be surpassed with a high level of suspicion, a good interview of the patient, an adequate understanding of psychopathology, and collateral information from the caregivers. Currently, there is no strong evidence that pharmacological interventions are effective. Psychosocial interventions are an essential aspect of an adequate treatment.

Important developments in this field are expected in the near future. Hopefully, as is happening now with AD, biomarkers or other specific techniques can be found for depression in AD. This will help to better understand its etiology, promote early detection, improve differential diagnosis, and monitor response to treatments. This can only lead to better diagnosis, treatment, and better quality of life for patients and their families.

Clinical case

Mr. N, age 83, attended the Memory Clinic accompanied by his wife. She convinced Mr. N to seek medical advice because she was worried about her husband's emotional state and memory loss.

Mr. N states that his wife is exaggerating. According to Mr. N, for the last 3 years he has sometimes been unable to remember names, objects, and places related to recent events. However, he feels that this has not interfered with his activities of daily living. He is a retired lawyer who until recently has been dedicated to reading, maintaining his garden, and participating in academic activities at the university where he used to teach.

His wife explained that during the last few months, Mr. N stopped going to the university because he could not concentrate and was unable to understand the subject discussed in these academic meetings. He had also stopped reading for the same reasons. He even got lost once while driving to the university. In the last few weeks, he had also stopped maintaining his garden, the stated reason being that he did not enjoy it like he used to. Mr. N was also complaining of feeling tired at all times. In fact, he recently spent many hours a day sleeping in an armchair in the living room. His wife gets very angry while mentioning that he lacks interest in doing any activities, saying, "Not even the visits from his favorite granddaughter could arouse his interest." He had experienced some weight loss due to a lack of appetite, eating only when his wife pressed him to do it. When asked to reveal his feelings, the patient answered that he was feeling unmotivated and was getting easily annoyed with his wife when she tried to help him.

Mr. N's lab tests results are normal. His brain magnetic resonance imaging (MRI) shows a generalized atrophy with moderate hippocampal atrophy. He performs different cognitive tests during the medical interview. The scores in episodic memory, language, and visuospatial abilities are lower than the values obtained 2 years ago and 2 standard deviations lower relative to the expected score for his age and level of education.

His wife reports that she has noticed a gradual decrease in functional and cognitive functions over the last 3 years. However, this decrease has accelerated in the last few weeks. Mr. N does not have a medical history of diabetes, hypercholesterolemia, or traumatic brain injury, and he has no family history of cognitive or psychiatric disorders. The only medication he takes is enalapril 10 mg/day to treat hypertension diagnosed 6 years ago.

Mr. N is diagnosed with depression in AD. He is prescribed a treatment with ACHIs, regular physical activity, and occupational therapy. He and his wife are also told about different safety measures to help them at home. Mr. N's wife is advised to attend a workshop for caregivers of patients with dementia. The clinical impression during the assessment was that she was suffering from caregiver's burden.

Two months later, Mr. N continues with a depressive episode and increasing symptoms of irritability. In this clinical context, an SSRI is added to the therapeutic dose of the ACHI. The following month, the patient shows a partial response of his depressive episode and a marked improvement in irritability. Two months later, Mr. N and his wife attend the clinic again and report an overall improvement in cognitive and psychiatric symptoms.

PEARLS TO TAKE HOME

- AD is the most prevalent type of dementia and has a devastating impact on patients' and families' quality of life.
- Of all psychiatric syndromes that may occur in AD, depression is the most common.
- Comorbid depression is associated with greater impairment in activities of daily

living, earlier placement in a nursing home, increased mortality risk, faster decline in cognitive functions, and poorer quality of life. It also increases stress and psychological morbidity of the patient's caregiver and family.

- Dysphoria, loss of interest, indecisiveness, and diminished ability to concentrate but with limited depressive ideation are the most common symptoms of depression in AD.
- Depression could be considered a risk factor for AD, a prodromal or early symptom of AD, a consequence of AD, or a differential diagnosis of AD.
- Given the modest efficacy of pharmacological interventions in depression in AD, nonpharmacological treatments are extremely relevant.

References

1. Alzheimer's Association. Changing the trajectory of Alzheimer's disease: a national imperative. http://www.alz.org/documents_custom/trajectory.pdf, 2010.
2. McKhann GM, Knopman DS, Chertkow H, et al. The diagnosis of dementia due to Alzheimer's disease: recommendations from the National Institute on Aging-Alzheimer's Association workgroups on diagnostic guidelines for Alzheimer's disease. *Alzheimers Dement*, 7: 263–269, 2011.
3. Lautenschlager NT. Under full sail. *Int Psychoger*, 23: 341–343, 2011.
4. Ballard C, Gauthier S, Corbett A, et al. Alzheimer's disease. *Lancet*, 377: 1019–1031, 2011.
5. Snowdon DA, Greiner LH, Mortimer JA, et al. Brain infarction and the clinical expression of Alzheimer disease: the Nun Study. *JAMA*, 277(10): 813–817, 1997.
6. Alzheimer's Association. Alzheimer's disease facts and figures. http://www.alz.org/downloads/Facts_Figures_2011.pdf, 2011.
7. Bond J. Inequalities in dementia care across Europe: key findings of the Facing Dementia Survey. *Int J Clin Pract*, 59, Suppl. 146: 8–14, 2005.
8. Kanner AM. Depression in Alzheimer's disease. In: *Depression in Neurological Disorders*. Cambridge Medical Communication Ltd, pp. 101–128, 2005.
9. Gauthier S, Ballard C. Behavioural disturbances. In: *Management of Dementia*, 2nd ed. Informa Healthcare USA, Inc, pp. 13–37, 2009.
10. Vilalta-Franch J, Garre-Olmo J, López-Pousa S, et al. Comparison of different clinical diagnostic criteria for depression in Alzheimer disease. *Am J Geriatr Psychiatry*, 14(7): 589–597, 2006.
11. Starkstein SE, Mizrahi R, Power BD. Depression in Alzheimer's disease: phenomenology, clinical correlates and treatment. *Int Rev Psychiatry*, 20(4): 382–388, 2008.
12. Gallo JJ, Rabins PV. Depression without sadness: alternative presentations of depression in late life. *Am Fam Physician*, 60: 820–826, 1999.
13. Olin JT, Katz IR, Meyers BS, et al. Provisional diagnostic criteria for depression of Alzheimer disease: rationale and background. *Am J Geriatr Psychiatry*, 10(2): 129–141, 2002.
14. Amore M, Tagariello P, Laterza C, et al. Subtypes of depression in dementia. *Arch Gerontol Geriatr*, 44, Suppl. 1: 23–33, 2007.
15. Schneider JA, Bennett DA. Where vascular meets neurodegenerative disease. *Stroke*, 41, 10 Suppl.: S144–S146, 2010.
16. Alexopoulos GS, Morimoto SS. The inflammation hypothesis in geriatric depression. *Int J Geriatr Psychiatry*, 26(11): 1109–1118, 2011. doi: 10.1002/gps.2672. [Epub ahead of print].
17. Landes AM, Sperry SD, Strauss ME. Prevalence of apathy, dysphoria, and depression in relation to dementia severity in Alzheimer's disease. *J Neuropsychiatry Clin Neurosci*, 17(3): 342–349, 2005.
18. Ownby RL, Crocco E, Acevedo A, et al. Depression and risk for Alzheimer disease: systematic review, meta-analysis, and metaregression analysis. *Arch Gen Psychiatry*, 63(5): 530–538, 2006.

19. Brommelhoff JA, Gatz M, Johansson B, et al. Depression as a risk factor or prodromal feature for dementia? Findings in a population-based sample of Swedish twins. *Psychol Aging*, 24(2): 373–384, 2009.

20. Panza F, Frisardi V, Capurso C, et al. Late-life depression, mild cognitive impairment, and dementia: possible continuum? *Am J Geriatr Psychiatry*, 18(2): 98–116, 2010.

21. Sun X, Steffens DC, Au R, et al. Amyloid-associated depression: a prodromal depression of Alzheimer disease? *Arch Gen Psychiatry*, 65(5): 542–550, 2008.

22. Wells CE. Pseudodementia. *Am J Psychiatry*, 136(7): 895–900, 1979.

23. Köhler S, Thomas AJ, Barnett NA, et al. The pattern and course of cognitive impairment in late-life depression. *Psychol Med*, 40: 591–602, 2010.

24. Kirsch I, et al. Initial severity and antidepressant benefits: a meta-analysis of data submitted to the Food and Drug Administration. *PLoS Med*, 5(2): e45, 2008.

25. Nelson JC, Devanand DP. A systematic review and meta-analysis of placebo-controlled antidepressant studies in people with depression and dementia. *J Am Geriatr Soc*, 59(4): 577–585, 2011.

26. Banerjee S, Hellier J, Dewey M, et al. Sertraline or mirtazapine for depression in dementia (HTA-SADD): a randomised, multicentre, double-blind, placebo-controlled trial. *Lancet*, 378(3789): 403–411, 2011. July 15. Epub ahead of print.

27. Baldwin RC. Assessment and management. In: *Depression in Later Life*. Oxford University Press, pp. 43–64, 2010.

28. Rozzini L, Vicini Chilovi B, Bertoletti E, et al. Acetylcholinesterase inhibitors and depressive symptoms in patients with mild to moderate Alzheimer's disease. *Aging Clin Exp Res*, 19(3): 220–223, 2007.

29. O'Neil ME, Freeman M, Christensen V, et al. A systematic evidence review of non-pharmacological interventions for behavioral symptoms of dementia. VA-ESP Project #05-225, 2011.

30. Rao V, Lyketsos CG. The benefits and risks of ECT for patients with primary dementia who also suffer from depression. *Int J Geriatr Psychiatry*, 15(8): 729–735, 2000.

Depression and Traumatic Brain Injury

Seth A. Mensah[1] and Michael P. Kerr[2]
[1]Welsh Neuropsychiatry Service, Whitchurch Hospital, Cardiff, UK
[2]Welsh Centre for Learning Disabilities, Cardiff University, Cardiff, UK

Introduction

Mood disorders are the most commonly reported psychiatric complication among survivors of traumatic brain injury (TBI) [1–3]. Of these disorders, depression is recognized as the most prevalent, with multiple biopsychosocial factors involved in its genesis, course, and maintenance. The presence of major depression has been shown to be associated with poor psychosocial and rehabilitation outcomes after TBI.

Unfortunately, both clinical practice and research regarding depression in patients with TBI have been hindered by controversies, ambiguities, and inconsistent data. As a result, there remains inadequate recognition of depression following TBI and disparate evidence on which to base treatment guidelines.

TBI is a major public health problem and a leading cause of morbidity worldwide, with over 2 million people hospitalized annually in the United States alone [4]. The legacies of all degrees of TBI are potentially lifelong and permeate every aspect of the life of the survivor, with consequent impact on psychosocial well-being. Therefore, it is imperative that depression preceding brain injury is carefully evaluated to avoid disruption of the functional and psychological recovery and overall outcome.

Depression in the general population has enormous financial cost and impact. In the authors' opinion, it is likely that this impact is even greater in individuals with TBI. The cost of depression to society was estimated by Chisholm [5], who included care costs, productivity costs, and psychosocial costs for the individual, the individual's families, friends, employers, and to society as a whole. The total estimated cost amounted to £3.4 billion in the United Kingdom and $44 billion in the United States [6] based on 1990 prices. Clearly, depression has a major international socioeconomic impact.

Asvall [7] further estimated that depression alone accounts for approximately 10% of life years lost to disability for the working population. Further, the cost to health-care services increases with the length of the illness.

This chapter explores the epidemiology, pathogenesis, assessment, and treatment of depression associated with TBI.

Epidemiologic data and bidirectional relation between depression and TBI

Prevalence of depression in the general population

The lifetime prevalence rates of depression have been found to vary widely. This disparity is caused by differing diagnostic categories, screening instruments, and case definitions among epidemiologic studies. The lifetime prevalence rates of depressive disorders have been estimated to be 4.4% (Epidemiological Catchment Area Study), 17.1% (National Co-morbidity Survey), and 30% (Kendler's Virginia Twin Survey of Women). It is

Depression in Neurologic Disorders: Diagnosis and Management, First Edition.
Edited by Andres M. Kanner.
© 2012 Blackwell Publishing Ltd. Published 2012 by Blackwell Publishing Ltd.

generally accepted that the current rate of major depression ranges from 2% to 5% [8].

Chronic or severe physical illness is associated with an increased risk of depression. It is believed that the stress associated with a serious or chronic physical illness may bring out an individual's vulnerability to depression. The literature suggests that the course of depression varies between individuals, as does the response to treatment.

Epidemiology

There are numerous studies exploring the epidemiology of depression in TBI. The reported frequency of depressive disorders following TBI has varied from 6% to 77%. Table 15.1 summarizes the prevalence rates of depression from various studies.

The variability in the reported frequency of depressive disorders, particularly major depression, may be due to the lack of uniformity in the psychiatric diagnosis.

Differences in methodology and limited sample sizes have contributed to differing descriptions of depression among patients with TBI. As a consequence, the field lacks a valid, comprehensive, and cohesive portrayal of depressive symptoms after brain injury.

Most epidemiologic studies have relied on rating scales or self-reports rather than on structured interviews and established diagnostic criteria (e.g., International Classification of Diseases, Tenth Edition [ICD-10], *Diagnostic and Statistical Manual of Mental Disorders*, Fourth Edition [DSM-IV]). Diagnosis is complicated by the fact that the expression of affective disorder in the population with brain injury is frequently atypical, and there is considerable overlap between the symptoms of brain injury and the symptoms of depression [9]. Depression may be overestimated if too much emphasis is placed on nonaffective symptoms (e.g., motivation, physical, sleep, and appetite disturbance), particularly when using cut-off scores on questionnaires, and underestimated if depressive symptoms are confused with other neuropsychiatric sequelae of TBI such as fatigue and apathy. The timing of the assessment following injury may also affect estimates of the severity and prevalence of depression.

Assessment instruments designed for psychiatric populations have frequently been used to describe depression after brain injury. Seel et al.

[10] and other researchers have employed the Neurobehavioral Functioning Inventory (NFI) to study the frequency and manifestations of depression in patients with TBI. Fedoroff et al. [11] observed that the Hamilton Rating Scale for Depression significantly differentiated between patients with and without depression. Lykouras et al. [12] suggested that Beck Depression Inventory scores of ≥29 are highly predictive of a diagnosis of major depressive episode in neurological inpatients.

McKinlay et al. [13] reported indirect evidence of depressed mood in approximately half of patients at 3, 6, or 12 months following severe brain injury.

In a series of 39 patients, Kinsella et al. [14] reported that 33% were classified as depressed within 2 years of severe brain injury. Schoenhuber and Gentilini [15] found depressive symptoms in 39% of 103 patients with mild head injury interviewed at a 1-year follow-up and concluded that these patients had an increased risk of developing depression compared with controls. Gualtieri and Cox [16] estimated that the frequency of major depression in patients with TBI lies between 25% and 50%. Hibbard et al. [17] used a structured interview and DSM-IV criteria to identify Axis I psychopathology in 100 adults with TBI who were evaluated an average of 8 years after trauma. The prevalence of major depression in this series was 61%. More recently, Kreutzer et al. [18] used the NFI to study the prevalence of major depressive disorder in a sample of 722 outpatients with TBI who were evaluated an average of 2.5 years following brain injury. Major depression, defined using DSM-IV criteria, was diagnosed in 303 patients (42%). In addition, Koponen et al. [19] reported that major depression had a lifetime prevalence of 26.7% in a group of 60 patients with TBI followed for an average of 30 years.

Variations in diagnostic criteria and assessment methods may best account for disparate prevalence reports. Small samples and variations in disease chronicity may also be contributory. For example, most brain injury studies examined fewer than 70 patients. The majority of studies described symptomatology at 12 months or less postinjury.

Equivocal findings regarding the identification of depressive symptoms are likely attributable to several factors:

Table 15.1 Prevalence of depression in TBI

Study	Number of Patients	Time Since TBI	Severity of TBI (Based on Coma Duration, GCS and PTA)	Diagnostic Tool/Criteria/Measure	Prevalence
1 Varney et al. (1987) [71]	120	2–8 years (mean 3.4 years)	Mild to severe	DSM-III	92/120 patients (pts) = 77%
2 Rutherford et al. (1977) [72]	145	1–2 months	Mild	Dichotomous scale—single item "Yes or No"	6%
3 McKinlay et al. (1981) [13]	55	3–12 months	Severe	Structured interview schedule for depressive symptoms	52–57%
4 Kinsella et al. (1988) [14]	39	Up to 24 months	Severe	General Health Questionnaire, the Leeds Scales of Depression and Anxiety, and Visual Analogue Scales of Depression and Anxiety	33%
5 Schoenhuber and Gentilini (1988) [15]	103	12 months	Mild	Self-Rating Depression Scale.	39%
6 Hibbard et al. (1998) [17]	100	8 years	Mild to severe	Structured Clinical Interview for DSM-IV (SCID) + DSM-IV	61%
7 Kreutzer et al. (2001) [18]	722	3 months–9 years (average 2.5 years)	Mild to severe	NFI (self-rated) + DSM-IV	42%
8 Koponen et al. (2002) [19]	60	30 years	Mild to severe	Schedules for Clinical Assessment in Neuropsychiatry (SCAN) + DSM-IV and SCID + DSM-III	26.7%
9 Jorge et al. (1993) [23]	66	1–12 months	Mild to severe	Structured Interview + DSM-III-R	28/66 pts = 42%

(Continued)

Table 15.1 (*Continued*)

Study	Number of Patients	Time Since TBI	Severity of TBI (Based on Coma Duration, GCS and PTA)	Diagnostic Tool/Criteria/ Measure	Prevalence
10 Deb et al. (1999) [73]	120	1 year	Mild to severe	Revised Clinical Interview Schedule (CIS-R) + ICD-10	14%
11 Robinson and Jorge (2005) [70]	89	1–24 months	Mild to severe	DSM-IV	40%
12 Holsinger et al. (2002) [74]	520	50 years	Mild to severe	Structured Interview (Diagnosis Interview Schedule, DIS) + DSM-IV	11.2%
13 Kersel et al. (2001) [75]	65	6–12 months	Severe	Beck Depression Inventory (BDI)	(70%) 24%; 24%
14 Kant et al. (1998) [76]	83	–	Mild to severe	BDI + DSM-III, Apathy Evaluation Scale	60%
15 Satz et al. (1998) [77]	100	6 months	Moderate to severe	1. Symptom Checklist ± 90, Revised 2. Neurobehavioral Rating Scale + DSM-III-R	18% 31%
16 Bowen et al. (1999) [78]	77	1.6 months 2.12 months	Mild to severe	Wimbledon Self-Report Scale (WSRS)	1. 39% 2. 35%
17 Brooks et al. (1983) [79]	55	1–12 months	Mild to severe	Dichotomous scale	57%
18 Hoofien et al. (2001) [21]	76	10–20 years (average 14.1 years)	Severe	Symptoms Checklist-90-Revised (SCR-90-R)	45%

	Study	N	Time post-injury	Severity	Measure	Prevalence
19	Douglas and Spellacy (2000) [80]	35	Average 7 years (3.5–10)	Severe	Self-Rating Depression Scale (SDS)	57%
20	Glenn et al. (2001) [42]	41	Average 3.4 years	Mild to severe	Beck Depression Inventory-II (BDI-II)	59%
21	Jorge et al. (2004) [81]	66	1. 1 month 2. 3 months 3. 6 month 4. 12 months	Mild to severe	Hamilton Rating Scale for Depression + DSM-III-R	1. 26% 2. 22.2% 3. 23.2% 4. 18.6%
22	Seel et al. (2003) [10]	666	10–126 months	Mild to severe	Neurobehavioral Functioning Inventory (NFI) + DSM-IV	27%
23	Dikmen et al. (1977) [44]	283	1. 1 month 2. 3–5 years	Moderate to severe	Center for Epidemiologic Studies Depression Scale (CES-D)	1. 31% 2. 17%
24	Bryant et al. (2010) [82]	817	12 months	Mild	Mini International Neuropsychiatric Interview (MINI)	9%
25	Atteberry-Bennett et al. (1986) [83]	37	Up to 9 months	Mild to severe	BDI	35%

1. Researchers have often relied on assessment tools with dichotomous (e.g., "Yes" or "No") response formats to identify the presence of symptoms. In the few studies where continuous rating scales were used, patients with very mild depression were classified in the same way as patients with severe symptoms.
2. Many studies have used samples restricted by size or by a single injury severity level, thereby limiting the findings.
3. A number of studies utilized assessment measures developed for other populations. Several researchers have suggested that the relevance of these measures to the brain injury population has yet to be demonstrated.

Despite the variability in estimated prevalence, it is clear that depression is common in the population with brain injury, may well be underdiagnosed [20], and may persist for many years postinjury [21, 22]. Data are lacking on other epidemiologic factors such as age, gender, socioeconomic status, employment, education, and marital status. These findings emphasize the need for careful psychiatric follow-up of patients with TBI.

Clinical manifestations

Diagnosis

Diagnostic criteria

Using DSM-IV diagnostic criteria, depressive disorders associated with TBI are categorized as *Mood Disorder due to TBI* with subtypes of (1) *with major depressive-like episode* (if the full criteria for a major depressive episode are met) or (2) *with depressive features* (prominent depressed mood, but full criteria for a major depressive episode are not met).

One of the fundamental challenges in the diagnosis of depression after TBI is the specificity of symptoms on which these diagnostic criteria are based. Symptoms of major depression such as sleep, appetite, or libido changes may occur in patients with TBI as a consequence of brain injury or as a nonspecific consequence of an acute medical illness. Thus, symptoms used to diagnose depressive disorders could be independent of the associated mood disturbance,

resulting in the overdiagnosis of major depressive disorder. On the other hand, patients may deny the presence of a depressed mood as part of their lack of awareness of deficit or a denial syndrome. This would result in underdiagnosis of depression.

Jorge et al. [23] examined the specificity of symptoms of depression after TBI and concluded that the standard DSM-based diagnostic criteria have a high sensitivity and specificity for identifying patients with depression when compared with alternative specific symptom diagnostic criteria. Therefore, they suggested that standard DSM-IV criteria are the most logical criteria for the diagnosis of major depression in the TBI population.

Other authors [24] lend further support to this claim by arguing that the use of categorical variables (e.g., depressed vs. nondepressed) may obscure important dimensional information regarding depressive phenomenology. The combination of structured diagnostic interviews and self-report and caregiver-based measures may represent a comprehensive approach to the assessment of depression following TBI.

Non-TBI

Before discussing depression in patients with brain injury, it is worth considering the disorder and its impact in noninjured individuals. The symptoms of depression fall into four categories:

1. Emotional (persistent sad mood)
2. Cognitive (feelings of worthlessness or inappropriate guilt)
3. Motivational (lack of interest)
4. Physical (appetite or sleep disturbance)

Clinical depression contrasts with the normal emotional experiences of sadness in being extreme, persistent, and disabling. Depression is one of the most common psychiatric illnesses and can have a major impact on people's health and quality of life. Depression also carries a high probability of relapse.

Coyne et al. [25] found that 85% of currently depressed individuals in primary care and 78% in psychiatric settings had had prior episodes of depression. Piccinelli and Wilkinson [26] found that 75% of individuals followed over 10 years had relapsed and 10% had experienced persistent depression.

TBI

Symptoms of depression after brain injury are found to be rather nonspecific, with no strong evidence of a clear pattern, which distinguishes them from depression in patients without TBI. Nevertheless, symptoms of disturbed interest and concentration are particularly prevalent, while guilt is less evident. Variability of mood is characteristic. Jorge et al. [23] demonstrated using *Diagnostic and Statistical Manual of Mental Disorders*, Third Edition, Revised (DSM-III-R) criteria that depressed mood, reduced energy, feelings of worthlessness, and suicidal ideation differentiated patients with depression from patients without depression in TBI populations.

Kreutzer et al. [18] showed that NFI items fatigue, frustration, poor concentration, boredom, and distractibility were commonly associated with DSM-IV depression, whereas feeling sad or blue was not. Kennedy et al. [27a] reported that NFI items reduced libido, reduced appetite, anhedonia, and lack of confidence were more predictive of DSM-IV major depression, while verbal and physical aggression, forgetfulness, and fatigue were the least important. Table 15.2 shows a comparison of NFI items with DSM-IV symptom domain.

Negative impact on quality of life

Depression has a negative impact on both lifespan and quality of life. Suicidal ideation in patients with TBI is of particular concern. Suicidal ideation, suicide attempts, and completed suicides have all been shown to be increased in survivors of TBI compared with populations without brain injury. Increased rates of suicide have been found in patients with relatively severe TBI. Approximately 1% of patients with TBI will commit suicide over a 15-year period, which is at least three times the standard suicide rate. Current evidence suggests that no small degree of this increase may be due to premorbid psychosocial factors since the increase is also present in patients with all types of cranial injury, including those with concussion and cranial fractures. Awareness of a suicide risk should be present in

the assessment of any TBI. In a discussion of completed suicide in patients with TBI, Tate et al. [27b] commented, "The small magnitude in no way corresponds to the seriousness of the problem."

The preferred method to determine whether brain injury is a risk factor for suicide would be to calculate the standardized mortality ratio (SMR) for suicide deaths in a large cohort of brain injury survivors. The SMR compares the rate of suicide in the index cohort with the expected rate of suicide in the population from which the cohort comes, taking into account that the risk of suicide is highly dependent on the age, sex, and sociocultural background of the subjects. It is most commonly expressed as a percentage; an SMR of 100% indicates that the risk of suicide is the same as in the control population.

Harris and Barraclough [28] performed a meta-analysis of suicide associated with various medical and psychiatric conditions. They found five studies of civilian brain injury with a total of five suicides, with an expected rate of 1.4%. For both civilian and war brain injuries, the SMR was in excess of 320%, indicating that the risk of suicide after brain injury was raised over threefold.

Tate et al. [27b] followed 896 patients admitted to a brain injury rehabilitation unit in Australia. Eight of these patients died from suicide, all of whom were male, over a follow-up period of up to 18 years. The time interval between injury and death ranged from 1 to 11 years. These patients had severe brain injuries with an average duration of posttraumatic amnesic periods of several weeks. Most of the patients had active psychiatric problems at the time of suicide, including five with mood disturbance and one with a psychotic disorder. Four of the patients had a history of previous suicide attempts following the brain injury, and in one the brain injury was itself a result of attempted suicide. In several cases, there had been repeated expressions of suicidal intent. Alcohol/drug abuse was not an associative factor. The findings clearly show a markedly increased suicide risk associated with TBI.

In a study in Denmark, Teasdale and Engberg [29] identified all cases admitted with a diagnosis of TBI between 1979 and 1993 and then screened the national register of deaths to identify those

Table 15.2 DSM-IV symptom domains and corresponding NFI items

DSM-IV Symptom Domain	NFI Item
Mood category	
Depressed mood	Sad, blue
	Feel hopeless
	Frustrated
	Easily angered or irritated
	Hit or push others
	Curse at others
	Scream or yell
	Argue
Diminished interest or pleasure	Bored
	Difficulty enjoying activities
	Sit with nothing to do
	Lonely
	Uncomfortable around others
	Loss of interest in sex
Feelings of worthlessness	Feel worthless
	No confidence
	Curse at self
Somatic category	
Weight change	Poor appetite
Sleep disturbance	Trouble falling asleep
Psychomotor agitation or retardation	Restless
	Talk too fast or slow
	Move slowly
Decreased energy	Weak
	Tire easily during physical activity
Cognitive category	
Diminished thinking ability	Cannot get mind off certain thoughts
	Concentration is poor
	Easily distracted
	Forget yesterday's events
	Forget to do chores or work
	Forget if I have done things
	Forget or miss appointments
Recurrent thoughts of death	Threaten to hurt self

Adapted from Seel et al. (2003) [10].

that had gone on to commit suicide. After a fol-low-up period of 15 years, suicide was identified in 750 (SMR: 300%), 46 (SMR: 270%), and 99 (SMR: 410%) cases of concussion, skull fracture, and intracerebral contusion or hemorrhage, respectively. The increased risk of suicide was sig-nificantly greater in the intracerebral contusion/hemorrhage group than in the other two groups. Suicide was associated with comorbid alcohol/drug abuse. Men were at slightly greater absolute risk; however, the lower absolute risk of suicide in women led to a higher SMR for all groups. A considerable proportion of the increased risk of suicide after brain injury is due to the preinjury personality and cultural factors of individuals who are at risk of sustaining brain injuries. Nevertheless, the greater risk in those with sig-nificant brain injury does indicate a specific con-tribution of brain injury and its disability [2].

In assessing and managing suicide risk in TBI, the following issues may need to be addressed: (1) lack of planning and problem solving for "getting out" of depressed moods, (2) poor memory that affects ability to cope with prob-lematic situations, (3) emotional lability and/or disinhibition and impulsiveness that may increase the risk of acting without considering the consequences of actions, (4) poor emotional expression leading to the depressed state going unnoticed, (5) perseveration over negative issues leading to a spiral of negative thinking, and (6) staff training and support regarding suicide risk.

Negative impact on the course and response to treatment of TBI

Depression after TBI increases the risk for devel-oping other neuropsychiatric problems, includ-ing increased suicidality, cognitive dysfunction, and aggressive behavior, and thereby contributes to morbidity and functional disability after TBI and interferes in the physical and cognitive reha-bilitation process. Major depression is a frequent complication of TBI that hinders a patient's recovery. It is associated with executive dysfunc-tion, negative affect, and prominent anxiety symptoms and has a negative impact on the short- and long-term course of TBI.

The negative impact of depression on TBI out-comes has been reported in the literature [30, 31].

Jorge et al. [32] showed that patients with depres-sion of at least 6-month duration had poorer psychosocial outcomes, whereas those with depression of less than 3 months recovered as well as patients without depression. Depression in TBI negatively influences patients' motivation and engagement in rehabilitation programs and social activities, and the current evidence sug-gests that these patients are not able to recover these losses even when the depression is over. Therefore, major depression has a deleterious effect on both the psychosocial and activities of daily living outcomes of patients with TBI.

Common pathogenic mechanisms operant in depression and TBI

Etiologic mechanisms

Biological

The pathophysiological and neuroanatomical basis of the association between depression and TBI remains to be fully explained. In recent years, a great deal of energy has been expended on unraveling the possible etiological correlates of depression in patients with brain injury, with particular focus placed on the relationship between lesion location and depression. However, progress in this field has been hindered by the difficulty in localizing the precise neuroanatomi-cal regions damaged by TBI. Typically, lesions associated with TBI are more diffuse than lesions observed in patients with stroke [24].

Various researchers have proposed that major depression is associated with lesions in the left hemisphere, specifically the anterior region [33, 34]. These assertions have caused many authors to attempt to replicate these findings, with some studies producing supportive evidence [35] and others not [36–39]. In a recent systematic review, Carson et al. [40] reported that the likelihood of post-TBI depression in a sample population was greater in patients with left anterior lesions, whereas according to a logistic regression model the likelihood of depression diminished with frontal lesions (i.e., right, left, or bilateral frontal, including orbitofrontal) or purely cortical lesions. Jorge et al. [23] followed Fedoroff et al.'s [11] sample of patients with TBI over a 12-month period, during which they were reassessed at 3-, 6-, and 12-month intervals. Only in the acute phase were lesions located in the left anterior head regions found to be significantly associated with major depression. An association was also found between right hemisphere lesions and depression with anxiety. The authors suggested that the findings were consistent with the hypothesis that major depression may be triggered by disruption of the ascending nonadrenergic and serotonergic pathways, resulting in depletion of these neurotransmitters. Disruption of other neurotransmitter systems (e.g., cholinergic, dopaminergic, and glutamatergic) have all been implicated in depression in patients with TBI.

Neuroimaging studies in patients with primary depression have found structural and metabolic abnormalities in regions of the prefrontal cortex, including dorsolateral prefrontal, anterior cingulate, and orbitofrontal cortices. Biological factors such as the involvement of the prefrontal cortex and probably other limbic and paralimbic structures may play a significant role in the complex pathophysiology of major depression. In a neuroimaging study of two groups with brain injury suitably matched for sociodemographic factors, Paradiso et al. [41] showed that at 3 months after injury, subjects with lateral damage had worse depressive features and apathy, with greater impairment of activities of daily living and social functioning. TBI is known by its very nature to result in specific damage and dysfunction to the neural systems implicated in the genesis and maintenance of depression.

Other factors found to be associated with depression in TBI populations include: sequelae of TBI, that is, cognitive dysfunction, posttraumatic epilepsy, and facial pain; writing impairment; thorax and other ongoing/chronic physical problems; and new trauma. The severity of TBI has not been shown convincingly to be associated with onset of depression, severity of depression, or its response to treatment.

In summary, it would appear that there is no good evidence for areas of specific vulnerability in terms of lesion location, and early suggestions of a specific association with injury to the left hemisphere have not been confirmed.

Psychosocial

Various psychosocial factors have been reported or suggested to be associated with post-TBI depression. These factors are also seen in the non-TBI depressed population. Glenn et al. [42] and Gomez-Hernandez et al. [43] are among researchers who have explored social factors contributing to the development of major depression after TBI. Risk factors associated with depression in TBI include:

1. Psychosocial pre- and postinjury stressors, including perceived subjective level of stress [43]
2. Poor premorbid social functioning and/or poverty [10]
3. Past psychiatric or brain injury history [11]
4. Alcohol abuse [44]
5. Fewer years of formal education [44]
6. Increased age [42, 45]
7. Lack of work/fear of job loss [43, 45]
8. Female gender [42]
9. Impaired close relationships (a sense of belonging was protective against depression) [43]

Psychosocial disability in TBI has been shown to be more strongly associated with depression than physical disability.

Treatment strategies

Treatment

As in the general mental health field, it is unlikely that one treatment option will be completely effective and efficient, particularly in terms of preventing relapse. More likely, a combination of approaches will be needed.

Recent developments suggest that people with TBI may require components of neurorehabilitation, pharmacological intervention, cognitive–behavioral therapy (CBT), and other treatment options through other modalities (from postacute outreach to community interventions) depending on their mental health status, cognitive profile, insight, and personal goals [46].

Treatment of psychiatric disorders occurring after TBI involves a range of different pharmacological and nonpharmacological strategies. Ideally, treatment of the neurobehavioral consequences of TBI should begin early in the acute phase following injury. If it is possible to modify the processes associated with neuronal damage, the intervention should be started as early as possible. This approach would presumably lead to the greatest amount of recovery of cognition, motivation, activity levels, and emotional disorder.

Pharmacologic

The progress made in recent years in elucidating neuronal pathologic mechanisms of both depression and TBI at the biomolecular level have rather disappointingly not translated into therapeutic interventions in the management of depression in the TBI population. Therefore, current treatment approaches are almost completely based on and supported by anecdotal case reports and clinical experience.

The selection of an antidepressant is guided by its side effect profile, potential for lowering seizure threshold, anticholinergic activity, sedative effects, and potential for interactions with other drugs through protein binding or enzyme induction. Patients with brain injury are more sensitive to the side effects of medications, especially psychotropics.

There have been no randomized controlled trials of antidepressant efficacy for depression after TBI [2], and to the best of the authors' knowledge, there have been no randomized double-blind placebo-controlled studies of the efficacy of pharmacological treatments of depression in patients with acute TBI. In a recent observational study of antidepressant use, Gainotti et al. [47] concluded that antidepressants are able to improve functional outcomes in patients with TBI who have depression. In a controlled comparison study of depression in groups with and without brain injury, Dinan and Mobayed [48] found that patients who were depressed following head injury responded less well than patients without brain injury (85% vs. 31%, respectively) to amitriptyline.

Wroblewski et al. [49] reported in a controlled prospective study that desipramine may be effective for treating depression in patients with severe TBI. Fann et al. [50] demonstrated the efficacy of sertraline in 15 patients with mild TBI, with statistically significant improvements in psychological distress, anger, and aggression as well as in the severity of postconcussive symptoms. Controversially, Fann et al. [51] also concluded in

a weakly powered trial that sertraline may also lead to a beneficial effect on visual and verbal memory and cognitive functioning.

These findings are consistent with the clinical impression that depression following brain injury may be more difficult to treat. Most neuropsychiatrists would recommend starting with a selective serotonin reuptake inhibitor (SSRI), partly because these drugs probably have a less adverse effect profile compared with tricyclic antidepressants (TCAs). Citalopram or sertraline would seem to be sensible choices.

The clinician should be guided by the fundamental principles of therapeutics. Doses of psychotropics must be prudently increased to minimize side effects (i.e., start low, go slow), with the patient receiving an adequate therapeutic trial with regard to dosage and duration of treatment. Patients with brain injury must be frequently reassessed to determine changes in treatment schedules and to receive special care in monitoring drug interactions. Depending on the augmenting drug's mechanism of action and potential side effects, augmentation therapy may be warranted if there is evidence of a partial response to a specific medication [23]. SSRIs appear to have a less adverse side effect profile. Their most commonly reported side effects include headache, gastrointestinal complaints, insomnia, diminished libido, and sexual dysfunction. Citalopram (starting at 10 mg/day), escitalopram (starting at 5–10 mg/day), sertraline (starting at 25–50 mg/day), or paroxetine (starting at 5–10 mg/day) are among the most useful drugs in this group. Fluoxetine has also been reported to be efficacious [52–54]. Fluvoxamine and trazodone are alternative antidepressants that also inhibit serotonin reuptake. For trazodone, treatment is started at low doses (50–100 mg). The dose may be gradually increased every 3–4 days up to 400 mg. TCAs have important anticholinergic effects that may interfere with cognitive and memory functions. In addition, clomipramine may lower the seizure threshold. If TCAs are used, however, nortriptyline (starting at 10 mg/day) constitutes a reasonable alternative provided that blood levels and toxic effects are carefully monitored. Data are lacking for novel and other antidepressants such as duloxetine, venlafaxine, and mirtazapine, but anecdotal accounts exist for their usefulness as second- or third-line drugs. The same applies to the use of lithium, carbamazepine, valproate, and lamotrigine.

There are case reports of successful treatments of depression in patients with TBI with psychostimulants, which are also used to treat concomitant deficits in attention and apathy [55]. These include dextroamphetamine (8–60 mg/day) and methylphenidate (10–60 mg/day). Treatment is begun at lower doses and then gradually increased. The recommendation for safe practice is for patients taking stimulants to be closely monitored to prevent abuse or toxic effects. The most common side effects are anxiety, dysphoria, headaches, irritability, anorexia, insomnia, cardiovascular symptoms, dyskinesias, or even psychotic symptoms.

Buspirone, a 5-HT1A agonist and D2 antagonist, has proved to be a safe and efficacious anxiolytic and has been used in post-TBI depression [56], but caution is advised in its use for people with epilepsy.

Nonpharmacologic

Psychotherapeutic treatment strategies

The role and usefulness of psychotherapeutic intervention, particularly CBT, has been mentioned by various researchers [57–59] in the management of comorbid depression in TBI. This type of therapy, which focuses on the present rather than the past, aims to understand, interpret, and break those underlying negative thoughts, dysfunctional beliefs, and assumptions along with any negative cognitive schemas and unhelpful behavior profiles that maintain the cycle of depression. CBT has been said to suit the management of depression following brain injury because it (1) accommodates and seeks to tackle the many personal and social sequelae that may contribute to psychological morbidity, both acutely and chronically; (2) provides the therapist with a wide range of tools with which to work; and (3) is inherently flexible with the potential for accommodating differences in individual circumstances and limitations [59]. CBT is advocated as particularly suited for people with TBI since it contains systems for managing the generalizability of "therapeutic work" from the treatment session, such as use of diaries and workbooks, and it promotes social and emotional control skills [60, 61]. Despite recent advances in CBT in the population without brain injury, there is still dearth of good quality research on its effectiveness in the population with brain injury. Even though there are no large and robust studies to establish an evidence base, the current evidence implies that treatment of depression in brain injury may be improved from the neuropsychological perspective. There is enough evidence, albeit based on just a few published studies, to support the use of CBT in comorbid depression in brain injury and to justify further research.

As mentioned earlier, depression in TBI can present with atypical clinical features and with considerable overlap between the apathy [62] and cognitive and neurobehavioral symptoms of brain injury and depression, which further complicates its recognition, diagnosis, and management. This led House [63] to suggest that difficulties with expressing and understanding emotion may be due to premorbid factors such as lack of psychological thinking, nonspecific motor effects impairing the expression of emotion, or difficulties in the perception of emotion, which may hinder the correct interpretation of depression. Focusing the CBT assessment and formulation on the individual patient is important, rather than rigidly applying diagnostic criteria designed for the population without brain injury with depression.

The individualized formulation should outline current problems, identify the extent of their impact on function, and develop an intervention according to the specific needs of the individual. It is important to identify any stressors and problems that the patient is experiencing and to understand their coping style as part of the assessment process [60]. Khan-Bourne and Brown [59] further stressed the importance of premorbid factors, such as significant life events that have occurred and how the individual coped with these events and the need to identify the individual's appraisal of the brain injury and the events surrounding it, so that core beliefs and dysfunctional assumptions can be assessed.

The following key features should characterize CBT assessment and formulation of depression in individuals with brain injury:

- CBT should be patient centered.
- CBT should clearly delineate the presenting problems.
- CBT should identify the extent of these problems' impact on function.
- CBT should identify precipitants and activating situations.
- CBT should consider premorbid factors.
- CBT should identify the individual's appraisal of the brain injury.

In addressing the deficiencies of psychotherapeutic interventions in survivors of TBI with depression, there is the need (1) to determine the relative efficacies of different psychotherapeutic approaches in different patient groups and at different phases of recovery, (2) to establish which components of effective therapies are responsible and their optimum modes of delivery, and (3) to determine the indicators of a successful outcome as well as ways of broadening access to other currently difficult-to-treat client groups, such as those with other forms of acquired brain injury.

Electroconvulsive therapy

Electroconvulsive therapy (ECT) remains a controversial yet effective therapeutic intervention within psychiatric practice. However, it appears that the use of ECT is declining in the United Kingdom and the United States [64, 65], with some researchers arguing that there is no clear exposition of a biological mechanism for supporting its use for purported mood disorder [66]. In contrast, ECT proponents argue that it may be effective for major depression and should remain a possible treatment option in such cases [67]. ECT is not contraindicated in survivors of TBI, as was demonstrated by Crow et al. [68] and Kant et al. [69], and should be considered when other treatment approaches have not resulted in improvements in depression. There have been no randomized controlled trials of ECT's effectiveness in brain injury [2].

It is recommended that ECT be administered with the lowest possible effective energy, using pulsatile, nondominant unilateral currents, with an interval of 2–5 days between treatments and four to six treatments for a complete course [70].

Conclusion and future directions

A strong body of evidence points to a close association between TBI and the development of depression. This association is influenced by premorbid factors and, it appears to a lesser extent, by the nature of the injury itself.

Identification of depression is complicated by the similarities in depressive symptomatology with features of the brain injury itself, which can lead to underrecognition of depression. Treatment options mirror those provided to the general population. The case for detailed assessment and treatment of depression associated with TBI is compelling. However, it is likely that many patients receive inadequate support for this comorbidity.

Future research should be directed toward prevention of and access to treatment for depression in people with TBI. Prevention-based research should involve the elucidation of the early features of depression and associated contributory factors. Treatment-based research should identify predictors of refractory depression and explore how treatment can be integrated at an early stage into the rehabilitation program.

Case history

A 36-year-old male suffered a severe head injury after falling from a ladder at his home. He was intubated following a deteriorating Glasgow Coma Scale score. He made good progress and was extubated. Magnetic resonance imaging (MRI) of the head showed a frontal contusion with cerebral edema.

Two weeks posttrauma he was discharged home to the care of the family with support from community physiotherapy and occupational therapy.

Initial home based-assessment showed him to have some continued confusion, poor attention, and irritability. By 8 weeks postinjury his family contacted emergency services with concerns over his mental state. He was described as confused, angry, aggressive, and irritable.

He was admitted to acute psychiatric services following an aggressive outburst; his behavior deteriorated in this setting and he was transferred to a neuropsychiatric ward.

Now 12 weeks postinjury the assessment showed continued confusion, apathy, and poor motivation. Initial formulation was of a dysexecutive syndrome related to frontal lobe trauma. A rehabilitative program was initiated to include regular physiotherapy, occupational therapy, and integration into the milieu of the ward.

While his confusion lifted he made little progress on the ward; in particular, his appetite and his motivation to participate in therapy were reduced. Following a case conference review a new formulation of depressive illness in addition to his frontal dysfunction was made.

It was felt that his current cognitive state would not support a formal application of CBT so treatment was initiated with an SSRI.

Over the proceeding 3 weeks an increase in appetite and motivation occurred. Concomitant improvement in irritability was noted.

At a further conference the initial response was noted and it was felt that his improvement was such that he would benefit from a CBT approach.

After a further 4 weeks he was discharged home on continued SSRI and with support from a neuropsychiatric day hospital.

It is likely that the early identification of a mood disorder in this man led to an earlier return to the home environment, reducing the impact of the injury on him and his family.

♀ PEARLS TO TAKE HOME

- Depression is a common and debilitating comorbidity of TBI.
- Skilled assessment is needed to tease out the co-occurrence of symptoms of TBI and depression, such as behavioral changes.
- There is increased depression after TBI compared with the population without TBI.
- Recognition is crucial to reduce the impact on quality of life and treatment outcome.
- Suicide is a rare but serious outcome, and particular attention must be made to premorbid factors during risk assessment.
- Treatment of depression with pharmacological and nonpharmacological approaches is essential to effective management. SSRIs remain the first line of pharmacotherapy.

References

1. Lishman WA. Brain damage in relation to psychiatric disability after head injury. *Br J Psychiatry*, 114: 373–410, 1968.
2. Fleminger S, Oliver DL, Williams WH, et al. The neuropsychiatry of depression after brain injury. *Neuropsychol Rehabil*, 13(1): 65–87, 2003.
3. Kim E, Lauterbach EC, Reeve A, et al. Neuropsychiatric complications of traumatic brain injury: a critical review of the literature (a report by the ANPA Committee on Research). *J Neuropsychiatry Clin Neurosci*, 19: 106–127, 2007.
4. Kraus JF, McArthur DL. Incidence and prevalence of, and costs associated with, traumatic brain injury. In: *Rehabilitation of the Adult and Child with Traumatic Brain Injury*, 3rd ed., eds. M Rosenthal, ER Griffith, JS Kreutzer, et al. Philadelphia: FA Davis Company, pp. 3–18, 1999.
5. Chisholm D. The economic consequences of depression. In: Depression: Social and Economic Timebomb: Strategies for Quality Care: Proceedings of an International Meeting Organized by the World Health Organization in Collaboration with the International Federation of Health Funds, Harvard Medical School and the Sir Robert Mond Memorial Trust, eds. A Dawson and A Tylee. London: BMJ Publishing Group, 2001.
6. Greenberg PE, Stiglin LE, Finkelstein SN, et al. The economic burden of depression in 1990. *J Clin Psychiatry*, 54: 405–418, 1993.
7. Asvall JE. Can we turn the table on depression? In: Depression: Social and Economic Timebomb: Strategies for Quality Care: Proceedings of an International Meeting Organized by the World Health Organization in Collaboration with the International Federation of Health Funds, Harvard Medical School and the Sir Robert Mond Memorial Trust, eds. A Dawson and A Tylee. London: BMJ Publishing Group, 2001.
8. Jenkins R, Bebbington P, Brugha T, et al. The national psychiatric morbidity surveys of Great Britain—initial findings from the household survey. *Psychol Med*, 27: 775–789, 1997.

9. Raskin SA, Stein PN. Depression. In: *Neuropsychological Management of Mild Traumatic Brain Injury*, eds. SA Raskin, C Mateer. New York: Oxford University Press, 2000.

10. Seel RT, Kreutzer JS, Rosenthal M, et al. Depression after traumatic brain injury: a National Institute on Disability and Rehabilitation Research Model Systems multicenter investigation. *Arch Phys Med Rehabil*, 84: 177–184, 2003.

11. Fedoroff JP, Starkstein SE, Forrester AW, et al. Depression in patients with acute traumatic brain injury. *Am J Psychiatry*, 149: 918–923, 1992.

12. Lykouras L, Oulis P, Adrachta D, et al. Beck Depression Inventory in the detection of depression among neurological inpatients. *Psychopathology*, 31: 213–219, 1998.

13. McKinlay WW, Brooks DN, Bond MR, et al. The short-term outcome of severe blunt head injury as reported by the relatives of the injured person. *J Neurol Neurosurg Psychiatry*, 44: 527–533, 1981.

14. Kinsella G, Moran C, Ford B, et al. Emotional disorder and its assessment within the severe head injured population. *Psychol Med*, 118: 57–63, 1988.

15. Schoenhuber R, Gentilini M. Anxiety and depression after mild head injury: a case control study. *J Neurol Neurosurg Psychiatry*, 51: 722–724, 1988.

16. Gualtieri CT, Cox DR. The neurobehavioral sequelae of traumatic brain injury. *Brain Inj*, 5: 219–232, 1991.

17. Hibbard MR, Uysal S, Kepler K, et al. Axis I psychopathology in individuals with traumatic brain injury. *J Head Trauma Rehabil*, 13: 24–39, 1998.

18. Kreutzer JS, Seel RT, Gourley E. The prevalence and symptom rates of depression after traumatic brain injury: a comprehensive examination. *Brain Inj*, 15: 563–576, 2001.

19. Koponen S, Taiminen T, Portin R, et al. Axis I and II psychiatric disorders after traumatic brain injury: a 30-year follow-up study. *Am J Psychiatry*, 159: 1315–1321, 2002.

20. Jean-Bay E. The biobehavioral correlates of post-traumatic brain injury depression. *J Neurosci Nursing*, 32: 169–176, 2000.

21. Hoofien D, Gilboa A, Vakil E, et al. Traumatic brain injury (TBI) 10–20 years later: a comprehensive outcome study of psychiatric symptomatology, cognitive abilities and psychosocial functioning. *Brain Inj*, 15(3): 189–209, 2001.

22. Linn RT, Allen K, Willer BS. Affective symptoms in the chronic stage of traumatic brain injury: a study of married couples. *Brain Inj*, 8: 135–147, 1994.

23. (a) Jorge RE, Robinson RG, Starkstein SE, et al. Depression and anxiety following traumatic brain injury. *J Neuropsychiatry Clin Neurosci*, 5: 369–374, 1993. (b) Jorge RE, Robinson RG, Arndt S. Are there symptoms that are specific for depressed mood in patients with traumatic brain injury? *J Nerv Ment Dis*, 181(2): 91–99, 1993.

24. Rosenthal M, Christensen BK, Ross TP. Depression following traumatic brain injury. *Arch Phys Med Rehabil*, 79(1): 90–103, 1998.

25. Coyne JC, Pepper CM, Flynn H. Significance of prior episodes of depression in two patient populations. *J Consult Clin Psychol*, 67: 76–81, 1999.

26. Piccinelli M, Wilkinson G. Outcome of depression in psychiatric settings. *Br J Psychiatry*, 164: 297–304, 1994.

27. (a) Kennedy RE, Livingston L, Riddick A, et al. Evaluation of the Neurobehavioral Functioning Inventory as a depression screening tool after traumatic brain injury. *J Head Trauma Rehabil*, 20: 512–526, 2005. (b) Tate R, Simpson G, Flanagan S, et al. Completed suicide after traumatic brain injury. *J Head Trauma Rehabil*, 12: 16–28, 1997.

28. Harris EC, Barraclough B. Suicide as an outcome for mental disorders: a meta-analysis. *Br J Psychiatry*, 170: 205–228, 1997.

29. Teasdale TW, Engberg AW. Suicide after traumatic brain injury: a population study. *J Neurol, Neurosurg, and Psychiatry*, 71: 436–440, 2001.

30. Gillen R, Tennen H, McKee TE, et al. Depressive symptoms and history of depression predict rehabilitation efficiency in stroke patients. *Arch Phys Med Rehabil*, 82: 1645–1649, 2001.

31. Rappaport MJ, McCullagh S, Streiner D, et al. The clinical significance of major

depression following mild traumatic brain injury. *Psychosomatics*, 44: 31–37, 2003.

32. Jorge RE, Robinson RG, Starkstein SE, et al. Influence of major depression on 1 year outcome in patients with traumatic brain injury. *J Neurosurg*, 81: 726–733, 1994.

33. Robinson RG, Szetela B. Mood change following left hemispheric brain injury. *Annals of Neurology*, 9(5): 447–453, 1981.

34. Robinson RG, Kubos KL, Starr LB, et al. Mood disorders in stroke patients. Importance of location of lesion. *Brain*, 107: 81–93, 1984.

35. Vataja R, Pohjasvaara T, Leppavuori A, et al. Magnetic resonance imaging correlates of depression after ischemic stroke. *Arch Gen Psychiatry*, 58(10): 925–931, 2001.

36. Gainotti G, Azzoni A, Marra C. Frequency, phenomenology and anatomical-clinical correlates of major post-stroke depression. *Br J Psychiatry*, 175: 163–167, 1999.

37. Herrmann M, Bartels C, Schumacher M, et al. Poststroke depression: is there a pathoanatomic correlate for depression in the postacute stage of stroke? *Stroke*, 26(5): 850–856, 1995.

38. House A, Dennis M, Warlow C, et al. Mood disorders after stroke and their relation to lesion location. A CT scan study. *Brain*, 113(Pt 4): 1113–1129, 1990.

39. Kim JS, Choi-Kwon S. Poststroke depression and emotional incontinence: correlation with lesion location. *Neurology*, 54(9): 1805–1810, 2000.

40. Carson AJ, MacHale S, Allen K, et al. Depression after stroke and lesion location: a systematic review. *Lancet*, 356(9224): 122–126, 2000.

41. Paradiso S, Chemerinski E, Yazici KM, et al. Frontal lobe syndrome reassessed: comparison of patients with lateral or medial frontal brain damage. *J Neurol Neurosurg Psychiatry*, 67: 664–667, 1999.

42. Glenn MB, O'Neil-Pirozzi T, Goldstein R, et al. Depression amongst outpatients with traumatic brain injury. *Brain Inj*, 15(9): 811–818, 2001.

43. Gomez-Hernandez R, Max JE, Kosier T, et al. Social impairment and depression after traumatic brain injury. *Arch Phys Med Rehabil*, 78: 1321–1136, 1997.

44. Dikmen S, Reitan RA. Emotional sequelae of head injury. *Ann Neurol*, 2: 492–494, 1977.

45. Levin HS, McCauley SR, Josic CP, et al. Predicting depression following mild traumatic brain injury. *Arch Gen Psychiatry*, 62: 523–528, 2005.

46. Ownsworth TL, Oei TP. Depression after traumatic brain injury: conceptualization and treatment considerations. *Brain Inj*, 12(9): 735–751, 1998.

47. Gainotti G, Antonucci G, Marra C, et al. Relation between depression after stroke, antidepressant medication and functional recovery. *J Neurol, Neurosurg Psychiatry*, 71: 258–261, 2001.

48. Dinan TG, Mobayed M. Treatment resistance of depression after head injury: a preliminary study of amitriptyline response. *Acta Psychiatr Scand*, 85(4): 292–294, 1992.

49. Wroblewski BA, Joseph AB, Cornblatt RR. Antidepressant pharmacotherapy and the treatment of depression in patients with severe traumatic brain injury: a controlled prospective study. *J Clin Psychiatry*, 57: 582–587, 1996.

50. Fann JR, Uomoto JM, Katon WJ. Cognitive improvement with treatment of depression following mild traumatic brain injury. *Psychosomatics*, 42: 48–54, 2001.

51. Fann JR, Uomoto JM, Katon WJ. Sertraline in the treatment of major depression following mild traumatic brain injury. *J Neuropsychiatry Clin Neurosci*, 12: 226–232, 2000.

52. Cassidy JW. Fluoxetine: a new serotonergically active antidepressant. *J Head Trauma Rehabil*, 4: 67–69, 1989.

53. Bessette RF, Peterson LG. Fluoxetine and organic mood syndrome. *Psychosomatics*, 33: 224–226, 1992.

54. Horsfield SA, Rosse RB, Tomasino V et al. Fluoxetine's effects on cognitive performance in patients with traumatic brain injury. *Int J Psychiatry Med*, 32: 337–344, 2002.

55. Gualtieri CT, Evans RW. Stimulant treatment for the neurobehavioural sequelae of traumatic brain injury. *Brain Inj*, 2: 273–290, 1988.

56. Gualtieri CT. Buspirone: neuropsychiatric effects. *J Head Trauma Rehabil*, 6: 90–92, 1991.

57. Prigatano GP. Disordered mind, wounded soul: the emerging role of psychotherapy in rehabilitation after brain injury. *J Head Trauma Rehabil*, 6: 1–10, 1991.

58. Sbordone RJ. Psychotherapeutic treatment of the client with traumatic brain injury: a conceptual model. In: *Community Integration Following Traumatic Brain Injury*, eds. JS Kreutzer, P Wehman, H Paul. Baltimore, MD: Brookes, 1990.

59. Khan-Bourne N, Brown RG. Cognitive behaviour therapy for the treatment of depression in individuals with brain injury. *Neuropsychol Rehabil*, 13(1): 89–107, 2003.

60. Ponsford JL, Sloan S, Snow P. *Traumatic Brain Injury: Rehabilitation for Everyday Adaptive Living*, Hove, UK: Psychology Press, 1995.

61. Williams WH, Jones RS. Teaching cognitive self-regulation of independence and emotion control skills. In: *Cognitive Therapy for People with Learning Disabilities*, eds. BS Kroese, D Dagnan, K Loumidis. London: Routledge, 1997.

62. Marin RS. Differential diagnosis of apathy and related disorders of diminished motivation. *Psychiatr Ann*, 27: 30–33, 1997.

63. House A. Management of mood disorder in adults with brain damage: can we improve what psychiatry has to offer? In: *Practical Problems in Clinical Psychiatry*, eds. K Hawton and PJ Cowen. New York: Oxford University Press, pp. 51–62, 1992.

64. Upadhyaya AK. Practice of ECT guidelines in the UK v. the USA. *Psychiatric Bulletin*, 17: 528–531, 1993.

65. Bhat M, Sibisi C. Electroconvulsive therapy practice in an inner city London teaching hospital over the last 3 years. In: Annual Meeting, Royal College of Psychiatry (UK) Conference, Edinburgh, 7th July, 2000.

66. Abrams D. *Electroconvulsive Therapy*, 2nd ed. Oxford: Oxford University Press, 1992.

67. Freeman C. *The ECT Handbook*. London: Royal College of Psychiatrists (UK) Publications, 1995.

68. Crow S, Meller W, Christenson G et al. Use of ECT after brain injury. *Convuls Ther*, 12: 113–116, 1996.

69. Kant R, Coffey CE, Bogyi AM. Safety and efficacy of ECT in patients with head injury: a case series. *J Neuropsychiatry Clin Neurosci*, 11: 32–37, 1999.

70. Robinson RG, Jorge RE. Mood disorders. In: *Textbook of Traumatic Brain Injury*, 1st ed., eds. JM Silver, TW McAllister, SC Yudofsky. Washington, DC: American Psychiatric Publishing Inc, pp. 201–212, 2005.

71. Varney NR, Martzke JS, Roberts RJ. Major depression in patients with closed head injury. *Neuropsychology*, 1: 7–9, 1987.

72. Rutherford WH, Merrett JD, McDonald JR. Sequelae of concussion caused by minor head injuries. *Lancet*, 1: 1–4, 1977.

73. Deb S, Lyons I, Koutzoukis C, et al. Rate of psychiatric illness 1 year after traumatic brain injury. *Am J Psychiatry*, 156: 374–378, 1999.

74. Holsinger T, Steffens DC, Phillips C, et al. Head injury in early adulthood and the lifetime risk of depression. *Arch Gen Psychiatry*, 59: 17–22, 2002.

75. Kersel DA, Marsh NV, Havill JH, et al. Psychosocial functioning during the year following severe traumatic brain injury. *Brain Inj*, 15(8): 683–696, 2001.

76. Kant R, Duffy JD, Pivovarnik A. Prevalence of apathy following head injury. *Brain Inj*, 12(1): 87–92, 1998.

77. Satz P, Forney DL, Zaucha K, et al. Depression, cognition, and functional correlates of recovery outcome after traumatic brain injury. *Brain Inj*, 12(7): 537–553, 1998.

78. Bowen A, Chamberlain MA, Tennant A, et al. The persistence of mood disorders following traumatic brain injury: a 1 year follow-up. *Brain Inj*, 13: 547–553, 1999.

79. Brooks DN, McKinlay W. Personality and behavioral change after severe blunt head injury—a relative's view. *J Neurol Neurosurg Psychiatry*, 46: 336–344, 1983.

80. Douglas JM, Spellacy FJ. Correlates of depression in adults with severe traumatic brain injury and their carers. *Brain Inj*, 14(1): 71–88, 2000.

81. Jorge RE, Robinson RG, Moser D, et al. Major depression following traumatic brain injury. *Arch Gen Psychiatry*, 61: 42–50, 2004.

82. Bryant RA, O'Donnell ML, Creamer M, et al. The psychiatric sequelae of traumatic injury. *Am J Psychiatry*, 167: 312–320, 2010.

83. Atteberry-Bennett J, Barth JT, Loyd BH, et al. The relationship between behavioral and cognitive deficits, demographics and depression in patients with minor head injuries. *Int J Clin Neuropsychol*, 8: 114–117, 1986.

Index

Depression in Neurologic Disorders: Diagnosis and Management, First Edition.
Edited by Andres M. Kanner.
© 2012 Blackwell Publishing Ltd. Published 2012 by Blackwell Publishing Ltd.